MW01109516

Minimum Data Set (MDS) 3.0 Coding Manual

item-by-item instructions for completing the MDS 3.0

Notice

This *Minimum Data Set (MDS) 3.0 Coding Manual* is designed to be an authoritative source of information for coding the MDS 3.0. The contents within this manual represent Chapter 3 of the Centers for Medicare & Medicaid Services' (CMS) *Long-Term Care Facility Resident Assessment Instrument (RAI) User's Manual Version 3.0.*

This manual is sold with the understanding that the CMS may update specific sections. This version reflects CMS changes through July 12, 2010. To stay current on any changes that occur, visit www.cms.hhs.gov.

Thank you for purchasing *Minimum Data Set (MDS) 3.0 Coding Manual*

Bulk order pricing information for this manual is available at:

www.ElderGuru.com/MDS

We can produce custom covers of this manual with custom, additional content for state or program specific trainings. Choose the service(s) that meet your needs.

About ElderGuru.com

ElderGuru.com provides professional level information on aging. Visit ElderGuru.com for aging information, news, downloads and professional writing services. ElderGuru.com is written and administered by Derrick Grant, a Licensed Social Worker extensive experience in aging services and public policy. To learn more visit: www.ElderGuru.com/about.

Copyright

The item-by-item instructions contained within this manual were developed by the CMS and are considered a public document.

Content outside CMS instructions is **Copyright 2010 Northern House Media, LLC**. All rights reserved.

Made in the United States of America.

ISBN 1451540736

EAN-13 9781451540734

Contents

CHAPTER 3: OVERVIEW TO THE ITEM-BY-ITEM GUIDE TO THE MDS 3.0

This chapter provides item-by-item coding instructions for all required sections and items in the comprehensive MDS Version 3.0 item set. The goal of this chapter is to facilitate the accurate coding of the MDS resident assessment and to provide assessors with the rationale and resources to optimize resident care and outcomes.

3.1 Using this Chapter

Throughout this chapter, MDS assessment sections are presented using a standard format for ease of review and instruction. In addition, screenshots of each section are available for illustration purposes. Note: There are images imbedded in this manual and if you are using a screen reader to access the content contained in the manual you should refer to the MDS 3.0 item set to review the referenced information. The order of the sections is as follows:

- **Intent.** The reason(s) for including this set of assessment items in the MDS.

- **Item Display.** To facilitate accurate resident assessment using the MDS, each assessment section is accompanied by screen shots, which display the item from the MDS 3.0 item set.

- **Item Rationale.** The purpose of assessing this aspect of a resident's clinical or functional status.

- **Health-related Quality of Life.** How the condition, impairment, improvement, or decline being assessed can affect a resident's quality of life, along with the importance of staff understanding the relationship of the clinical or functional issue related to quality of life.

- **Planning for Care.** How assessment of the condition, impairment, improvement, or decline being assessed can contribute to appropriate care planning.

- **Steps for Assessment.** Sources of information and methods for determining the correct response for coding each MDS item.

- **Coding Instructions.** The proper method of recording each response, with explanations of individual response categories.

- **Coding Tips and Special Populations.** Clarifications, issues of note, and conditions to be considered when coding individual MDS items.

- **Examples.** Case examples of appropriate coding for most, if not all, MDS sections/items.

Additional layout issues to note include (1) the ⏯ symbol is displayed in all MDS 3.0 sections/items that require a resident interview, and (2) important definitions are highlighted in the columns, and these and other definitions of interest may be found in the glossary.

3.2 Becoming Familiar with the MDS-recommended Approach

1. **First, reading the Manual is essential.**

   - **The CMS Long-Term Care Facility Resident Assessment Instrument User's Manual is the <u>primary</u> source of information for completing an MDS assessment.**

   - Notice how the manual is organized.

   - Using it correctly will increase the accuracy of your assessments.

   - While it is important to understand and apply the information in Chapter 3, facilities should also become familiar with Chapters 1, 2, 4, 5 and 6. These Chapters provide the framework and supporting information for data collected on the item set as well as the process for further assessment and care planning.

   - It is important to understand the entire process of the RAI in conjunction with the intent and rationale for coding items on the MDS 3.0 item set.

   - Check the MDS 3.0 Web site regularly for updates at: http://www.cms.gov/NursingHomeQualityInits/25_NHQIMDS30.asp.

   - If you require further assistance, submit your question to your State RAI Coordinator listed in Appendix B or to the MDS 3.0 Q&A mailbox at MDSQuestions@cms.gov.

2. **Second, review the MDS item set.**

   - Notice how sections are organized and where information should be recorded.

   - Work through one section at a time.

   - Examine item definitions and response categories as provided on the form, realizing that more detailed definitions and coding information is found in each Section of Chapter 3.

3. **Complete a thorough review of Chapter 3.**

   - Review procedural instructions, time frames, and general coding conventions.

   - Become familiar with the intent of each item, rationale and steps for assessment.

   - Become familiar with the item itself with its coding choices and responses, keeping in mind the clarifications, issues of note, and other pertinent information needed to understand how to code the item.

   - Do the definitions and instructions differ from current practice at your facility? Does your facility processes require updating to comply with MDS requirements?

   - Complete a test MDS assessment for a resident at your facility. Enter the appropriate codes on the MDS.

- Make a note where your review could benefit from additional information, training, and using the varying skill sets of the interdisciplinary team. Be certain to explore resources available to you.

- As you are completing this test case, read through the instructions that apply to each section as you are completing the MDS. Work through the Manual and item set one section at a time until you are comfortable coding items. Make sure you understand this information before going on to another section.

- Review the test case you completed. Would you still code it the same way? Are you surprised by any definitions, instructions, or case examples? For example, do you understand how to code ADLs?

- As you review the coding choices in your test case against the manual, make notations corresponding to the section(s) of this Manual where you need further clarification, or where questions arose. Note sections of the manual that help to clarify these coding and procedural questions.

- Would you now complete your initial case differently?

- It will take time to go through all this material. Do it slowly and carefully without rushing. Discuss any clarifications, questions or issues with your State RAI Coordinator (see Appendix B)

4. **Use of information in this chapter:**

  - Keep this chapter with you during the assessment process.

  - Where clarification is needed, review the intent, rationale and specific coding instructions for each item in question.

3.3 Coding Conventions

There are several standard conventions to be used when completing the MDS assessment, as follows.

- Unlike the MDS 2.0, the standard look-back period for the MDS 3.0 is **7 days**, unless otherwise stated.

- **With the exception of certain items in Sections K and O, the look-back period generally <u>does not</u> include a hospital stay.**

- There are a few instances in which scoring on one item will govern how scoring is completed for one or more additional items. This is called a skip pattern. The instructions direct the assessor to "skip" over the next item (or several items) and go on to another. When you encounter a skip pattern, leave the item blank and move on to the next item as directed (e.g., item B0100, **Comatose**, directs the assessor to skip to item G0110, **Activities of Daily Living Assistance**, if B0100 is answered **code 1, yes.** The intervening items from B0200-F0800 would not be coded (i.e. left blank). If B0100 was recorded as **code 0, no,** then the assessor would continue to code the MDS at the next item, B0200).

- Use a check mark for boxes with where the instructions state to "check all that apply," if specified condition is met; otherwise these boxes remain blank (e.g., F0800, **Staff Assessment of Daily and Activity Preferences**, boxes A-Z).

- Use a numeric response (a number or pre-assigned value) for blank boxes (e.g., D0350, **Safety Notification**).

- When completing hard copy forms to be used for data entry, capital letters may be easiest to read. Print legibly.

- When recording month, day, and year for dates, enter two digits for the month and the day and four digits for the year. For example, the third day of January in the year 2011 is recorded as:

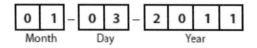

- Almost all MDS 3.0 items allow a dash (-) value to be entered and submitted to the MDS QIES ASAP system.

    - A dash value indicates that an item was not assessed. This most often occurs when a resident is discharged before the item could be assessed.
    - Dash values allow a partial assessment to be submitted when an assessment is required for payment purposes.
    - There are five date items (A2400C, M0300B3, O0400A6, O0400B6, and O0400C6) that use a dash-filled value to indicate that the event has not yet occurred. For example, if there is an ongoing Medicare stay, then the end date for that Medicare stay (A2400C) has not occurred, therefore, this item would be dash-filled.
    - The few items that do not allow dash values include identification items in Section A (e.g., reasons for assessment, resident name, assessment reference date) and ICD-9 diagnosis codes (Item I8000).
    - To determine whether a specific item allows a dash value or not, refer to the MDS 3.0 Data Submission Specifications at: http://www.cms.gov/NursingHomeQualityInits/25_NHQIMDS30.asp#TopOfPage

- When the term "physician" is used in this manual, it should be interpreted as including nurse practitioners, physician assistants, or clinical nurse specialists, if allowable under state licensure laws and Medicare.

- Residents should be the primary source of information for resident assessment items. Should the resident not be able to participate in the assessment, the resident's family, significant other, and guardian or legally authorized representative should be consulted.

- Several times throughout the manual the word "significant" is used. The term may have different connotations depending on the circumstance in which it is used. For the MDS 3.0 , the term "significant" when discussing clinical, medical, or laboratory findings refers to measures of supporting evidence that are considered when developing or assigning a diagnosis, and therefore reflects clinical judgment. When the term "significant" is used in discussing relationships between people, as in "significant other," it means a person, who may be a family member or a close friend that is important or influential in the life of the resident.

Section	Title	Intent
A	Identification Information	Obtain key information to uniquely identify each resident, nursing home, and reasons for assessment.
B	Hearing, Speech, and Vision	Document the resident's ability to hear, understand, and communicate with others and whether the resident experiences visual, hearing or speech limitations and/or difficulties.
C	Cognitive Patterns	Determine the resident's attention, orientation, and ability to register and recall information.
D	Mood	Identify signs and symptoms of mood distress.
E	Behavior	Identify behavioral symptoms that may cause distress or are potentially harmful to the resident, or may be distressing or disruptive to facility residents, staff members or the environment.
F	Preferences for Customary Routine and Activities	Obtain information regarding the resident's preferences for his or her daily routine and activities.
G	Functional Status	Assess the need for assistance with activities of daily living (ADLs), altered gait and balance, and decreased range of motion.
H	Bladder and Bowel	Gather information on the use of bowel and bladder appliances, the use of and response to urinary toileting programs, urinary and bowel continence, bowel training programs, and bowel patterns.
I	Active Disease Diagnosis	Code diseases that have a relationship to the resident's current functional, cognitive, mood or behavior status, medical treatments, nursing monitoring, or risk of death.
J	Health Conditions	Document health conditions that impact the resident's functional status and quality of life.
K	Swallowing/Nutritional Status	Assess conditions that could affect the resident's ability to maintain adequate nutrition and hydration.
L	Oral/Dental Status	Record any oral or dental problems present.
M	Skin Conditions	Document the risk, presence, appearance, and change of pressure ulcers as well as other skin ulcers, wounds or lesions. Also includes treatment categories related to skin injury or avoiding injury.
N	Medications	Record the number of days that any type of injection, insulin, and/or select medications was received by the resident.
O	Special Treatments and Procedures	Identify any special treatments, procedures, and programs that the resident received during the specified time periods.
P	Restraints	Record the frequency that the resident was restrained by any of the listed devices at any time during the day or night.
Q	Participation in Assessment and Goal Setting	Record the participation of the resident, family and/or significant others in the assessment, and to understand the resident's overall goals.
V	Care Area Assessment (CAA) Summary	Document triggered care areas, whether or not a care plan has been developed for each triggered area, and the location of care area assessment documentation.
X	Correction Request	Indicate whether an MDS record is a new record to be added to the QIES ASAP system or a request to modify or inactivate a record already present in the QIES ASAP database.
Z	Assessment Administration	Provide billing information and signatures of persons completing the assessment.

SECTION A: IDENTIFICATION INFORMATION

Intent: The intent of this section is to obtain key information to uniquely identify each resident, the home in which he or she resides, and the reasons for assessment.

A0100: Facility Provider Numbers

A0100. Facility Provider Numbers
A. National Provider Identifier (NPI): ☐☐☐☐☐☐☐☐☐☐
B. CMS Certification Number (CCN): ☐☐☐☐☐☐☐☐☐☐☐☐
C. State Provider Number: ☐☐☐☐☐☐☐☐☐☐☐☐☐☐

Item Rationale

- Allows the identification of the nursing home submitting assessment.

Coding Instructions

- Nursing homes must have a National Provider Number (NPI) and a CMS Certified Number (CCN).
- Enter the nursing home provider numbers:
    - A. National Provider Identifier (NPI)
    - B. CMS Certified Number (CCN)
    - C. State Provider Number (optional)

DEFINITIONS

NATIONAL PROVIDER IDENTIFIER (NPI) A unique Federal number that identifies providers of health care services. The NPI applies to the nursing home for all of its residents.

CMS CERTIFICATION NUMBER (CCN) Replaces the term "Medicare/Medicaid Provider Number" in survey, certification, and assessment-related activities.

STATE PROVIDER NUMBER Medicaid Provider Number established by a state.

A0200: Type of Provider

A0200. Type of Provider	
Enter Code ☐	**Type of provider** 1. **Nursing home (SNF/NF)** 2. **Swing Bed**

Item Rationale

- Allows designation of type of provider.

Coding Instructions

- **Code 1, nursing home (SNF/NF):** if a Medicare skilled nursing facility (SNF) or Medicaid nursing facility (NF).
- **Code 2, swing bed:** if a distinct swing bed unit.

> **DEFINITION**
>
> **SWING BED**
> A rural hospital with less than 100 beds that participates in the Medicare program that has CMS approval to provide post-hospital SNF care. The hospital may use its beds, as needed, to provide either acute or SNF care.

A0310: Type of Assessment

For Comprehensive, Quarterly, and PPS Assessments, Entry and Discharge Records.

A0310. Type of Assessment	
Enter Code ☐☐	**A. Federal OBRA Reason for Assessment** 01. **Admission** assessment (required by day 14) 02. **Quarterly** review assessment 03. **Annual** assessment 04. **Significant change in status** assessment 05. **Significant correction** to **prior comprehensive** assessment 06. **Significant correction** to **prior quarterly** assessment 99. **Not OBRA required** assessment
Enter Code ☐☐	**B. PPS Assessment** <u>**PPS Scheduled Assessments for a Medicare Part A Stay**</u> 01. **5-day** scheduled assessment 02. **14-day** scheduled assessment 03. **30-day** scheduled assessment 04. **60-day** scheduled assessment 05. **90-day** scheduled assessment 06. **Readmission/return** assessment <u>**PPS Unscheduled Assessments for a Medicare Part A Stay**</u> 07. **Unscheduled assessment used for PPS** (OMRA, significant or clinical change, or significant correction assessment) <u>**Not PPS Assessment**</u> 99. **Not PPS** assessment
Enter Code ☐	**C. PPS Other Medicare Required Assessment - OMRA** 0. **No** 1. **Start of therapy** assessment 2. **End of therapy** assessment 3. **Both Start and End of therapy** assessment
Enter Code ☐	**D. Is this a Swing Bed clinical change assessment?** Complete only if A0200 = 2 0. **No** 1. **Yes**
Enter Code ☐	**E. Is this assessment the first assessment** (OBRA, PPS, or Discharge) **since the most recent admission?** 0. **No** 1. **Yes**
Enter Code ☐☐	**F. Entry/discharge reporting** 01. **Entry** record 10. **Discharge** assessment-**return not anticipated** 11. **Discharge** assessment-**return anticipated** 12. **Death in facility** record 99. **Not entry/discharge** record

A0310: Type of Assessment (cont.)

Item Rationale

- Allows identification of needed assessment content.

Coding Instructions for A0310, Type of Assessment

Enter the code corresponding to the reason or reasons for completing this assessment.

If the assessment is being completed for both Omnibus Budget Reconciliation Act (OBRA)–required clinical reasons (A0310A) and Prospective Payment System (PPS) reasons (A0310B and A0310C) all requirements for both types of assessments must be met. See Chapter 2 on assessment schedules for details of these requirements.

Coding Instructions for A0310A, Federal OBRA Reason for Assessment

- Document the reason for completing the assessment, using the categories of assessment types. For detailed information on the requirements for scheduling and timing of the assessments, see Chapter 2 on assessment schedules.
- Enter the number corresponding to the OBRA reason for assessment. This item contains 2 digits. For codes 01-06, enter "0" in the first box and place the correct number in the second box. If the assessment is not coded 01-06, enter code "99".
  - **01.** Admission assessment (required by day 14)
  - **02.** Quarterly review assessment
  - **03.** Annual assessment
  - **04.** Significant change in status assessment
  - **05.** Significant correction to prior comprehensive assessment
  - **06.** Significant correction to prior quarterly assessment
  - **99.** Not OBRA required assessment

Coding Tips and Special Populations

- If a nursing home resident elects the Medicare hospice benefit, the nursing home is required to complete an MDS significant change in status assessment. See Chapter 2 for details on this requirement.
- It is CMS' intent to have a significant change in status assessment completed EVERY time the hospice benefit has been elected, even if a recent MDS was done and the only change is the election of the hospice benefit.

A0310: Type of Assessment (cont.)

Coding Instructions for A0310B, **PPS Assessment**

- Enter the number corresponding to the PPS reason for completing this assessment. This item contains 2 digits. For codes 01-07, enter "0" in the first box and place the correct number in the second box. If the assessment is not coded as 01-07, enter code "99".

- See Chapter 2 on assessment schedules for detailed information on the scheduling and timing of the assessments.

PPS Scheduled Assessments for a Medicare Part A Stay

01.	5-day scheduled assessment
02.	14-day scheduled assessment
03.	30-day scheduled assessment
04.	60-day scheduled assessment
05.	90-day scheduled assessment
06.	Readmission/return assessment

> **DEFINITION**
>
> **PROSPECTIVE PAYMENT SYSTEM (PPS)**
> Method of reimbursement in which Medicare payment is made based on the classification system of that service (e.g., resource utilization groups, RUGs, for skilled nursing facilities).

PPS Unscheduled Assessments for Medicare Part A Stay

| **07.** | Unscheduled assessment used for PPS (OMRA, significant change, or significant correction assessment) |

Not PPS Assessment

| **99.** | Not PPS assessment |

Coding Instructions for A0310C, **PPS Other Medicare Required Assessment—OMRA**

- **Code 0, no:** if this assessment is not an OMRA.

- **Code 1, start of therapy assessment:** with an assessment reference date (ARD) that is 5 to 7 days after the first day therapy services are provided (except when the assessment is used as a short stay assessment, see Chapter 6).

- **Code 2, end of therapy assessment:** with an ARD that is 1 to 3 days after the last day therapy services were provided.

- **Code 3, both the start and end of therapy assessment:** with an ARD that is both 5 to 7 days after the first day therapy services were provided and that is 1 to 3 days after the last day therapy services were provided (except when the assessment is used as a short stay assessment, see Chapter 6).

Coding Instructions for A0310D, **Is This a Swing Bed Clinical Change Assessment?**

- **Code 0, no:** if this assessment is not a swing bed clinical change assessment.

- **Code 1, yes:** if this assessment is a swing bed clinical change assessment.

A0310: Type of Assessment (cont.)

Coding Instructions for A0310E, Is This Assessment the First Assessment (OBRA, PPS, or Discharge) since the Most Recent Admission?

- **Code 0, no:** if this assessment is not the first assessment since the most recent entry of any kind (admission or reentry).
- **Code 1, yes:** if this assessment is the first assessment since the most recent entry of any kind (admission or reentry).

Coding Tips and Special Populations

- A0310E = 0 for any tracking record (entry or death in facility).

Coding Instructions for A0310F, Entry/Discharge Reporting

- Enter the number corresponding to the reason for completing this assessment or tracking record. This item contains 2 digits. For code 01, enter "0" in the first box and place "1" in the second box. If the assessment is not coded as "01" or "10-12," enter "99":
  - **01.** Entry record (tracking record)
  - **10.** Discharge assessment-return not anticipated
  - **11.** Discharge assessment-return anticipated
  - **12.** Death in facility record (tracking record)
  - **99.** Not entry/discharge

A0410: Submission Requirement

A0410. Submission Requirement	
Enter Code ☐	1. **Neither federal nor state required submission** 2. **State but not federal required submission** (FOR NURSING HOMES ONLY) 3. **Federal required submission**

Item Rationale

- There must be a Federal and/or State authority to submit MDS assessment data to the MDS National Repository.
- Nursing homes must be certain they are submitting MDS assessments under the appropriate authority. With this item, the nursing home indicates the submission authority.

Steps for Assessment

1. Ask the nursing home administrator or representative which units in the nursing home are Medicare certified, if any, and which units are Medicaid certified, if any.
2. Identify all units in the nursing home that are not certified, if any.

A0410: Submission Requirement (cont.)

- If some or all of the units in the nursing home are neither Medicare nor Medicaid certified, ask the nursing home administrator or representative whether the State has authority to collect MDS information for residents on units that are neither Medicare nor Medicaid certified.

Coding Instructions

- **Code 1, neither Federal nor State required submission:** if the MDS record is for a resident on a unit that is neither Medicare nor Medicaid certified, and the State does not have authority to collect MDS information for residents on this unit. If the record is submitted, it will be rejected and all information from that record will be purged.
- **Code 2, State but not Federal required submission:** if the MDS record is for a resident on a unit that is neither Medicare nor Medicaid certified, but the State has authority, under State licensure or other requirements, to collect MDS information for these residents.
- **Code 3, Federal required submission:** if the MDS record is for a resident on a Medicare and/or Medicaid certified unit. There is CMS authority to collect MDS information for residents on this unit.

A0500: Legal Name of Resident

A0500. Legal Name of Resident	
A. First name: ☐☐☐☐☐☐☐☐☐☐	B. Middle initial: ☐
C. Last name: ☐☐☐☐☐☐☐☐☐☐☐☐☐☐☐☐☐☐	D. Suffix: ☐☐☐

Item Rationale

- Allows identification of resident
- Also used for matching of records for resident

Steps for Assessment

1. Ask resident, family, significant other, guardian, or legally authorized representative.
2. Check the resident's name on his or her Medicare card, or if not in the program, check a Medicaid card or other government-issued document.

> **DEFINITION**
>
> **LEGAL NAME**
> Resident's name as it appears on the Medicare card. If the resident is not enrolled in the Medicare program, use the resident's name as it appears on a Medicaid card or other government-issued document.

A0500: Legal Name of Resident (cont.)

Coding Instructions

Use printed letters. Enter in the following order:

A. First Name
B. Middle Initial (if the resident has no middle initial, leave Item A0500B blank; if the resident has two or more middle names, use the initial of the first middle name)
C. Last Name
D. Suffix (e.g., Jr./Sr.)

A0600: Social Security and Medicare Numbers

A0600. Social Security and Medicare Numbers
A. **Social Security Number:**
☐☐☐ – ☐☐ – ☐☐☐☐
B. **Medicare number** (or comparable railroad insurance number):
☐☐☐☐☐☐☐☐☐☐☐☐

Item Rationale

- Allows identification of the resident.
- Allows records for resident to be matched in system.

Coding Instructions

- Enter the Social Security Number (SSN) in A0600A, one number per space starting with the leftmost space. If no social security number is available for the resident (e.g., if the resident is a recent immigrant or a child) the item may be left blank.
- Enter Medicare number in A0600B exactly as it appears on the resident's documents.
- If the resident does not have a Medicare number, a Railroad Retirement Board (RRB) number may be substituted. These RRB numbers contain both letters and numbers. To enter the RRB number, enter the first letter of the code in the leftmost space followed by one letter/digit per space. If no Medicare number or RRB number is known or available, the item may be left blank.
- For PPS assessments (A0310B = 01, 02, 03, 04, 05, 06, and 07), either the SSN (A0600A) or Medicare number/RRB number (A0600B) must be present and both may not be blank.

> **DEFINITIONS**
>
> **SOCIAL SECURITY NUMBER**
> A tracking number assigned to an individual by the U.S. Federal government for taxation, benefits, and identification purposes.
>
> **MEDICARE NUMBER (OR COMPARABLE RAILROAD INSURANCE NUMBER)**
> An identifier assigned to an individual for participation in national health insurance program. The Medicare Health Insurance identifier may be different from the resident's social security number (SSN), and may contain both letters and numbers. For example, many residents may receive Medicare benefits based on a spouse's Medicare eligibility.

A0600: Social Security and Medicare Numbers (cont.)

- A0600B can only be a Medicare number or a Railroad Retirement Board number.

A0700: Medicaid Number

A0700. Medicaid Number - Enter "+" if pending, "N" if not a Medicaid recipient
☐☐☐☐☐☐☐☐☐☐☐☐☐☐

Item Rationale

- Assists in correct resident identification.

Coding Instructions

- Record this number if the resident is a Medicaid recipient.
- Enter one number per box beginning in the leftmost box.
- Recheck the number to make sure you have entered the digits correctly.
- Enter a "+" in the leftmost box if the number is pending. If you are notified later that the resident does have a Medicaid number, just include it on the next assessment.
- If not applicable because the resident is not a Medicaid recipient, enter "N" in the leftmost box.

Coding Tips and Special Populations

- To obtain the Medicaid number, check the resident's Medicaid card, admission or transfer records, or medical record.
- Confirm that the resident's name on the MDS matches the resident's name on the Medicaid card.
- It is not necessary to process an MDS correction to add the Medicaid number on a prior assessment. However, a correction may be a State-specific requirement.

A0800: Gender

A0800. Gender	
Enter Code ☐	1. Male 2. Female

Item Rationale

- Assists in correct identification.
- Provides demographic gender specific health trend information.

Coding Instructions

- **Code 1:** if resident is male.
- **Code 2:** if resident is female.

A0800: Gender (cont.)

Coding Tips and Special Populations

- Resident gender on the MDS must match what is in the Social Security system.

A0900: Birth Date

A0900. Birth Date
☐☐ - ☐☐ - ☐☐☐☐ Month   Day   Year

Item Rationale

- Assists in correct identification.
- Allows determination of age.

Coding Instructions

- Fill in the boxes with the appropriate birth date. If the complete birth date is known, do not leave any boxes blank. If the month or day contains only a single digit, fill the first box in with a "0." For example: January 2, 1918, should be entered as 01-02-1918.
- Sometimes, only the birth year or the birth year and birth month will be known. These situations are handled as follows:
  — If only the birth year is known (e.g., 1918), then enter the year in the "year" portion of A0900, and leave the "month" and "day" portions blank. If the birth year and birth month are known, but the day of the month is not known, then enter the year in the "year" portion of A0900, enter the month in the "month" portion of A0900, and leave the "day" portion blank.

A1000: Race/Ethnicity

A1000. Race/Ethnicity
↓ Check all that apply
☐   A. American Indian or Alaska Native
☐   B. Asian
☐   C. Black or African American
☐   D. Hispanic or Latino
☐   E. Native Hawaiian or Other Pacific Islander
☐   F. White

A1000: Race/Ethnicity (cont.)

Item Rationale

- This item uses the common uniform language approved by the Office of Management and Budget (OMB) to report racial and ethnic categories. The categories in this classification are social-political constructs and should not be interpreted as being scientific or anthropological in nature.
- Provides demographic race/ethnicity specific health trend information.
- These categories are NOT used to determine eligibility for participation in any Federal program.

Steps for Assessment: Interview Instructions

1. Ask the resident to select the category or categories that most closely correspond to his or her race/ethnicity from the list in A1000.

   - Individuals may be more comfortable if this and the preceding question are introduced by saying, "We want to make sure that all our residents get the best care possible, regardless of their race or ethnic background. We would like you to tell us your ethnic and racial background so that we can review the treatment that all residents receive and make sure that everyone gets the highest quality of care" (Baker et al., 2005).

2. If the resident is unable to respond, ask a family member or significant other.
3. Category definitions are provided to resident or family only if requested by them in order to answer the item.
4. Respondents should be offered the option of selecting one or more racial designations.

DEFINITIONS

RACE/ETHNICITY

AMERICAN INDIAN OR ALASKA NATIVE
A person having origins in any of the original peoples of North and South America (including Central America), and who maintains tribal affiliation or community attachment.

ASIAN
A person having origins in any of the original peoples of the Far East, Southeast Asia, or the Indian subcontinent including, for example, Cambodia, China, India, Japan, Korea, Malaysia, Pakistan, the Philippine Islands, Thailand, Vietnam.

BLACK OR AFRICAN AMERICAN
A person having origins in any of the black racial groups of Africa. Terms such as "Haitian" or "Negro" can be used in addition to "Black or African American."

HISPANIC OR LATINO
A person of Cuban, Mexican, Puerto Rican, South or Central American or other Spanish culture or origin regardless of race. The term Spanish Origin can be used in addition to Hispanic or Latino.

NATIVE HAWAIIAN OR OTHER PACIFIC ISLANDER
A person having origins in any of the original peoples of Hawaii, Guam, Samoa, or other Pacific Islands.

WHITE
A person having origins in any of the original peoples of Europe, the Middle East, or North Africa.

A1000: Race/Ethnicity (cont.)

5. Only if the resident is unable to respond and no family member or significant other is available, observer identification or medical record documentation may be used.

Coding Instructions

Check all that apply.

- Enter the race or ethnic category or categories the resident, family or significant other uses to identify him or her.

A1100: Language

A1100. Language	
Enter Code ⬚	**A. Does the resident need or want an interpreter to communicate with a doctor or health care staff?** 0. **No** 1. **Yes** → Specify in A1100B, Preferred language 9. **Unable to determine**
	B. Preferred language:

Item Rationale

Health-related Quality of Life

- Inability to make needs known and to engage in social interaction because of a language barrier can be very frustrating and can result in isolation, depression, and unmet needs.
- Language barriers can interfere with accurate assessment.

Planning for Care

- When a resident needs or wants an interpreter, the nursing home should ensure that an interpreter is available.
- An alternate method of communication also should be made available to help to ensure that basic needs can be expressed at all times, such as a communication board with pictures on it for the resident to point to (if able).
- Identifies residents who need interpreter services in order to answer interview items or participate in consent process.

Steps for Assessment

1. Ask the resident if he or she needs or wants an interpreter to communicate with a doctor or health care staff.
2. If the resident is unable to respond, a family member or significant other should be asked.
3. If neither source is available, review record for evidence of a need for an interpreter.
4. If an interpreter is wanted or needed, ask for preferred language.

A1100: Language (cont.)

5. It is acceptable for a family member or significant other to be the interpreter if the resident is comfortable with it and if the family member or significant other will translate exactly what the resident says without providing his or her interpretation.

Coding Instructions for A1100A

- **Code 0, no:** if the resident (or family or medical record if resident unable to communicate) indicates that the resident does not want or need an interpreter to communicate with a doctor or health care staff.
- **Code 1, yes:** if the resident (or family or medical record if resident unable to communicate) indicates that he or she needs or wants an interpreter to communicate with a doctor or health care staff. Specify preferred language. Proceed to 1100B and enter the resident's preferred language.
- **Code 9, unable to determine:** if no source can identify whether the resident wants or needs an interpreter.

Coding Instructions for A1100B

- Enter the preferred language the resident primarily speaks or understands after interviewing the resident and family, observing the resident and listening, and reviewing the medical record.

Coding Tips and Special Populations

- An organized system of signing such as American Sign Language (ASL) can be reported as the preferred language if the resident needs or wants to communicate in this manner.

A1200: Marital Status

A1200. Marital Status	
Enter Code ☐	1. Never married 2. Married 3. Widowed 4. Separated 5. Divorced

Item Rationale

- Allows understanding of the formal relationship the resident has and can be important for care and discharge planning.
- Demographic information.

Steps for Assessment

1. Ask the resident about his or her marital status.
2. If the resident is unable to respond, ask a family member or other significant other.
3. If neither source can report, review the medical record for information.

A1200: Marital Status (cont.)

Coding Instructions

- Choose the answer that best describes the current marital status of the resident and enter the corresponding number in the code box:
  1. Never Married
  2. Married
  3. Widowed
  4. Separated
  5. Divorced

A1300: Optional Resident Items

A1300. Optional Resident Items
A. Medical record number:
⬚⬚⬚⬚⬚⬚⬚⬚⬚⬚
B. Room number:
⬚⬚⬚⬚⬚⬚⬚⬚
C. Name by which resident prefers to be addressed:
⬚⬚⬚⬚⬚⬚⬚⬚⬚⬚⬚⬚⬚⬚⬚⬚⬚⬚⬚⬚
D. Lifetime occupation(s) - put "/" between two occupations:
⬚⬚⬚⬚⬚⬚⬚⬚⬚⬚⬚⬚⬚⬚⬚⬚⬚⬚⬚⬚

Item Rationale

- Some facilities prefer to include the nursing home medical record number on the MDS to facilitate tracking.
- Some facilities conduct unit reviews of MDS items in addition to resident and nursing home level reviews. The unit may be indicated by the room number.
- Preferred name and lifetime occupation help nursing home staff members personalize their interactions with the resident.
- Many people are called by a nickname or middle name throughout their life. It is important to call residents by the name they prefer in order to establish comfort and respect between staff and resident. Also, some cognitively impaired or hearing impaired residents might have difficulty responding when called by their legal name, if it is not the name most familiar to them.
- Others may prefer a more formal and less familiar address. For example, a physician might appreciate being referred to as "Doctor."
- Knowing a person's lifetime occupation is also helpful for care planning and conversation purposes. For example, a carpenter might enjoy pursuing hobby shop activities.
- These are optional items because they are not needed for CMS program function.

A1300: Optional Resident Items (cont.)

Coding Instructions for A1300A, Medical Record Number

- Enter the resident's medical record number (from the nursing home medical record, admission office or Health Information Management Department) if the nursing home chooses to exercise this option.

Coding Instructions for A1300B, Room Number

- Enter the resident's room number if the nursing home chooses to exercise this option.

Coding Instructions for A1300C, Name by Which Resident Prefers to Be Addressed

- Enter the resident's preferred name. This field captures a preferred nickname, middle name, or title that the resident prefers staff use.
- Obtained from resident self-report or family or significant other if resident is unable to respond.

Coding Instructions for A1300D, Lifetime Occupation(s)

- Enter the job title or profession that describes the resident's main occupation(s) before retiring or entering the nursing home. When two occupations are identified, place a slash (/) between each occupation.
- The lifetime occupation of a person whose primary work was in the home should be recorded as "homemaker." For a resident who is a child or a mentally retarded/developmentally delayed adult resident who has never had an occupation, record as "none."

A1500: Preadmission Screening and Resident Review (PASRR)

A1500. Preadmission Screening and Resident Review (PASRR)	
Complete only if A0310A = 01	
Enter Code ☐	Has the resident been evaluated by Level II PASRR and determined to have a serious mental illness and/or mental retardation or a related condition? 0. No 1. Yes 9. Not a Medicaid certified unit

Item Rationale

Health-related Quality of Life

- All individuals who are admitted to a Medicaid certified nursing facility must have a Level I PASRR completed to screen for possible mental illness, mental retardation (MI/MR) or related conditions regardless of the resident's method of payment (please contact your local State Medicaid Agency for details regarding PASRR requirements and exemptions).

- Individuals who have or are suspected to have MI/MR or related conditions may not be admitted to a Medicaid-certified nursing facility unless approved through Level II PASRR determination. Those residents covered by Level II PASRR process may require certain care and services provided by the nursing home, and/or specialized services provided by the State.

- A resident with MI or MR must have a Resident Review (RR) conducted when there is a significant change in the resident's physical or mental condition. Therefore, when a significant change in status MDS assessment is completed for a resident with MI or MR, the nursing home is required to notify the State mental health authority, mental retardation or developmental disability authority (depending on which operates in their State) in order to notify them of the resident's change in status. Section 1919(e)(7)(B)(iii) of the Social Security Act requires the notification or referral for a significant change.[1]

- Each State Medicaid agency might have specific processes and guidelines for referral, and which types of significant changes should be referred. Therefore, facilities should become acquainted with their own State requirements.

- Please see https://www.cms.gov/PASRR/01_Overview.asp for CMS information on PASRR.

Planning for Care

- The Level II PASRR determination and the evaluation report specify services to be provided by the nursing home and/or specialized services defined by the State.

- The State is responsible for providing specialized services to individuals with MI/MR. In some States specialized services are provided to residents in Medicaid-certified facilities (in other States specialized services are only provided in other facility types such as a psychiatric hospital). The nursing home is required to provide all other care and services appropriate to the resident's condition.

- The services to be provided by the nursing home and/or specialized services provided by the State that are specified in the Level II PASRR determination and the evaluation report should be addressed in the plan of care.

- Identifies individuals who are subject to Resident Review upon change in condition.

Steps for Assessment

1. Complete if A0310A = 01 (Admission Assessment).

2. Review the Level I PASRR form to determine whether a Level II PASRR was required.

3. Review the PASRR report provided by the State if Level II screening was required.

---

[1] The statute may also be referenced as 42 USC 1396r(e)(7)(B)(iii). Note that as of this revision date the statute supersedes Federal regulations at 42 CFR 483.114(c), which still reads as requiring annual resident review. The regulation has not yet been updated to reflect the statutory change to resident review upon significant change in condition.

A1500: Preadmission Screening and Resident Review (PASRR) (cont.)

Coding Instructions

- **Code 0, no:** if any of the following apply:
  - — PASRR Level I screening did not result in a referral for Level II screening, or
  - — Level II screening determined that the resident does not have a serious mental illness and/or mental retardation-related condition, or
  - — PASRR screening is not required because the resident was admitted from a hospital after requiring acute inpatient care, is receiving services for the condition for which he or she received care in the hospital, and the attending physician has certified before admission that the resident is likely to require less than 30 days of nursing home care.

- **Code 1, yes:** if PASRR Level II screening determined that the resident has a serious mental illness and/or mental retardation-related condition.

- **Code 9, not a Medicaid-certified unit:** if bed is not in a Medicaid-certified nursing home. The PASRR process does not apply to nursing home units that are not certified by Medicaid (unless a State requires otherwise) and therefore the question is not applicable.

  - — Note that the requirement is based on the certification of the part of the nursing home the resident will occupy. In a nursing home in which some parts are Medicaid certified and some are not, this question applies when a resident is admitted, or transferred to, a Medicaid certified part of the building.

A1550: Conditions Related to Mental Retardation/Developmental Delay (MR/DD) Status

	A1550. Conditions Related to MR/DD Status
	If the resident is 22 years of age or older, complete only if A0310A = 01
	If the resident is 21 years of age or younger, complete only if A0310A = 01, 03, 04, or 05
↓	Check all conditions that are related to MR/DD status that were manifested before age 22, and are likely to continue indefinitely
	MR/DD With Organic Condition
☐	A. Down syndrome
☐	B. Autism
☐	C. Epilepsy
☐	D. Other organic condition related to MR/DD
	MR/DD Without Organic Condition
☐	E. MR/DD with no organic condition
	No MR/DD
☐	Z. None of the above

A1550: Conditions Related to MR/DD Status (cont.)

Item Rationale

- To document conditions associated with mental retardation or developmental disabilities.

Steps for Assessment

1. If resident is 22 years of age or older on the assessment date, complete only if A0310A = 01 (admission assessment).

2. If resident is 21 years of age or younger on the assessment date, complete if A0310A = 01, 03, 04, or 05 (admission assessment, annual assessment, significant change in status assessment, significant correction to prior comprehensive assessment).

Coding Instructions

- Check all conditions related to MR/DD status that were present before age 22.

- When age of onset is not specified, assume that the condition meets this criterion AND is likely to continue indefinitely.

- **Code A:** if Down syndrome is present.

- **Code B:** if autism is present.

- **Code C:** if epilepsy is present.

- **Code D:** if other organic condition related to MR/DD is present.

- **Code E:** if an MR/DD condition is present but the resident does not have any of the specific conditions listed.

- **Code Z:** if MR/DD condition is not present.

DEFINITION

DOWN SYNDROME
A common genetic disorder in which a child is born with 47 rather than 46 chromosomes, resulting in developmental delays, mental retardation, low muscle tone, and other possible effects.

AUTISM
A developmental disorder that is characterized by impaired social interaction, problems with verbal and nonverbal communication, and unusual, repetitive, or severely limited activities and interests.

EPILEPSY
A common chronic neurological disorder that is characterized by recurrent unprovoked seizures.

DEFINITION

OTHER ORGANIC CONDITION RELATED TO MR/DD
Examples of diagnostic conditions include congenital syphilis, maternal intoxication, mechanical injury at birth, prenatal hypoxia, neuronal lipid storage diseases, phenylketonuria (PKU), neurofibromatosis, microcephalus, macroencephaly, meningomyelocele, congenital hydrocephalus, etc.

A1600: Entry Date (date of this entry into the facility)

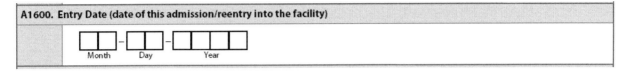

A1600. Entry Date (date of this admission/reentry into the facility)

☐☐ - ☐☐ - ☐☐☐☐	
Month Day Year	

Item Rationale

- To document the date of admission or reentry into the nursing home.

Coding Instructions

- Enter the most recent date of entry to this nursing home. Use the format: Month-Day-Year: XX-XX-XXXX. For example, October 12, 2010, would be entered as 10-12-2010.

> **DEFINITIONS**
>
> **ENTRY DATE**
> The initial date of admission to the nursing home, or the date the resident most recently returned to your nursing home after being discharged (whether or not the return was anticipated).

A1700: Type of Entry

Appears on Entry Tracking Record

A1700. Type of Entry

Enter Code	
☐	1. Admission
	2. Reentry

Item Rationale

- Captures whether date in A1600 is an admission date or a reentry date.

Coding Instructions

- **Code 1, admission:** when one of the following occurs:
    1. resident has never been admitted to this facility before; OR
    2. resident has been in this facility previously and was discharged prior to completion of the OBRA admission assessment; OR
    3. resident has been in this facility previously and was discharged return not anticipated; OR
    4. resident has been in this facility previously and was discharged return anticipated and did not return within 30 days of discharge.
- **Code 2, reentry:** when all 3 of the following occurred prior to the this entry, the resident was:
    1. admitted to this nursing home (i.e., OBRA admission assessment was completed), AND
    2. discharged return anticipated, AND
    3. returned to facility within 30 days of discharge.

23

A1700: Type of Entry (cont.)

Coding Tips and Special Populations

- Swing bed facilities will always code the resident's entry as an admission, '1', since an OBRA Admission assessment must have been completed to code as a reentry. OBRA Admission assessments are not completed for swing bed residents.
- In determining if a resident returns to the facility within 30 days, the day of discharge from the facility is not counted in the 30 days. For example, a resident is discharged return anticipated on December 1 would need to return to the facility December 31 to meet the "within 30 day" requirement.

A1800: Entered From

Appears on Entry Tracking Record.

A1800. Entered From	
Enter Code	01. **Community** (private home/apt., board/care, assisted living, group home)
	02. **Another nursing home or swing bed**
	03. **Acute hospital**
	04. **Psychiatric hospital**
	05. **Inpatient rehabilitation facility**
	06. **MR/DD facility**
	07. **Hospice**
	99. **Other**

Item Rationale

- Understanding the setting that the individual was in immediately prior to nursing home admission informs care planning and may also inform discharge planning and discussions.
- Demographic information.

Steps for Assessment

1. Review transfer and admission records.
2. Ask the resident and/or family or significant others.

Coding Instructions

Enter the 2-digit code that corresponds to the location or program the resident was admitted from for this admission.

- **Code 01, community (private home/apt, board/care, assisted living, group home):** if the resident was admitted from a private home, apartment, board and care, assisted living facility or group home.

DEFINITIONS

PRIVATE HOME OR APARTMENT Any house, condominium, or apartment in the community whether owned by the resident or another person. Also included in this category are retirement communities and independent housing for the elderly.

BOARD AND CARE/ ASSISTED LIVING/ GROUP HOME
A non-institutional community residential setting that includes services of the following types: home health services, homemaker/ personal care services, or meal services.

A1800: Entered From (cont.)

- **Code 02, another nursing home or swing bed:** if the resident was admitted from an institution (or a distinct part of an institution) that is primarily engaged in providing skilled nursing care and related services for residents who require medical or nursing care or rehabilitation services for injured, disabled, or sick persons. Includes swing beds.

- **Code 03, acute hospital:** if the resident was admitted from an institution that is engaged in providing, by or under the supervision of physicians for inpatients, diagnostic services, therapeutic services for medical diagnosis, and the treatment and care of injured, disabled, or sick persons.

- **Code 04, psychiatric hospital:** if the resident was admitted from an institution that is engaged in providing, by or under the supervision of a physician, psychiatric services for the diagnosis and treatment of mentally ill residents.

- **Code 05, inpatient rehabilitation facility (IRF):** if the resident was admitted from an institution that is engaged in providing, under the supervision of physicians, services for the rehabilitation of injured, disabled or sick persons. Includes IRFs that are units within acute care hospitals.

- **Code 06, MR/DD facility:** if the resident was admitted from an institution that is engaged in providing, under the supervision of a physician, any health and rehabilitative services for individuals who are mentally retarded or who have developmental disabilities.

- **Code 07, hospice:** if the resident was admitted from a program for terminally ill persons where an array of services is necessary for the palliation and management of terminal illness and related conditions. The hospice must be licensed by the State as a hospice provider and/or certified under the Medicare program as a hospice provider. Includes community-based or inpatient hospice programs.

- **Code 99, other:** if the resident was admitted from none of the above.

Coding Tips and Special Populations

- If an individual was enrolled in a home-based hospice program enter **07, Hospice**, instead of **01, Community**.

A2000: Discharge Date

Appears on Discharge Assessments and Death in Facility Tracking Record.

A2000. Discharge Date
Complete only if A0310F = 10, 11, or 12
☐☐ - ☐☐ - ☐☐☐☐
Month   Day   Year

Item Rationale

- Closes case in system.

A2000: Discharge Date (cont.)

Coding Instructions

- Enter the date the resident was discharged (whether or not return is anticipated). This is the date the resident leaves the facility.
- For discharge assessments, the discharge date (A2000) and ARD (A2300) must be the same date.
- Do not include leave of absence or hospital observational stays less than 24 hours unless admitted to the hospital.
- Obtain data from the medical, admissions or transfer records.

Coding Tips and Special Populations

- If a resident was receiving services under SNF Part A PPS, the discharge date may be later than the end of Medicare stay date (A2400C).

A2100: Discharge Status

Appears on Discharge Assessments and Death in Facility Tracking Record.

A2100. Discharge Status
Complete only if A0310F = 10, 11, or 12
Enter Code [ ][ ]   01. **Community** (private home/apt., board/care, assisted living, group home)   02. **Another nursing home or swing bed**   03. **Acute hospital**   04. **Psychiatric hospital**   05. **Inpatient rehabilitation facility**   06. **MR/DD facility**   07. **Hospice**   08. **Deceased**   99. **Other**

Item Rationale

- Demographic and outcome information.

Steps for Assessment

1. Review the medical record including the discharge plan and discharge orders for documentation of discharge location.

Coding Instructions

Select the 2-digit code that corresponds to the resident's discharge status.

- **Code 01, community (private home/apt., board/care, assisted living, group home):** if discharge location is a private home, apartment, board and care, assisted living facility, or group home.

A2100: Discharge Status (cont.)

- **Code 02, another nursing home or swing bed:** if discharge location is an institution (or a distinct part of an institution) that is primarily engaged in providing skilled nursing care and related services for residents who require medical or nursing care or rehabilitation services for injured, disabled, or sick persons. Includes swing beds.

- **Code 03, acute hospital:** if discharge location is an institution that is engaged in providing, by or under the supervision of physicians for inpatients, diagnostic services, therapeutic services for medical diagnosis, and the treatment and care of injured, disabled, or sick persons.

- **Code 04, psychiatric hospital:** if discharge location is an institution that is engaged in providing, by or under the supervision of a physician, psychiatric services for the diagnosis and treatment of mentally ill residents.

- **Code 05, inpatient rehabilitation facility:** if discharge location is an institution that is engaged in providing, under the supervision of physicians, rehabilitation services for the rehabilitation of injured, disabled or sick persons. Includes IRFs that are units within acute care hospitals.

- **Code 06, MR/DD facility:** if discharge location is an institution that is engaged in providing, under the supervision of a physician, any health and rehabilitative services for individuals who are mentally retarded or who have developmental delay.

- **Code 07, hospice:** if discharge location is a program for terminally ill persons where an array of services is necessary for the palliation and management of terminal illness and related conditions. The hospice must be licensed by the State as a hospice provider and/or certified under the Medicare program as a hospice provider. Includes community-based (e.g., home) or inpatient hospice programs.

- **Code 08, deceased:** if resident is deceased.

- **Code 99, other:** if discharge location is none of the above.

A2200: Previous Assessment Reference Date for Significant Correction

A2200. Previous Assessment Reference Date for Significant Correction
Complete only if A0310A = 05 or 06
☐☐ - ☐☐ - ☐☐☐☐
Month   Day   Year

Item Rationale

- To identify the ARD of a previous comprehensive or quarterly assessment (A0310A = 05 or 06) in which a significant error is discovered.

A2200: Previous Assessment Reference Date for Significant Correction (cont.)

Coding Instructions

- Complete only if A0310A = 05 (Significant correction to prior comprehensive assessment) or A0310A = 06 (Significant correction to prior quarterly assessment).
- Enter the ARD of the prior comprehensive or quarterly assessment in which a significant error has been identified and a correction is required.

A2300: Assessment Reference Date

A2300. Assessment Reference Date
Observation end date:
☐☐ - ☐☐ - ☐☐☐☐
Month   Day   Year

Item Rationale

- Designates the end of the look-back period so that all assessment items refer to the resident's status during the same period of time.
- As the last day of the look-back period, the ARD serves as the reference point for determining the care and services captured on the MDS assessment. Anything that happens after the ARD will not be captured on that MDS. For example, for a MDS item with a 7-day look-back period, assessment information is collected for a 7-day period ending on and including the ARD which is the 7th day of this look-back period. For an item with a 14-day look-back period, the information is collected for a 14-day period ending on and including the ARD. The look-back period includes observations and events through the end of the day (midnight) of the ARD.

Steps for Assessment

1. Interdisciplinary team members should select the ARD based on the reason for the assessment and compliance with all timing and scheduling requirements outlined in Chapter 2.

Coding Instructions

- Enter the appropriate date on the lines provided. Do not leave any spaces blank. If the month or day contains only a single digit, enter a "0" in the first space. Use four digits for the year. For example, October 2, 2010, should be entered as: 10-02-2010..

> **DEFINITIONS**
>
> **ASSESSMENT REFERENCE DATE (ARD)**
> The specific end-point for look-back periods in the MDS assessment process. Almost all MDS items refer to the resident's status over a designated time period referring back in time from the Assessment Reference Date (ARD). Most frequently, this look-back period, also called the observation or assessment period, is a 7-day period ending on the ARD. Look-back periods may cover the 7 days ending on this date, 14 days ending on this date, etc.

A2300: Assessment Reference Date (cont.)

- For detailed information on the timing of the assessments, see Chapter 2 on assessment schedules.
- For discharge assessments, the discharge date item (A2000) and the ARD item (A2300) must contain the same date.

Coding Tips and Special Populations

- When the resident dies or is discharged prior to the end of the look-back period for a required assessment, the ARD must be adjusted to equal the discharge date.
- The look-back period may not be extended simply because a resident was out of the nursing home during part of the look-back period (e.g., a home visit, therapeutic leave, or hospital observation stay less than 24 hours when resident is not admitted). For example, if the ARD is set at day 13 and there is a 2-day temporary leave during the look-back period, the 2 leave days are still considered part of the look-back period.
- When collecting assessment information, data from the time period of the leave of absence is captured as long as the particular MDS item permits. For example, if the family takes the resident to the physician during the leave, the visit would be counted in Item O0600, **Physician Examination** (if criteria are otherwise met).

  This requirement applies to all assessments, regardless of whether they are being completed for clinical or payment purposes.

A2400: Medicare Stay

A2400. Medicare Stay	
Enter Code ☐	**A. Has the resident had a Medicare-covered stay since the most recent entry?** 　0. **No** → Skip to B0100, Comatose 　1. **Yes** → Continue to A2400B, Start date of most recent Medicare stay **B. Start date of most recent Medicare stay:** 　☐☐ – ☐☐ – ☐☐☐☐ 　Month　　Day　　　Year **C. End date of most recent Medicare stay** - Enter dashes if stay is ongoing: 　☐☐ – ☐☐ – ☐☐☐☐ 　Month　　Day　　　Year

Item Rationale

- Identifies when a resident is receiving services under the SNF PPS.
- Identifies when a resident's Medicare Part A stay begins and ends.
- The end date is used to determine if the resident's stay qualifies for the short stay assessment.

A2400: Medicare Stay (cont.)

Coding Instructions for A2400A, Has the Resident Had a Medicare-covered Stay since the Most Recent Entry?

- **Code 0, no:** if the resident has not had a covered Medicare Part A covered stay since the most recent entry. Skip to B0100, Comatose.
- **Code 1, yes:** if the resident has had a Medicare Part A covered stay since the most recent entry. Continue to A2400B.

Coding Instructions for A2400B, Start of Most Recent Medicare Stay

- **Code the date of day 1** of this Medicare stay if A2400A is **coded 1, yes**.

Coding Instructions for A2400C, End Date of Most Recent Medicare Stay

- **Code the date of last day** of this Medicare stay if A2400A is **coded 1, yes**.
- If the Medicare Part A stay is ongoing there will be no end date to report. Enter dashes to indicate that the stay is ongoing.
- The end of Medicare date is coded as follows, whichever occurs first:
  — Date SNF benefit exhausts (i.e., the 100th day of the benefit); or
  — Date of last day covered as recorded on the Advance Beneficiary Notice of Noncoverage (ABN); or
  — Date the resident's payer source changes from Medicare A to another payer (regardless if the resident was moved to another bed or not); or
  — Date the resident was discharged from the facility (see Item A2000, Discharge date).

> **DEFINITIONS**
>
> **MOST RECENT MEDICARE STAY**
> This is a Medicare Part A covered stay that has started on or after the most recent entry (admission or reentry) to the nursing home.
>
> **MEDICARE-COVERED STAY**
> Skilled Nursing Facility stays billable to Medicare Part A. Does not include stays billable to Medicare Advantage HMO plans.
>
> **CURRENT MEDICARE STAY**
> NEW ADMISSION: Day 1 of Medicare Part A stay.
>
> READMISSION: Day 1 of Medicare Part A coverage after readmission following a discharge.

Coding Tips and Special Populations

- When a resident on Medicare Part A returns following a therapeutic leave of absence or a hospital observation stay of less than 24 hours (without hospital admission), this is a continuation of the Medicare Part A stay, not a new Medicare Part A stay.
- The end date of the Medicare stay may be earlier than actual discharge date from the facility (Item A2000).

Examples

1. Mrs. G. began receiving services under Medicare Part A on October 14, 2010. Due to her stable condition and ability to manage her medications and dressing changes, the facility determined that she no longer qualified for Part A SNF coverage and issued an ABN with the last day of coverage as November 23, 2010. Mrs. G. was discharged from the facility on November 24, 2010. Code the following on her discharge assessment:

   - A2000 = 11-24-2010
   - A2400A = 1
   - A2400B = 10-14-2010
   - A2400C = 11-23-2010

2. Mr. N began receiving services under Medicare Part A on December 11, 2010. He was sent to the ER on December 19, 2010 at 8:30pm and was not admitted to the hospital. He returned to the facility on December 20, 2010, at 11:00 am. The facility completed his 14-day PPS assessment with an ARD of December 23, 2010. Code the following on his 14-day PPS assessment:

   - A2400A = 1
   - A2400B = 12-11-2010
   - A2400C = ----------

3. Mr. R. began receiving services under Medicare Part A on October 15, 2010. He was discharged return anticipated on October 20, 2010, to the hospital. Code the following on his discharge assessment:

   - A2000 = 10-20-2010
   - A2400A = 1
   - A2400B = 10-15-2010
   - A2400C = 10-20-2010

SECTION B: HEARING, SPEECH, AND VISION

Intent: The intent of items in this section is to document the resident's ability to hear (with assistive hearing devices, if they are used), understand, and communicate with others and whether the resident experiences visual limitations or difficulties related to diseases common in aged persons.

B0100: Comatose

B0100. Comatose	
Enter Code [ ]	**Persistent vegetative state/no discernible consciousness** 0. **No** → Continue to B0200, Hearing 1. **Yes** → Skip to G0110, Activities of Daily Living (ADL) Assistance

Item Rationale

Health-related Quality of Life

- Residents who are in a coma or persistent vegetative state are at risk for the complications of immobility, including skin breakdown and joint contractures.

Planning for Care

- Care planning should center on eliminating or minimizing complications and providing care consistent with the resident's health care goals.

> **DEFINITIONS**
>
> **COMATOSE (coma)**
> A pathological state in which neither arousal (wakefulness, alertness) nor awareness exists. The person is unresponsive and cannot be aroused; he/she does not open his/her eyes, does not speak and does not move his/her extremities on command or in response to noxious stimuli (e.g., pain).

Steps for Assessment

1. Review the medical record to determine if a neurological diagnosis of comatose or persistent vegetative state has been documented by a physician, or nurse practitioner, physician assistant, or clinical nurse specialist if allowable under state licensure laws.

Coding Instructions

- **Code 0, no:** if a diagnosis of coma or persistent vegetative state is not present during the 7-day look-back period. Continue to B0200 **Hearing**.

- **Code 1, yes:** if the record indicates that a physician, nurse practitioner or clinical nurse specialist has documented a diagnosis of coma or persistent vegetative state that is applicable during the 7-day look-back period. Skip to Section G0110, **Activities of Daily Living (ADL) Assistance**.

B0100: Comatose (cont.)

Coding Tips

- Only code if a diagnosis of coma or persistent vegetative state has been assigned. For example, some residents in advanced stages of progressive neurologic disorders such as Alzheimer's disease may have severe cognitive impairment, be non-communicative and sleep a great deal of time; however, they are usually not comatose or in a persistent vegetative state, as defined here.

DEFINITIONS

PERSISTENT VEGETATIVE STATE
Sometimes residents who were comatose after an anoxic-ischemic injury (i.e., not enough oxygen to the brain) from a cardiac arrest, head trauma, or massive stroke, regain wakefulness but do not evidence any purposeful behavior or cognition. Their eyes are open, and they may grunt, yawn, pick with their fingers, and have random body movements. Neurological exam shows extensive damage to both cerebral hemispheres.

B0200: Hearing

B0200. Hearing	
Enter Code ☐	**Ability to hear** (with hearing aid or hearing appliances if normally used) 0. **Adequate** - no difficulty in normal conversation, social interaction, listening to TV 1. **Minimal difficulty** - difficulty in some environments (e.g., when person speaks softly or setting is noisy) 2. **Moderate difficulty** - speaker has to increase volume and speak distinctly 3. **Highly impaired** - absence of useful hearing

Item Rationale

Health-related Quality of Life

- Problems with hearing can contribute to sensory deprivation, social isolation, and mood and behavior disorders.

- Unaddressed communication problems related to hearing impairment can be mistaken for confusion or cognitive impairment.

Planning for Care

- Address reversible causes of hearing difficulty (such as cerumen impaction).

- Evaluate potential benefit from hearing assistance devices.

- Offer assistance to residents with hearing difficulties to avoid social isolation.

B0200: Hearing (cont.)

- Consider other communication strategies for persons with hearing loss that is not reversible or is not completely corrected with hearing devices.

- Adjust environment by reducing background noise by lowering the sound volume on televisions or radios, because a noisy environment can inhibit opportunities for effective communication.

Steps for Assessment

1. Ensure that the resident is using his or her normal hearing appliance if they have one. Hearing devices may not be as conventional as a hearing aid. Some residents by choice may use hearing amplifiers or a microphone and headphones as an alternative to hearing aids. Ensure whatever hearing appliance is used, it is operational.

2. Interview the resident and ask about hearing function in different situations (e.g. hearing staff members, talking to visitors, using telephone, watching TV, attending activities).

3. Observe the resident during your verbal interactions and when he or she interacts with others throughout the day.

4. Think through how you can best communicate with the resident. For example, you may need to speak more clearly, use a louder tone, speak more slowly or use gestures. The resident may need to see your face to understand what you are saying, or you may need to take the resident to a quieter area for them to hear you. All of these are cues that there is a hearing problem.

5. Review the medical record.

6. Consult the resident's family, direct care staff, activities personnel, and speech or hearing specialists.

Coding Instructions

- **Code 0, adequate:** No difficulty in normal conversation, social interaction, or listening to TV. The resident hears all normal conversational speech and telephone conversation and announcements in group activities.

- **Code 1, minimal difficulty:** Difficulty in some environments (e.g., when a person speaks softly or the setting is noisy). The resident hears speech at conversational levels but has difficulty hearing when not in quiet listening conditions or when not in one-on-one situations. The resident's hearing is adequate after environmental adjustments are made, such as reducing background noise by moving to a quiet room or by lowering the volume on television or radio.

- **Code 2, moderate difficulty:** Speaker has to increase volume and speak distinctly. Although hearing-deficient, the resident compensates when the speaker adjusts tonal quality and speaks distinctly; or the resident can hear only when the speaker's face is clearly visible.

B0200: Hearing (cont.)

- **Code 3, highly impaired:** Absence of useful hearing. The resident hears only some sounds and frequently fails to respond even when the speaker adjusts tonal quality, speaks distinctly, or is positioned face-to-face. There is no comprehension of conversational speech, even when the speaker makes maximum adjustments.

Coding Tips for Special Populations

- Residents who are unable to respond to a standard hearing assessment due to cognitive impairment will require alternate assessment methods. The resident can be observed in their normal environment. Does he or she respond (e.g., turn his or her head) when a noise is made at a normal level? Does the resident seem to respond only to specific noise in a quiet environment? Assess whether the resident responds only to loud noise or do they not respond at all.

B0300: Hearing Aid

B0300. Hearing Aid	
Enter Code ☐	**Hearing aid or other hearing appliance used** in completing B0200, Hearing 0. **No** 1. **Yes**

Item Rationale

Health-related Quality of Life

- Problems with hearing can contribute to social isolation and mood and behavior disorders.

- Many residents without hearing aids or other hearing appliances could benefit from them.

- Many persons who benefit from and own hearing aids do not have them on arrival at the nursing home or the hearing aid is not functional.

Planning for Care

- Knowing if a hearing aid was used when determining hearing ability allows better identification of evaluation and management needs.

- For residents with hearing aids, use and maintenance should be included in care planning.

- Residents who do not have adequate hearing without a hearing aid should be asked about history of hearing aid use.

- Residents who do not have adequate hearing despite wearing a hearing aid might benefit from a re-evaluation of the device or assessment for new causes of hearing impairment.

Steps for Assessment

1. Prior to beginning the hearing assessment, ask the resident if he or she owns a hearing aid or other hearing appliance and, if so, whether it is at the nursing home.

2. If the resident cannot respond, write the question down and allow the resident to read it.

B0300: Hearing Aid (cont.)

3. If the resident is still unable, check with family and care staff about hearing aid or other hearing appliances.

4. Check the medical record for evidence that the resident had a hearing appliance in place when hearing ability was recorded.

5. Ask staff and significant others whether the resident was using a hearing appliance when they observed hearing ability (above).

Coding Instructions

- **Code 0, no:** if the resident did not use a hearing aid (or other hearing appliance) for the 7-day hearing assessment coded in **B0200, Hearing.**

- **Code 1, yes:** if the resident did use a hearing aid (or other hearing appliance) for the hearing assessment coded in **B0200, Hearing.**

B0600: Speech Clarity

B0600. Speech Clarity	
Enter Code [ ]	**Select best description of speech pattern** 0. **Clear speech** - distinct intelligible words 1. **Unclear speech** - slurred or mumbled words 2. **No speech** - absence of spoken words

Item Rationale

Health-related Quality of Life

> **DEFINITIONS**
>
> **SPEECH**
> The verbal expression of articulate words.

- Unclear speech or absent speech can hinder communication and be very frustrating to an individual.

- Unclear speech or absent speech can result in physical and psychosocial needs not being met and can contribute to depression and social isolation.

Planning for Care

- If speech is absent or is not clear enough for the resident to make needs known, other methods of communication should be explored.

- Lack of speech clarity or ability to speak should not be mistaken for cognitive impairment.

Steps for Assessment

1. Listen to the resident.

2. Ask primary assigned caregivers about the resident's speech pattern.

3. Review the medical record.

B0600: Speech Clarity (cont.)

4. Determine the quality of the resident's speech, not the content or appropriateness—just words spoken.

Coding Instructions

- **Code 0, clear speech:** if the resident usually utters distinct, intelligible words.

- **Code 1, unclear speech:** if the resident usually utters slurred or mumbled words.

- **Code 2, no speech:** if there is an absence of spoken words.

B0700: Makes Self Understood

B0700. Makes Self Understood	
Enter Code	**Ability to express ideas and wants**, consider both verbal and non-verbal expression 0. **Understood** 1. **Usually understood** - difficulty communicating some words or finishing thoughts **but** is able if prompted or given time 2. **Sometimes understood** - ability is limited to making concrete requests 3. **Rarely/never understood**

Item Rationale

Health-related Quality of Life

- Problems making self understood can be very frustrating for the resident and can contribute to social isolation and mood and behavior disorders.

- Unaddressed communication problems can be inappropriately mistaken for confusion or cognitive impairment.

Planning for Care

- Ability to make self understood can be optimized by not rushing the resident, breaking longer questions into parts and waiting for reply, and maintaining eye contact (if appropriate).

- If a resident has difficulty making self understood:

  — Identify the underlying cause or causes.

  — Identify the best methods to facilitate communication for that resident.

> **DEFINITIONS**
>
> **MAKES SELF UNDERSTOOD**
> Able to express or communicate requests, needs, opinions, and to conduct social conversation in his or her primary language, whether in speech, writing, sign language, gestures, or a combination of these. Deficits in the ability to make one's self understood (expressive communication deficits) can include reduced voice volume and difficulty in producing sounds, or difficulty in finding the right word, making sentences, writing, and/or gesturing.

B0700: Makes Self Understood (cont.)

Steps for Assessment

1. Assess using the resident's preferred language.

2. Interact with the resident. Be sure he or she can hear you or have access to his or her preferred method for communication. If the resident seems unable to communicate, offer alternatives such as writing, pointing or using cue cards.

3. Observe his or her interactions with others in different settings and circumstances.

4. Consult with the primary nurse assistant (over all shifts), if available, the resident's family, and speech-language pathologist.

Coding Instructions

- **Code 0, understood:** if the resident expresses requests and ideas clearly.

- **Code 1, usually understood:** if the resident has difficulty communicating some words or finishing thoughts **but** is able if prompted or given time. He or she may have delayed responses or may require some prompting to make self understood.

- **Code 2, sometimes understood:** if the resident has limited ability but is able to express concrete requests regarding at least basic needs (e.g., food, drink, sleep, toilet).

- **Code 3, rarely or never understood:** if, at best, the resident's understanding is limited to staff interpretation of highly individual, resident-specific sounds or body language (e.g., indicated presence of pain or need to toilet).

B0800: Ability to Understand Others

B0800. Ability To Understand Others	
Enter Code [ ]	**Understanding verbal content, however able** (with hearing aid or device if used) 0. **Understands** - clear comprehension 1. **Usually understands** - misses some part/intent of message **but** comprehends most conversation 2. **Sometimes understands** - responds adequately to simple, direct communication only 3. **Rarely/never understands**

Item Rationale

Health-related Quality of Life

- Inability to understand direct person-to-person communication

  — Can severely limit association with others.

  — Can inhibit the individual's ability to follow instructions that can affect health and safety.

38

Planning for Care

- Thorough assessment to determine underlying cause or causes is critical in order to develop a care plan to address the individual's specific deficits and needs.

- Every effort should be made by the facility to provide information to the resident in a consistent manner that he or she understands based on an individualized assessment.

Steps for Assessment

1. Assess in the resident's preferred language.

2. If the resident uses a hearing aid, hearing device or other communications enhancement device, the resident should use that device during the evaluation of the resident's understanding of person-to-person communication.

3. Interact with the resident and observe his or her understanding of other's communication.

4. Consult with direct care staff over all shifts, if possible, the resident's family, and speech-language pathologist (if involved in care).

5. Review the medical record for indications of how well the resident understands others.

> **DEFINITIONS**
>
> **ABILITY TO UNDERSTAND OTHERS**
> Comprehension of direct person-to-person communication whether spoken, written, or in sign language or Braille. Includes the resident's ability to process and understand language. Deficits in one's ability to understand (receptive communication deficits) can involve declines in hearing, comprehension (spoken or written) or recognition of facial expressions.

Coding Instructions

- **Code 0, understands:** if the resident clearly comprehends the message(s) and demonstrates comprehension by words or actions/behaviors.

- **Code 1, usually understands:** if the resident misses some part or intent of the message **but** comprehends most of it. The resident may have periodic difficulties integrating information but generally demonstrates comprehension by responding in words or actions.

- **Code 2, sometimes understands:** if the resident demonstrates frequent difficulties integrating information, and responds adequately only to simple and direct questions or instructions. When staff rephrase or simplify the message(s) and/or use gestures, the resident's comprehension is enhanced.

- **Code 3, rarely/never understands:** if the resident demonstrates very limited ability to understand communication. Or, if staff have difficulty determining whether or not the resident comprehends messages, based on verbal and nonverbal responses. Or, the resident can hear sounds but does not understand messages.

B1000: Vision

B1000. Vision	
Enter Code ☐	**Ability to see in adequate light** (with glasses or other visual appliances) 0. **Adequate** - sees fine detail, including regular print in newspapers/books 1. **Impaired** - sees large print, but not regular print in newspapers/books 2. **Moderately impaired** - limited vision; not able to see newspaper headlines but can identify objects 3. **Highly impaired** - object identification in question, but eyes appear to follow objects 4. **Severely impaired** - no vision or sees only light, colors or shapes; eyes do not appear to follow objects

Item Rationale

Health-related Quality of Life

- A person's reading vision often diminishes over time.

- If uncorrected, vision impairment can limit the enjoyment of everyday activities such as reading newspapers, books or correspondence, and maintaining and enjoying hobbies and other activities. It also limits the ability to manage personal business, such as reading and signing consent forms.

- Moderate, high or severe impairment can contribute to sensory deprivation, social isolation, and depressed mood.

> ### DEFINITIONS
>
> **ADEQUATE LIGHT**
> Lighting that is sufficient or comfortable for a person with normal vision to see fine detail.

Planning for Care

- Reversible causes of vision impairment should be sought.

- Consider whether simple environmental changes such as better lighting or magnifiers would improve ability to see.

- Consider large print reading materials for persons with impaired vision.

- For residents with moderate, high, or severe impairment, consider alternative ways of providing access to content of desired reading materials or hobbies.

Steps for Assessment

1. Ask direct care staff over all shifts if possible about the resident's usual vision patterns during the 7-day look-back period (e.g., is the resident able to see newsprint, menus, greeting cards?).

2. Then ask the resident about his or her visual abilities.

3. Test the accuracy of your findings:

   - Ensure that the resident's customary visual appliance for close vision is in place (e.g., eyeglasses, magnifying glass).

   - Ensure adequate lighting.

B1000: Vision (cont.)

- Ask the resident to look at regular-size print in a book or newspaper. Then ask the resident to read aloud, starting with larger headlines and ending with the finest, smallest print. If the resident is unable to read a newspaper, provide material with larger print, such as a flyer or large textbook.

- When the resident is unable to read out loud (e.g. due to aphasia, illiteracy), you should test this by another means such as, but not limited to:

- Substituting numbers or pictures for words that are displayed in the appropriate print size (regular-size print in a book or newspaper)

Coding Instructions

- **Code 0, adequate:** if the resident sees fine detail, including regular print in newspapers/books.

- **Code 1, impaired:** if the resident sees large print, but not regular print in newspapers/books.

- **Code 2, moderately impaired:** if the resident has limited vision and is not able to see newspaper headlines but can identify objects in his or her environment.

- **Code 3, highly impaired:** if the resident's ability to identify objects in his or her environment is in question, but the resident's eye movements appear to be following objects (especially people walking by).

- **Code 4, severely impaired:** if the resident has no vision, sees only light, colors or shapes, or does not appear to follow objects with eyes.

Coding Tips and Special Populations

- Some residents have never learned to read or are unable to read English. In such cases, ask the resident to read numbers, such as dates or page numbers, or to name items in small pictures. Be sure to display this information in two sizes (equivalent to regular and large print).

- If the resident is unable to communicate or follow your directions for testing vision, observe the resident's eye movements to see if his or her eyes seem to follow movement of objects or people. These gross measures of visual acuity may assist you in assessing whether or not the resident has any visual ability. For residents who appear to do this, **code 3, highly impaired.**

B1200: Corrective Lenses

B1200. Corrective Lenses	

Enter Code
☐
	Corrective lenses (contacts, glasses, or magnifying glass) used in completing B1000, Vision
	  0. **No**
	  1. **Yes**

B1200: Corrective Lenses (cont.)

Item Rationale

Health-related Quality of Life

- Decreased ability to see can limit the enjoyment of everyday activities and can contribute to social isolation and mood and behavior disorders.

- Many residents who do not have corrective lenses could benefit from them, and others have corrective lenses that are not sufficient.

- Many persons who benefit from and own visual aids do not have them on arrival at the nursing home.

Planning for Care

- Knowing if corrective lenses were used when determining ability to see allows better identification of evaluation and management needs.

- Residents with eyeglasses or other visual appliances should be assisted in accessing them. Use and maintenance should be included in care planning.

- Residents who do not have adequate vision without eyeglasses or other visual appliances should be asked about history of corrective lens use.

- Residents who do not have adequate vision, despite using a visual appliance, might benefit from a re-evaluation of the appliance or assessment for new causes of vision impairment.

Steps for Assessment

1. Prior to beginning the assessment, ask the resident whether he or she uses eyeglasses or other vision aids and whether the eyeglasses or vision aids are at the nursing home. Visual aids do not include surgical lens implants.

2. If the resident cannot respond, check with family and care staff about the resident's use of vision aids during the 7-day look-back period.

3. Observe whether the resident used eyeglasses or other vision aids during reading vision test (B1000).

4. Check the medical record for evidence that the resident used corrective lenses when ability to see was recorded.

5. Ask staff and significant others whether the resident was using corrective lenses when they observed the resident's ability to see.

B1200: Corrective Lenses (cont.)

Coding Instructions

- **Code 0, no:** if the resident did not use eyeglasses or other vision aid during the **B1000, Vision** assessment.

- **Code 1, yes:** if corrective lenses or other visual aids were used when visual ability was assessed in completing **B1000, Vision.**

SECTION C: COGNITIVE PATTERNS

Intent: The items in this section are intended to determine the resident's attention, orientation and ability to register and recall new information. These items are crucial factors in many care-planning decisions.

C0100: Should Brief Interview for Mental Status Be Conducted?

C0100. Should Brief Interview for Mental Status (C0200-C0500) be Conducted?
Attempt to conduct interview with all residents

Enter Code
0. **No** (resident is rarely/never understood) → Skip to and complete C0700-C1000, Staff Assessment for Mental Status
1. **Yes** → Continue to C0200, Repetition of Three Words

Item Rationale

Health-related Quality of Life

- This information identifies if the interview will be attempted.
- Most residents are able to attempt the Brief Interview for Mental Status (BIMS).
- A structured cognitive test is more accurate and reliable than observation alone for observing cognitive performance.
  — Without an attempted structured cognitive interview, a resident might be mislabeled based on his or her appearance or assumed diagnosis.
  — Structured interviews will efficiently provide insight into the resident's current condition that will enhance good care.

Planning for Care

- Structured cognitive interviews assist in identifying needed supports.
- The structured cognitive interview is helpful for identifying possible delirium behaviors (C1300).

Steps for Assessment

1. Determine if the resident is rarely/never understood verbally or in writing. If rarely/never understood, skip to C0700 - C0100, Staff Assessment of Mental Status.
2. Review **Language** item (A1100), to determine if the resident needs or wants an interpreter.
   - If the resident needs or wants an interpreter, complete the interview with an interpreter.

Coding Instructions

Record whether the cognitive interview should be attempted with the resident.

- **Code 0, no:** if the interview should not be attempted because the resident is rarely/never understood or an interpreter is needed but not available. Skip to C0700, **Staff Assessment of Mental Status**.
- **Code 1, yes:** if the interview should be attempted because the resident is at least sometimes understood verbally or in writing, and if an interpreter is needed, one is available. Proceed to C0200, **Repetition of Three Words**.

44

C0100: Should Brief Interview for Mental Status Be Conducted? (cont.)

Coding Tips

- If the resident needs an interpreter, every effort should be made to have an interpreter present for the BIMS. If it is not possible for a needed interpreter to participate on the day of the interview, code C0100 = 0 to indicate interview not attempted and complete C0700-C1000, **Staff Assessment of Mental Status**, instead of C0200-C0500, **Brief Interview for Mental Status**.

C0200-C0500: Brief Interview for Mental Status (BIMS)

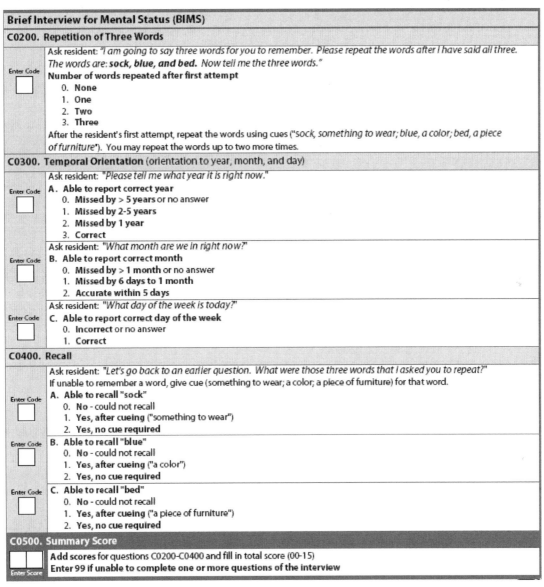

Brief Interview for Mental Status (BIMS)	
C0200. Repetition of Three Words	
Enter Code	Ask resident: *"I am going to say three words for you to remember. Please repeat the words after I have said all three. The words are: **sock, blue, and bed.** Now tell me the three words."* **Number of words repeated after first attempt** 0. None 1. One 2. Two 3. Three After the resident's first attempt, repeat the words using cues (*"sock, something to wear; blue, a color; bed, a piece of furniture"*). You may repeat the words up to two more times.
C0300. Temporal Orientation (orientation to year, month, and day)	
Enter Code	Ask resident: *"Please tell me what year it is right now."* **A. Able to report correct year** 0. Missed by > 5 years or no answer 1. Missed by 2-5 years 2. Missed by 1 year 3. Correct
Enter Code	Ask resident: *"What month are we in right now?"* **B. Able to report correct month** 0. Missed by > 1 month or no answer 1. Missed by 6 days to 1 month 2. Accurate within 5 days
Enter Code	Ask resident: *"What day of the week is today?"* **C. Able to report correct day of the week** 0. Incorrect or no answer 1. Correct
C0400. Recall	
Enter Code	Ask resident: *"Let's go back to an earlier question. What were those three words that I asked you to repeat?"* If unable to remember a word, give cue (something to wear; a color; a piece of furniture) for that word. **A. Able to recall "sock"** 0. No - could not recall 1. Yes, after cueing ("something to wear") 2. Yes, no cue required
Enter Code	**B. Able to recall "blue"** 0. No - could not recall 1. Yes, after cueing ("a color") 2. Yes, no cue required
Enter Code	**C. Able to recall "bed"** 0. No - could not recall 1. Yes, after cueing ("a piece of furniture") 2. Yes, no cue required
C0500. Summary Score	
Enter Score	Add scores for questions C0200-C0400 and fill in total score (00-15) **Enter 99 if unable to complete one or more questions of the interview**

Item Rationale

Health-related Quality of Life

- Direct or performance-based testing of cognitive function decreases the chance of incorrect labeling of cognitive ability and improves detection of delirium.
- Cognitively intact residents may appear to be cognitively impaired because of extreme frailty, hearing impairment or lack of interaction.
- Some residents may appear to be more cognitively intact than they actually are.
- When cognitive impairment is incorrectly diagnosed or missed, appropriate communication, worthwhile activities and therapies may not be offered.
- A resident's performance on cognitive tests can be compared over time.
  — If performance worsens, then an assessment for delirium and or depression should be considered.
- The BIMS is an opportunity to observe residents for signs and symptoms of delirium (C1300).

Planning for Care

- Assessment of a resident's mental state provides a direct understanding of resident function that may:
  — enhance future communication and assistance and
  — direct nursing interventions to facilitate greater independence such as posting or providing reminders for self-care activities.
- A resident's performance on cognitive tests can be compared over time.
  — An abrupt change in cognitive status may indicate delirium and may be the only indication of a potentially life threatening illness.
  — A decline in mental status may also be associated with a mood disorder.
- Awareness of possible impairment may be important for maintaining a safe environment and providing safe discharge planning.

Steps for Assessment: Basic Interview Instructions for BIMS (C0200-C0500)

1. Refer to Appendix D for a review of basic approaches to effective interviewing techniques.
2. Interview any resident not screened out by **Should Brief Interview for Mental Status Be Conducted?** item (C0100).
3. Conduct the interview in a private setting.
4. Be sure the resident can hear you.

- Residents with hearing impairment should be tested using their usual communication devices/techniques, as applicable.

- Try an external assistive device (headphones or hearing amplifier) if you have any doubt about hearing ability.
- Minimize background noise.

5. Sit so that the resident can see your face. Minimize glare by directing light sources away from the resident's face.

6. Give an introduction before starting the interview.

   Suggested language: "I would like to ask you some questions. We ask everyone these same questions. This will help us provide you with better care. Some of the questions may seem very easy, while others may be more difficult."

7. If the resident expresses concern that you are testing his or her memory, he or she may be more comfortable if you reply: "We ask these questions of everyone so we can make sure that our care will meet your needs."

8. Directly ask the resident each item in C0200 through C0400 at one sitting and in the order provided.

9. If the resident chooses not to answer a particular item, accept his or her refusal and move on to the next questions. For C0200 through C0400, code refusals as incorrect.

Coding Instructions

See coding instructions for individual items.

Coding Tips

- On occasion, the interviewer may not be able to state the items clearly because of an accent. If the interviewer is unable to pronounce any cognitive items clearly, have a different staff member complete the BIMS.
- Nonsensical responses should be coded as zero.
- Rules for stopping the interview before it is complete:
  — Stop the interview after completing (C0300C) "Day of the Week" if:
    1. all responses have been nonsensical (i.e., any response that is unrelated, incomprehensible, or incoherent; not informative with respect to the item being rated), OR
    2. there has been no verbal or written response to any of the questions up to this point, OR
    3. there has been no verbal or written response to some questions up to this point and for all others, the resident has given a nonsensical response.
- If the interview is stopped, do the following:
    1. Code **-, dash** in C0400A, C0400B, and C0400C.
    2. Code **99** in the summary score in C0500.
    3. Code **1, yes** in C0600 Should the Staff Assessment for Mental Status (C0700-C1000) be Conducted?
    4. Complete the **Staff Assessment for Mental Status**.

- When staff identify that the resident's primary method of communication is in written format, the BIMS can be administered in writing. **The administration of the BIMS in writing should be limited to this circumstance.**
- See Appendix E for details regarding how to administer the BIMS in writing.

Examples of Incorrect and Nonsensical Responses

> **DEFINITIONS**
>
> **NONSENSICAL RESPONSE** Any response that is unrelated, incomprehensible, or incoherent; it is not informative with respect to the item being rated.

1. Interviewer asks resident to state the year. The resident replies that it is 1935. This answer is incorrect but related to the question.

   Coding: This answer is **coded 0, incorrect** but would NOT be considered a nonsensical response.

   Rationale: The answer is wrong, but it is logical and relates to the question.

2. Interviewer asks resident to state the year. The resident says, "Oh what difference does the year make when you're as old as I am?" The interviewer asks the resident to try to name the year, and the resident shrugs.

   Coding: This answer is **coded 0, incorrect** but would NOT be considered a nonsensical response.

   Rationale: The answer is wrong because refusal is considered a wrong answer, but the resident's comment is logical and clearly relates to the question.

3. Interviewer asks the resident to name the day of the week. Resident answers, "Sylvia, she's my daughter."

   Coding: The answer is **coded 0, incorrect**; the response is illogical and nonsensical.

   Rationale: The answer is wrong, and the resident's comment clearly does not relate to the question; it is nonsensical.

C0200: Repetition of Three Words

Brief Interview for Mental Status (BIMS)

C0200. Repetition of Three Words

Enter Code
☐
	Ask resident: *"I am going to say three words for you to remember. Please repeat the words after I have said all three. The words are: **sock, blue, and bed.** Now tell me the three words."*
	Number of words repeated after first attempt
	   0. **None**
	   1. **One**
	   2. **Two**
	   3. **Three**
	After the resident's first attempt, repeat the words using cues (*"sock, something to wear; blue, a color; bed, a piece of furniture"*). You may repeat the words up to two more times.

Item Rationale

Health-related Quality of Life

- Inability to repeat three words on first attempt may indicate:
  — a hearing impairment,
  — a language barrier, or
  — inattention that may be a sign of delirium.

Planning for Care

- A cue can assist learning.
- Cues may help residents with memory impairment who can store new information in their memory but who have trouble retrieving something that was stored (e.g., not able to remember someone's name but can recall if given part of the first name).
- Staff can use cues when assisting residents with learning and recall in therapy, and in daily and restorative activities.

Steps for Assessment

> | DEFINITIONS |
> |---|
> | **CATEGORY CUE**
Phrase that puts a word in context to help with learning and to serve as a hint that helps prompt the resident. The category cue for sock is "something to wear." The category cue for blue is "a color." For bed, the category cue is "a piece of furniture." |

Basic BIMS interview instructions are shown on page C-5. In addition, for repetition of three words:

1. Say to the resident: "I am going to say three words for you to remember. Please repeat the words after I have said all three. The words are: sock, blue, and bed."
2. Immediately after presenting the three words, say to the resident: "Now please tell me the three words."
3. After the resident's first attempt to repeat the items:

   - If the resident correctly stated all three words, say, "That's right, the words are sock, something to wear; blue, a color; and bed, a piece of furniture" [category cues].

- Category cues serve as a hint that helps prompt residents' recall ability. Putting words in context stimulates learning and fosters memory of the words that residents will be asked to recall in item C0400, even among residents able to repeat the words immediately.

- If the resident recalled two or fewer words, say to the resident: "Let me say the three words again. They are sock, something to wear; blue, a color; and bed, a piece of furniture. Now tell me the three words." If the resident still does not recall all three words correctly, you may repeat the words and category cues one more time.

- If the resident does not repeat all three words after three attempts, re-assess ability to hear. If the resident can hear, move on to the next question. If he or she is unable to hear, attempt to maximize hearing (alter environment, use hearing amplifier) before proceeding.

Coding Instructions

*Record the maximum number of words that the resident correctly repeated on the **first** attempt. This will be any number between 0 and 3.*

- The words may be recalled in any order and in any context. For example, if the words are repeated back in a sentence, they would be counted as repeating the words.
- Do not score the number of repeated words on the second or third attempt. These attempts help with learning the item, but only the number correct on the first attempt go into the total score. Do not record the number of attempts that the resident needed to complete.
- **Code 0, none:** if the resident did not repeat any of the 3 words on the first attempt.
- **Code 1, one:** if the resident repeated only 1 of the 3 words on the first attempt.
- **Code 2, two:** if the resident repeated only 2 of the 3 words on the first attempt.
- **Code 3, three:** if the resident repeated all 3 words on the first attempt.

Coding Tips

- On occasion, the interviewer may not be able to state the words clearly because of an accent or slurred speech. If the interviewer is unable to pronounce any of the 3 words clearly, have a different staff member conduct the interview.

Examples

1. The interviewer says, "The words are sock, blue, and bed. Now please tell me the three words." The resident replies, "Bed, sock, and blue." The interviewer repeats the three words with category cues, by saying, "That's right, the words are sock, something to wear; blue, a color; and bed, a piece of furniture."

    Coding: C0200 would be **coded 3, three** words correct.
    Rationale: The resident repeated all three items on the first attempt. The order of repetition does not affect the score.

2. The interviewer says, "The words are sock, blue, and bed. Now please tell me the three words." The resident replies, "Sock, bed, black." The interviewer repeats the three words plus the category cues, saying, "Let me say the three words again. They are sock, something to wear; blue, a color; and bed, a piece of furniture. Now tell me the three words." The resident says, "Oh yes, that's right, sock, blue, bed."

    Coding: C0200 would be **coded 2, two** of three words correct.
    Rationale: The resident repeated two of the three items on the first attempt. Residents are scored based on the first attempt.

C0200: Repetition of Three Words (cont.)

3. The interviewer says, "The words are sock, blue, and bed. Now please tell me the three words." The resident says, "Blue socks belong in the dresser." The interviewer repeats the three words plus the category cues.

   Coding: C0200 would be **coded 2, two** of the three words correct.
   Rationale: The resident repeated two of the three items—blue and sock. The resident put the words into a sentence, resulting in the resident repeating two of the three words.

4. The interviewer says, "The words are sock, blue, and bed. Now please tell me the three words." The resident replies, "What were those three words?" The interviewer repeats the three words plus the category cues.

   Coding: C0200 would be **coded 0, none** of the words correct.
   Rationale: The resident did not repeat any of the three words after the first time the interviewer said them.

C0300: Temporal Orientation (Orientation to Year, Month, and Day)

C0300.	Temporal Orientation (orientation to year, month, and day)
Enter Code ☐	Ask resident: *"Please tell me what year it is right now."* **A. Able to report correct year** 0. **Missed by > 5 years** or no answer 1. **Missed by 2-5 years** 2. **Missed by 1 year** 3. **Correct**
Enter Code ☐	Ask resident: *"What month are we in right now?"* **B. Able to report correct month** 0. **Missed by > 1 month** or no answer 1. **Missed by 6 days to 1 month** 2. **Accurate within 5 days**
Enter Code ☐	Ask resident: *"What day of the week is today?"* **C. Able to report correct day of the week** 0. **Incorrect** or no answer 1. **Correct**

Item Rationale

Health-related Quality of Life

- A lack of temporal orientation may lead to decreased communication or participation in activities.
- Not being oriented may be frustrating or frightening.

Planning for Care

- If staff know that a resident has a problem with orientation, they can provide reorientation aids and verbal reminders that may reduce anxiety.

DEFINITIONS

TEMPORAL ORIENTATION
In general, the ability to place oneself in correct time. For the BIMS, it is the ability to indicate the correct date in current surroundings.

C0300: Temporal Orientation (Orientation to Year, Month, and Day) (cont.)

- Reorienting those who are disoriented or at risk of disorientation may be useful in treating symptoms of delirium.
- Residents who are not oriented may need further assessment for delirium, especially if this fluctuates or is recent in onset.

Steps for Assessment

Basic BIMS interview instructions are shown on page C-5.

1. Ask the resident each of the 3 questions in Item C0300 separately.
2. Allow the resident up to 30 seconds for each answer and do not provide clues.
3. If the resident specifically asks for clues (e.g., "is it bingo day?") respond by saying, "I need to know if you can answer this question without any help from me."

Coding Instructions for C0300A, Able to Report Correct Year

- **Code 0, missed by >5 years or no answer:** if the resident's answer is incorrect and is greater than 5 years from the current year or the resident chooses not to answer the item.
- **Code 1, missed by 2-5 years:** if the resident's answer is incorrect and is within 2 to 5 years from the current year.
- **Code 2, missed by 1 year:** if the resident's answer is incorrect and is within one year from the current year.
- **Code 3, correct:** if the resident states the correct year.

Examples

1. The date of interview is May 5, 2011. The resident, responding to the statement, "Please tell me what year it is right now," states that it is 2011.

   Coding: C0300A would be **coded 3, correct.**
   Rationale: 2011 is the current year.

2. The date of interview is June 16, 2011. The resident, responding to the statement, "Please tell me what year it is right now," states that it is 2007.

   Coding: C0300A would be **coded 1, missed by 2-5 years.**
   Rationale: 2007 is within 2 to 5 years of 2011.

3. The date of interview is January 10, 2011. The resident, responding to the statement, "Please tell me what year it is right now," states that it is 1911.

   Coding: C0300A would be **coded 0, missed by more than 5 years.**
   Rationale: Even though the '11 part of the year would be correct, 1911 is more than 5 years from 2011.

C0300: Temporal Orientation (Orientation to Year, Month, and Day) (cont.)

4. The date of interview is April 1, 2011. The resident, responding to the statement, "Please tell me what year it is right now," states that it is "'11". The interviewer asks, "Can you tell me the full year?" The resident still responds "'11," and the interviewer asks again, "Can you tell me the full year, for example, nineteen-eighty-two." The resident states, "2011."

    Coding: C0300A would be **coded 3, correct.**

    Rationale: Even though '11 is partially correct, the only correct answer is the exact year. The resident must state "2011," not "'11" or "1811" or "1911."

Coding Instructions for C0300B, Able to Report Correct Month

Count the current day as day 1 when determining whether the response was accurate within 5 days or missed by 6 days to 1 month.

-   **Code 0, missed by >1 month or no answer:** if the resident's answer is incorrect by more than 1 month or if the resident chooses not to answer the item.
-   **Code 1, missed by 6 days to 1 month:** if the resident's answer is accurate within 6 days to 1 month.
-   **Code 2, accurate within 5 days:** if the resident's answer is accurate within 5 days, count current date as day 1.

Coding Tips

-   In most instances, it will be immediately obvious which code to select. In some cases, you may need to write the resident's response in the margin and go back later to count days if you are unsure whether the date given is within 5 days.

Examples

1. The date of interview is June 25, 2011. The resident, responding to the question, "What month are we in right now?" states that it is June.

    Coding: C0300B would be **coded 2, accurate within 5 days.**

    Rationale: The resident correctly stated the month.

2. The date of interview is June 28, 2011. The resident, responding to the question, "What month are we in right now?" states that it is July.

    Coding: C0300B would be **coded 2, accurate within 5 days.**

    Rationale: The resident correctly stated the month within 5 days, even though the correct month is June. June 28th (day 1) + 4 more days is July 2nd, so July is within 5 days of the interview.

3. The date of interview is June 25, 2011. The resident, responding to the question, "What month are we in right now?" states that it is July.

> **Coding:** C0300B would be **coded 1, missed by 6 days to 1 month**.
>
> **Rationale:** The resident missed the correct month by six days. June 25th (day 1) + 5 more days = June 30th. Therefore, the resident's answer is incorrect within 6 days to 1 month.

4. The date of interview is June 30, 2011. The resident, responding to the question, "What month are we in right now?" states that it is August.

> **Coding:** C0300B would be **coded 0, missed by more than 1 month**.
>
> **Rationale:** The resident missed the month by more than 1 month.

5. The date of interview is June 2, 2011. The resident, responding to the question, "What month are we in right now?" states that it is May.

> **Coding:** C0300B would be **coded 2, accurate within 5 days.**
>
> **Rationale:** June 2 minus 5 days = May 29th. The resident correctly stated the month within 5 days even though the current month is June.

Coding Instructions for C0300C. **Able to Report Correct Day of the Week**

- **Code 0, incorrect, or no answer:** if the answer is incorrect or the resident chooses not to answer the item.
- **Code 1, correct:** if the answer is correct.

Examples

1. The day of interview is Monday, June 25, 2011. The interviewer asks: "What day of the week is it today?" The resident responds, "It's Monday."

> **Coding:** C0300C would be **coded 1, correct**.
>
> **Rationale:** The resident correctly stated the day of the week.

2. The day of interview is Monday, June 25, 2011. The resident, responding to the question, "What day of the week is it today?" states, "Tuesday."

> **Coding:** C0300C would be **coded 0, incorrect**.
>
> **Rationale:** The resident incorrectly stated the day of the week.

3. The day of interview is Monday, June 25, 2011. The resident, responding to the question, "What day of the week is it today?" states, "Today is a good day."

> **Coding:** C0300C would be **coded 0, incorrect**.
>
> **Rationale:** The resident did not answer the question correctly.

C0400: Recall

C0400. Recall	
	Ask resident: *"Let's go back to an earlier question. What were those three words that I asked you to repeat?"* If unable to remember a word, give cue (something to wear; a color; a piece of furniture) for that word.

Enter Code
 ☐
	A. Able to recall "sock"
	   0. **No** - could not recall
	   1. **Yes, after cueing** ("something to wear")
	   2. **Yes, no cue required**

Enter Code
 ☐
	B. Able to recall "blue"
	   0. **No** - could not recall
	   1. **Yes, after cueing** ("a color")
	   2. **Yes, no cue required**

Enter Code
 ☐
	C. Able to recall "bed"
	   0. **No** - could not recall
	   1. **Yes, after cueing** ("a piece of furniture")
	   2. **Yes, no cue required**

Item Rationale

Health-related Quality of Life

- Many persons with cognitive impairment can be helped to recall if provided cues.
- Providing memory cues can help maximize individual function and decrease frustration for those residents who respond.

Planning for Care

- Care plans should maximize use of cueing for resident who respond to recall cues. This will enhance independence.

Steps for Assessment

Basic BIMS interview instructions are shown on page C-5.

1. Ask the resident the following: "Let's go back to an earlier question. What were those three words that I asked you to repeat?"
2. Allow up to 5 seconds for spontaneous recall of each word.
3. For any word that is not correctly recalled after 5 seconds, provide a category cue (refer to "Steps for Assessment," pages C-7–C-8 for the definition of category cue). Category cues should be used only after the resident is unable to recall one or more of the three words.
4. Allow up to 5 seconds after category cueing for each missed word to be recalled.

Coding Instructions

*For **each** of the three words the resident is asked to remember:*

- **Code 0, no—could not recall:** if the resident cannot recall the word even after being given the category cue or if the resident responds with a nonsensical answer or chooses not to answer the item.
- **Code 1, yes, after cueing:** if the resident requires the category cue to remember the word.
- **Code 2, yes, no cue required:** if the resident correctly remembers the word spontaneously without cueing.

55

C0400: Recall (cont.)

Coding Tips

- If on the first try (without cueing), the resident names multiple items in a category, one of which is correct, they should be coded as correct for that item.
- If, however, the interviewer gives the resident the cue and the resident then names multiple items in that category, the item is coded as could not recall, even if the correct item was in the list.

Examples

1. The resident is asked to recall the three words that were initially presented. The resident chooses not to answer the question and states, "I'm tired, and I don't want to do this anymore."

   Coding: C0400A-C0400C would be **coded 0, no—could not recall**, could not recall for each of the three words.
   Rationale: Choosing not to answer a question often indicates an inability to answer the question, so refusals are **coded 0, no—could not recall**. This is the most accurate way to score cognitive function, even though, on occasion, residents might choose not to answer for other reasons.

2. The resident is asked to recall the three words. The resident replies, "Socks, shoes, and bed." The examiner then cues, "One word was a color." The resident says, "Oh, the shoes were blue."

   Coding: C0400A, sock, would be **coded 2, yes, no cue required**.
   Rationale: The resident's initial response to the question included "sock." He is given credit for this response, even though he also listed another item in that category (shoes), because he was answering the initial question, without cueing.
   Coding: C0400B, blue, would be **coded 1, yes, after cueing.**
   Rationale: The resident did not recall spontaneously, but did recall after the category cue was given. Responses that include the word in a sentence are acceptable.
   Coding: C0400C, bed, would be **coded 2, yes, no cue required.**
   Rationale: The resident independently recalled the item on the first attempt.

3. The resident is asked to recall the three words. The resident answers, "I don't remember." The assessor then says, "One word was something to wear." The resident says, "Clothes." The assessor then says, "OK, one word was a color." The resident says, "Blue." The assessor then says, "OK, the last word was a piece of furniture." The resident says, "Couch."

   Coding: C0400A, sock, would be **coded 0, no—could not recall.**
   Rationale: The resident did not recall the item, even with a cue.
   Coding: C0400B, blue, would be **coded 1, yes, after cueing.**
   Rationale: The resident did recall after being given the cue.
   Coding: C0400C, bed, would be **coded 0, no—could not recall.**
   Rationale: The resident did not recall the item, even with a cue.

C0400: Recall (cont.)

4. The resident is asked to recall the three words. The resident says, "I don't remember." The assessor then says, "One word was something to wear." The resident says, "Hat, shirt, pants, socks, shoe, belt."

> **Coding:** C0400A, sock, would be **coded 0, no—could not recall.**
>
> **Rationale:** After getting the category cue, the resident named more than one item (i.e., a laundry list of items) in the category. The resident's response is coded as incorrect, even though one of the items was correct, because the resident did not demonstrate recall and likely named the item by chance.

C0500: Summary Score

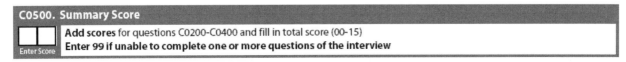

C0500. Summary Score	
Enter Score	**Add scores** for questions C0200-C0400 and fill in total score (00-15) **Enter 99 if unable to complete one or more questions of the interview**

Item Rationale

Health-related Quality of Life

- The total score:
  - Allows comparison with future and past performance.
  - Decreases the chance of incorrect labeling of cognitive ability and improves detection of delirium.
  - Provides staff with a more reliable estimate of resident function and allows staff interactions with residents that are based on more accurate impressions about resident ability.

Planning for Care

- The BIMS is a brief screener that aids in detecting cognitive impairment. It does not assess all possible aspects of cognitive impairment. A diagnosis of dementia should only be made after a careful assessment for other reasons for impaired cognitive performance. The final determination of the level of impairment should be made by the resident's physician or mental health care specialist; however, these practitioners can be provided specific BIMS results and the following guidance:

The BIMS total score is highly correlated with Mini-Mental State Exam (MMSE; Folstein, Folstein, & McHugh, 1975) scores. Scores from a carefully conducted BIMS assessment where residents can hear all questions and the resident is not delirious suggest the following distributions:

> 13-15: cognitively intact
>
> 8-12: moderately impaired
>
> 0-7: severe impairment

C0500: Summary Score (cont.)

- Abrupt changes in cognitive status (as indicative of a delirium) often signal an underlying potentially life threatening illness and a change in cognition may be the only indication of an underlying problem.

- Care plans can be more individualized based upon reliable knowledge of resident function.

Steps for Assessment

After completing C0200-C0400:

1. Add up the values for all questions from C0200 through C0400.
2. Do not add up the score while you are interviewing the resident. Instead, focus your full attention on the interview.

Coding Instructions

Enter the total score as a two-digit number. The total possible BIMS score ranges from 00 to 15.

- If the resident chooses not to answer a specific question(s), that question is coded as incorrect and the item(s) counts in the total score. If, however, the resident chooses not to answer four or more items, then the interview is coded as incomplete and a staff assessment is completed.

- To be considered a completed interview, the resident had to attempt and provide relevant answers to at least four of the questions included in C0200-C0400. To be relevant, a response only has to be related to the question (logical); it does not have to be correct. See general coding tips on page C-6 for residents who choose not to participate at all.

- **Code 99, unable to complete interview:** if (a) the resident chooses not to participate in the BIMS, (b) if four or more items were coded 0 because the resident chose not to answer or gave a nonsensical response, *or* (c) if any of the BIMS items is coded with a dash.
  - — Note: a zero score does not mean the BIMS was incomplete. To be incomplete, a resident had to choose not to answer or give completely unrelated, nonsensical responses to four or more items.

Coding Tips

- Occasionally, a resident can communicate but chooses not to participate in the BIMS and therefore does not attempt any of the items in the section. This would be considered an incomplete interview; enter 99 for C0500, **Summary Score**, and complete the staff assessment of mental status.

C0500: Summary Score (cont.)

Example

1. The resident's scores on items C0200-C0400 were as follows:

C0200 (repetition)	3
C0300A (year)	2
C0300B (month)	2
C0300C (day)	1
C0400A (recall "sock")	2
C0400B (recall "blue")	2
C0400C (recall "bed")	0

   Coding: C0500 would be **coded 12**.

C0600: Should the Staff Assessment for Mental Status (C0700-C1000) Be Conducted?

C0600. Should the Staff Assessment for Mental Status (C0700 - C1000) be Conducted?
Enter Code [ ]   0. **No** (resident was able to complete interview) → Skip to C1300, Signs and Symptoms of Delirium   1. **Yes** (resident was unable to complete interview) → Continue to C0700, Short-term Memory OK

Item Rationale

Health-related Quality of Life

- Direct or performance-based testing of cognitive function using the BIMS is preferred as it decreases the chance of incorrect labeling of cognitive ability and improves detection of delirium. However, a minority of residents are unable or unwilling to participate in the BIMS.
- Mental status can vary among persons unable to communicate or who do not complete the interview.
  — Therefore, report of observed behavior is needed for persons unable to complete the BIMS interview.
  — When cognitive impairment is incorrectly diagnosed or missed, appropriate communication, activities, and therapies may not be offered.

Planning for Care

- Abrupt changes in cognitive status (as indicative of delirium) often signal an underlying potentially life-threatening illness and a change in cognition may be the only indication of an underlying problem.
  — This remains true for persons who are unable to communicate or to complete the BIMS.
- Specific aspects of cognitive impairment, when identified, can direct nursing interventions to facilitate greater independence and function.

C0600: Should the Staff Assessment for Mental Status (C0700-C1000) Be Conducted? (cont.)

Steps for Assessment

1. Review whether **Summary Score** item (C0500), is **coded 99**, unable to complete interview.

Coding Instructions

- **Code 0, no:** if the BIMS was completed and scored between 00 and 15. Skip to C1300.
- **Code 1, yes:** if the resident chooses not to participate in the BIMS or if four or more items were **coded 0** because the resident chose not to answer or gave a nonsensical response. Continue to C0700-C1000 and perform the Staff Assessment for Mental Status. Note: C0500 should be **coded 99**.

Coding Tips

- If a resident is scored 00 on C0500, C0700-C1000, Staff Assessment, should not be completed. **00** is a legitimate value for C0500 and indicates that the interview was complete. To have an incomplete interview, a resident had to choose not to answer or had to give completely unrelated, nonsensical responses to four or more BIMS items.

C0700-C1000: Staff Assessment of Mental Status Item

Staff Assessment for Mental Status	
Do not conduct if Brief Interview for Mental Status (C0200-C0500) was completed	
C0700. Short-term Memory OK	
Enter Code ☐	**Seems or appears to recall after 5 minutes** 0. **Memory OK** 1. **Memory problem**
C0800. Long-term Memory OK	
Enter Code ☐	**Seems or appears to recall long past** 0. **Memory OK** 1. **Memory problem**
C0900. Memory/Recall Ability	
↓ Check all that the resident was normally able to recall	
☐	A. **Current season**
☐	B. **Location of own room**
☐	C. **Staff names and faces**
☐	D. **That he or she is in a nursing home**
☐	Z. **None of the above** were recalled
C1000. Cognitive Skills for Daily Decision Making	
Enter Code ☐	**Made decisions regarding tasks of daily life** 0. **Independent** - decisions consistent/reasonable 1. **Modified independence** - some difficulty in new situations only 2. **Moderately impaired** - decisions poor; cues/supervision required 3. **Severely impaired** - never/rarely made decisions

C0700-C1000: Staff Assessment of Mental Status Item (cont.)

Item Rationale

Health-related Quality of Life

- Cognitive impairment is prevalent among some groups of residents, but not all residents are cognitively impaired.
- Many persons with memory problems can function successfully in a structured, routine environment.
- Residents may appear to be cognitively impaired because of communication challenges or lack of interaction but may be cognitively intact.
- When cognitive impairment is incorrectly diagnosed or missed, appropriate communication, worthwhile activities, and therapies may not be offered.

Planning for Care

- Abrupt changes in cognitive status (as indicative of a delirium) often signal an underlying potentially life-threatening illness and a change in cognition may be the only indication of an underlying problem.
- The level and specific areas of impairment affect daily function and care needs. By identifying specific aspects of cognitive impairment, nursing interventions can be directed toward facilitating greater function.
- Probing beyond first, perhaps mistaken, impressions is critical to accurate assessment and appropriate care planning.

C0700: Short-term Memory OK

C0700. Short-term Memory OK	
Enter Code [ ]	Seems or appears to recall after 5 minutes 0. Memory OK 1. Memory problem

Item Rationale

Health-related Quality of Life

- To assess the mental state of residents who cannot be interviewed, an intact 5-minute recall ("short-term memory OK") indicates greater likelihood of normal cognition.
- An observed "memory problem" should be taken into consideration in Planning for Care.

Planning for Care

- Identified memory problems typically indicate the need for:

C0700: Short-term Memory OK (cont.)

— Assessment and treatment of an underlying related medical problem (particularly if this is a new observation) or adverse medication effect, or

— possible evaluation for other problems with thinking

— additional nursing support

— at times frequent prompting during daily activities

— additional support during recreational activities.

Steps for Assessment

1. Determine the resident's short-term memory status by asking him or her:

   - to describe an event 5 minutes after it occurred if you can validate the resident's response, or

   - to follow through on a direction given 5 minutes earlier.

2. Observe how often the resident has to be re-oriented to an activity or instructions.
3. Staff members also should observe the resident's cognitive function in varied daily activities.
4. Observations should be made by staff across all shifts and departments and others with close contact with the resident.
5. Ask direct care staff across all shifts and family or significant others about the resident's short-term memory status.
6. Review the medical record for clues to the resident's short-term memory during the look-back period.

Coding Instructions

Based on all information collected regarding the resident's short-term memory during the 7-day look-back period, identify and code according to the most representative level of function.

- **Code 0, memory OK:** if the resident recalled information after 5 minutes.
- **Code 1, memory problem:** if the most representative level of function shows the absence of recall after 5 minutes.

Coding Tips

- If the test cannot be conducted (resident will not cooperate, is non-responsive, etc.) and staff members were unable to make a determination based on observing the resident, use the standard "no information" code (a dash, "-") to indicate that the information is not available because it could not be assessed.

C0700: Short-term Memory OK (cont.)

Example

1. A resident has just returned from the activities room where she and other residents were playing bingo. You ask her if she enjoyed herself playing bingo, but she returns a blank stare. When you ask her if she was just playing bingo, she says, "no." **Code 1, memory problem.**

> **Coding:** C0700, would be **coded 1, memory problem.**
>
> **Rationale:** The resident could not recall an event that took place within the past 5 minutes.

C0800: Long-term Memory OK

C0800. Long-term Memory OK	
Enter Code ☐	Seems or appears to recall long past 0. Memory OK 1. Memory problem

Item Rationale

Health-related Quality of Life

- An observed "long-term memory problem" may indicate the need for emotional support, reminders, and reassurance. It may also indicate delirium if this represents a change from the resident's baseline.
- An observed "long-term memory problem" should be taken into consideration in Planning for Care.

Planning for Care

- Long-term memory problems indicate the need for:
  — Exclusion of an underlying related medical problem (particularly if this is a new observation) or adverse medication effect, or
  — possible evaluation for other problems with thinking
  — additional nursing support
  — at times frequent prompting during daily activities
  — additional support during recreational activities.

Steps for Assessment

1. Determine resident's long-term memory status by engaging in conversation, reviewing memorabilia (photographs, memory books, keepsakes, videos, or other recordings that are meaningful to the resident) with the resident or observing response to family who visit.
2. Ask questions for which you can validate the answers from review of the medical record, general knowledge, the resident's family, etc.

   - Ask the resident, "Are you married?" "What is your spouse's name?" "Do you have any children?" "How many?" "When is your birthday?"

C0800: Long-term Memory OK (cont.)

3. Observe if the resident responds to memorabilia or family members who visit.
4. Observations should be made by staff across all shifts and departments and others with close contact with the resident.
5. Ask direct care staff across all shifts and family or significant others about the resident's memory status.
6. Review the medical record for clues to the resident's long-term memory during the look-back period.

Coding Instructions

- **Code 0, memory OK:** if the resident accurately recalled long past information.
- **Code 1, memory problem:** if the resident did not recall long past information or did not recall it correctly.

Coding Tips

- If the test cannot be conducted (resident will not cooperate, is non-responsive, etc.) and staff were unable to make a determination based on observation of the resident, use the standard "no information" code (a dash, "-"), to indicate that the information is not available because it could not be assessed.

C0900: Memory/Recall Ability

C0900. Memory/Recall Ability	
↓ Check all that the resident was normally able to recall	
☐	A. Current season
☐	B. Location of own room
☐	C. Staff names and faces
☐	D. That he or she is in a nursing home
☐	Z. None of the above were recalled

Item Rationale

Health-related Quality of Life

- An observed "memory/recall problem" with these items may indicate:
  — cognitive impairment and the need for additional support with reminders to support increased independence; or
  — delirium, if this represents a change from the resident's baseline.

Planning for Care

- An observed "memory/recall problem" with these items may indicate the need for:
  — Exclusion of an underlying related medical problem (particularly if this is a new observation) or adverse medication effect; or
  — possible evaluation for other problems with thinking;
  — additional signs, directions, pictures, verbal reminders to support the resident's independence;

C0900: Memory/Recall Ability (cont.)

— an evaluation for acute delirium if this represents a change over the past few days to weeks;

— an evaluation for chronic delirium if this represents a change over the past several weeks to months; or

— additional nursing support;

— the need for emotional support, reminders and reassurance to reduce anxiety and agitation.

Steps for Assessment

1. Ask the resident about each item. For example, "What is the current season? Is it fall, winter, spring, or summer?" "What is the name of this place?" If the resident is not in his or her room, ask, "Will you show me to your room?" Observe the resident's ability to find the way.

2. For residents with limited communication skills, in order to determine the most representative level of function, ask direct care staff across all shifts and family or significant other about recall ability.

   - Ask whether the resident gave indications of recalling these subjects or recognizing them during the look-back period.

3. Observations should be made by staff across all shifts and departments and others with close contact with the resident.

4. Review the medical record for indications of the resident's recall of these subjects during the look-back period.

Coding Instructions

*For each item that the resident recalls, check the corresponding answer box. If the resident recalls none, check **none of above**.*

- **Check C0900A, current season:** if resident is able to identify the current season (e.g., correctly refers to weather for the time of year, legal holidays, religious celebrations, etc.).

- **Check C0900B, location of own room:** if resident is able to locate and recognize own room. It is not necessary for the resident to know the room number, but he or she should be able to find the way to the room.

- **Check C0900C, staff names and faces:** if resident is able to distinguish staff members from family members, strangers, visitors, and other residents. It is not necessary for the resident to know the staff member's name, but he or she should recognize that the person is a staff member and not the resident's son or daughter, etc.

- **Check C0900D, that he or she is in a nursing home:** if resident is able to determine that he or she is currently living in a nursing home. To check this item, it is not necessary that the resident be able to state the name of the nursing home, but he or she should be able to refer to the nursing home by a term such as a "home for older people," a "hospital for the elderly," "a place where people who need extra help live," etc.

- **Check C0900Z, none of above was recalled.**

C1000: Cognitive Skills for Daily Decision Making

C1000. Cognitive Skills for Daily Decision Making	
Enter Code ☐	**Made decisions regarding tasks of daily life** 0. **Independent** - decisions consistent/reasonable 1. **Modified independence** - some difficulty in new situations only 2. **Moderately impaired** - decisions poor; cues/supervision required 3. **Severely impaired** - never/rarely made decisions

Item Rationale

Health-related Quality of Life

- An observed "difficulty with daily decision making" may indicate:
  — underlying cognitive impairment and the need for additional coaching and support or
  — possible anxiety or depression.

Planning for Care

- An observed "difficulty with daily decision making" may indicate the need for:
  — a more structured plan for daily activities and support in decisions about daily activities,
  — encouragement to participate in structured activities, or
  — an assessment for underlying delirium and medical evaluation.

Steps for Assessment

1. Review the medical record. Consult family and direct care staff across all shifts. Observe the resident.
2. Observations should be made by staff across all shifts and departments and others with close contact with the resident.
3. The intent of this item is to record what the resident is doing (performance). Focus on whether or not the resident is actively making these decisions and not whether staff believes the resident might be capable of doing so.
4. Focus on the resident's actual performance. Where a staff member takes decision-making responsibility away from the resident regarding tasks of everyday living, or the resident does not participate in decision making, whatever his or her level of capability may be, the resident should be coded as impaired performance in decision making.

DEFINITIONS

DAILY DECISION MAKING
Includes: choosing clothing; knowing when to go to meals; using environmental cues to organize and plan (e.g., clocks, calendars, posted event notices); in the absence of environmental cues, seeking information appropriately (i.e. not repetitively) from others in order to plan the day; using awareness of one's own strengths and limitations to regulate the day's events (e.g., asks for help when necessary); acknowledging need to use appropriate assistive equipment such as a walker.

C1000: Cognitive Skills for Daily Decision Making (cont.)

Coding Instructions

Record the resident's actual performance in making everyday decisions about tasks or activities of daily living. Enter one number that corresponds to the most correct response.

- **Code 0, independent:** if the resident's decisions in organizing daily routine and making decisions were consistent, reasonable and organized reflecting lifestyle, culture, values.
- **Code 1, modified independence:** if the resident organized daily routine and made safe decisions in familiar situations, but experienced some difficulty in decision making when faced with new tasks or situations.
- **Code 2, moderately impaired:** if the resident's decisions were poor; the resident required reminders, cues, and supervision in planning, organizing, and correcting daily routines.
- **Code 3, severely impaired:** if the resident's decision making was severely impaired; the resident never (or rarely) made decisions.

Coding Tips

- If the resident "rarely or never" made decisions, despite being provided with opportunities and appropriate cues, Item C1000 would be **coded 3, severely impaired**. If the resident makes decisions, although poorly, **code 2, moderately impaired**.
- A resident's considered decision to exercise his or her right to decline treatment or recommendations by interdisciplinary team members should **not** be captured as impaired decision making in Item C1000, **Cognitive Skills for Daily Decision Making**.

Examples

1. Mr. B. seems to have severe cognitive impairment and is non-verbal. He usually clamps his mouth shut when offered a bite of food.
2. Mrs. C. does not generally make conversation or make her needs known, but replies "yes" when asked if she would like to take a nap.

> **Coding:** For the examples listed in 1A and 1B, Item C1000 would be **coded 3, severe impairment.**
>
> **Rationale:** In both examples, the residents are primarily non-verbal and do not make their needs known, but they do give basic verbal or non-verbal responses to simple gestures or questions regarding care routines. More information about how the residents function in the environment is needed to definitively answer the questions. From the limited information provided it appears that their communication of choices is limited to very particular circumstances, which would be regarded as "rarely/never" in the relative number of decisions a person could make during the course of a week on the MDS. If such decisions are more frequent or involved more activities, the resident may be only moderately impaired or better.

C1000: Cognitive Skills for Daily Decision Making (cont.)

3. A resident makes her own decisions throughout the day and is consistent and reasonable in her decision-making except that she constantly walks away from the walker she has been using for nearly 2 years. Asked why she doesn't use her walker, she replies, "I don't like it. It gets in my way, and I don't want to use it even though I know all of you think I should."

   Coding: C1000 would be **coded 0, independent.**

   Rationale: This resident is making and expressing understanding of her own decisions, and her decision is to decline the recommended course of action – using the walker. Other decisions she made throughout the look-back period were consistent and reasonable.

4. A resident routinely participates in coffee hour on Wednesday mornings, and often does not need a reminder. Due to renovations, however, the meeting place was moved to another location in the facility. The resident was informed of this change and was accompanied to the new location by the activities director. Staff noticed that the resident was uncharacteristically agitated and unwilling to engage with other residents or the staff. She eventually left and was found sitting in the original coffee hour room. Asked why she came back to this location, she responded, "the aide brought me to the wrong room, I'll wait here until they serve the coffee."

   Coding: C1000 would be **coded 1, modified independent.**

   Rationale: The resident is independent under routine circumstances. However, when the situation was new or different, she had difficulty adjusting.

5. Mr. G. enjoys congregate meals in the dining and is friendly with the other residents at his table. Recently, he has started to lose weight. He appears to have little appetite, rarely eats without reminders and willingly gives his food to other residents at the table. Mr. G. requires frequent cueing from staff to eat and supervision to prevent him from sharing his food.

   Coding: C1000 would be **coded 2, moderately impaired.**

   Rationale: The resident is making poor decisions by giving his food away. He requires cueing to eat and supervision to be sure that he is eating the food on his plate.

C1300: Signs and Symptoms of Delirium*

Delirium		
C1300. Signs and Symptoms of Delirium (from CAM©)		
Code **after completing** Brief Interview for Mental Status or Staff Assessment, and reviewing medical record		
Coding: 0. **Behavior not present** 1. **Behavior continuously present, does not fluctuate** 2. **Behavior present, fluctuates** (comes and goes, changes in severity)	↓ **Enter Codes in Boxes**	
	☐	A. **Inattention** - Did the resident have difficulty focusing attention (easily distracted, out of touch or difficulty following what was said)?
	☐	B. **Disorganized thinking** - Was the resident's thinking disorganized or incoherent (rambling or irrelevant conversation, unclear or illogical flow of ideas, or unpredictable switching from subject to subject)?
	☐	C. **Altered level of consciousness** - Did the resident have altered level of consciousness (e.g., **vigilant** - startled easily to any sound or touch; **lethargic** - repeatedly dozed off when being asked questions, but responded to voice or touch; **stuporous** - very difficult to arouse and keep aroused for the interview; **comatose** - could not be aroused)?
	☐	D. **Psychomotor retardation** - Did the resident have an unusually decreased level of activity such as sluggishness, staring into space, staying in one position, moving very slowly?

*Item C1300 is adapted from the Confusion Assessment Method (CAM; Inouye et al., 1990) that has copyright protection and cannot be modified. The reference to "comatose" in response C (Altered level of consciousness) is not applicable as Section C would be skipped if the resident was comatose (i.e., B0100 = 1).

Item Rationale

Health-related Quality of Life

- Delirium is associated with:
  — increased mortality,
  — functional decline,
  — development or worsening of incontinence,
  — behavior problems,
  — withdrawal from activities
  — rehospitalizations and increased length of nursing home stay.
- Delirium can be misdiagnosed as dementia.
- A recent deterioration in cognitive function may indicate delirium, which may be reversible if detected and treated in a timely fashion.

Planning for Care

- Delirium may be a symptom of an acute, treatable illness such as infection or reaction to medications.
- Prompt detection is essential in order to identify and treat or eliminate the cause.

C1300: Signs and Symptoms of Delirium (cont.)

Steps for Assessment

1. Observe resident behavior during the **BIMS** items (C0200-C0400) for the signs and symptoms of delirium. Some experts suggest that increasing the frequency of assessment (as often as daily for new admissions) will improve the level of detection.
2. If the **Staff Assessment for Mental Status** items (C0700-C1000) was completed instead of the BIMS, ask staff members who conducted the interview about their observations of signs and symptoms of delirium.
3. Review medical record documentation during the 7-day look-back period to determine the resident's baseline status, fluctuations in behavior, and behaviors that might have occurred during the 7-day look-back period that were not observed during the BIMS.
4. Interview staff, family members and others in a position to observe the resident's behavior during the 7-day look-back period.

For additional guidance on the signs and symptoms of delirium can be found in Appendix C.

DEFINITIONS
DELIRIUM A mental disturbance characterized by new or acutely worsening confusion, disordered expression of thoughts, change in level of consciousness or hallucinations.

Steps for Assessment for C1300A, **Inattention**

Basic delirium assessment instructions are on page C-33. In addition, for C1300 (Inattention):

1. Assess attention separately from level of consciousness. Evidence of inattention may be found during the resident interview, in the medical record, or from family or staff reports of inattention during the 7-day look-back period.
2. An additional step to identify difficulty with attention is to ask the resident to count backwards from 20.

Coding Instructions for C1300A, **Inattention**

- **Code 0, behavior not present:** if the resident remains focused during the interview and all other sources agree that the resident was attentive during other activities.

- **Code 1, behavior continuously present, did not fluctuate:** if the resident had difficulty focusing attention, was easily distracted, or had difficulty keeping track of what was said AND the inattention did not vary during the look-back period. All sources must agree that inattention was consistently present to select this code.

DEFINITIONS
INATTENTION Reduced ability to maintain attention to external stimuli and to appropriately shift attention to new external stimuli. Resident seems unaware or out of touch with environment (e.g., dazed, fixated or darting attention).
FLUCTUATION The behavior tends to come and go and/or increase or decrease in severity. The behavior may fluctuate over the course of the interview or during the 7-day look-back period. Fluctuating behavior may be noted by the interviewer, reported by staff or family or documented in the medical record.

70

C1300: Signs and Symptoms of Delirium (cont.)

- **Code 2, behavior present, fluctuates:** if inattention is noted during the interview or any source reports that the resident had difficulty focusing attention, was easily distracted, or had difficulty keeping track of what was said AND the inattention varied during interview or during the look-back period or if information sources disagree in assessing level of attention.

Examples

1. The resident tries to answer all questions during the BIMS. Although she answers several items incorrectly and responds "I don't know" to others, she pays attention to the interviewer. Medical record and staff indicate that this is her consistent behavior.

    Coding: Item C1300A would be **coded 0, behavior not present.**
    Rationale: The resident remained focused throughout the interview and this was constant during the look-back period.

2. Questions during the BIMS must be frequently repeated because resident's attention wanders. This behavior occurs throughout the interview and medical records and staff agree that this behavior is consistently present. The resident has a diagnosis of dementia.

    Coding: Item C1300A would be **coded 1, behavior continuously present, does not fluctuate.**
    Rationale: The resident's attention consistently wandered throughout the 7-day look-back period. The resident's dementia diagnosis does not affect the coding.

3. During the BIMS interview, the resident was not able to focus on all questions asked and his gaze wandered. However, several notes in the resident's medical record indicate that the resident was attentive when staff communicated with him.

    Coding: Item C1300A would be **coded 2, behavior present, fluctuates.**
    Rationale: Evidence of inattention was found during the BIMS but was noted to be absent in the medical record. This disagreement shows possible fluctuation in the behavior. If any information source reports the symptom as present, C1300A **cannot be coded as 0, Behavior not present.**

4. Resident is dazedly staring at the television for the first several questions. When you ask a question, she looks at you momentarily but does not answer. Midway through questioning, she seems to pay more attention and tries to answer.

    Coding: Item C1300A would be **coded 2, behavior present, fluctuates.**
    Rationale: Resident's attention fluctuated during the interview. If as few as one source notes fluctuation, then the behavior should be **coded 2.**

C1300: Signs and Symptoms of Delirium (cont.)

Coding Instructions for C1300B, Disorganized Thinking

DEFINITIONS

DISORGANIZED THINKING Evidenced by rambling, irrelevant, or incoherent speech.

- **Code 0, behavior not present:** if all sources agree that the resident's thinking was organized and coherent, even if answers were inaccurate or wrong.

- **Code 1, behavior continuously present, did not fluctuate:** if, during the interview and according to other sources, the resident's responses were consistently disorganized or incoherent, conversation was rambling or irrelevant, ideas were unclear or flowed illogically, or the resident unpredictably switched from subject to subject.

- **Code 2, behavior present, fluctuates:** if, during the interview or according to other data sources, the resident's responses fluctuated between disorganized/incoherent and organized/clear. Also code as fluctuating if information sources disagree.

Examples

1. The interviewer asks the resident, who is often confused, to give the date, and the response is: "Let's go get the sailor suits!" The resident continues to provide irrelevant or nonsensical responses throughout the interview, and medical record and staff indicate this is constant.

    Coding: C1300B would be **coded 1, behavior continuously present, does not fluctuate.**

    Rationale: All sources agree that the disorganized thinking is constant.

2. The resident responds that the year is 1837 when asked to give the date. The medical record and staff indicate that the resident is never oriented to time but has coherent conversations. For example, staff reports he often discusses his passion for baseball.

    Coding: C1300B would be **coded 0, behavior not present.**

    Rationale: The resident's answer was related to the question, even though it was incorrect. No other sources report disorganized thinking.

3. The resident was able to tell the interviewer her name, the year and where she was. She was able to talk about the activity she just attended and the residents and staff that also attended. Then the resident suddenly asked the interviewer, "Who are you? What are you doing in my daughter's home?"

    Coding: C1300B would be **coded 2, behavior present, fluctuates.**

    Rationale: The resident's thinking fluctuated between coherent and incoherent at least once. If as few as one source notes fluctuation, then the behavior should be **coded 2.**

C1300: Signs and Symptoms of Delirium (cont.)

Coding Instructions for C1300C, **Altered Level of Consciousness**

- **Code 0, behavior not present:** if all sources agree that the resident was alert and maintained wakefulness during conversation, interview(s), and activities.

- **Code 1, behavior continuously present, did not fluctuate:** if, during the interview and according to other sources, the resident was consistently lethargic (difficult to keep awake), stuporous (very difficult to arouse and keep aroused), vigilant (startles easily to any sound or touch), or comatose.

- **Code 2, behavior present, fluctuates:** if, during the interview or according to other sources, the resident varied in levels of consciousness. For example, was at times alert and responsive, while at other times resident was lethargic, stuporous, or vigilant. Also code as fluctuating if information sources disagree.

Coding Tips

- A diagnosis of coma or stupor does not have to be present for staff to note the behavior in this section.

> **DEFINITIONS**
>
> **ALTERED LEVEL OF CONSCIOUSNESS**
>
> **VIGILANT** - startles easily to any sound or touch;
>
> **LETHARGIC** - repeatedly dozes off when you are asking questions, but responds to voice or touch;
>
> **STUPOR** - very difficult to arouse and keep aroused for the interview;
>
> **COMATOSE** - cannot be aroused despite shaking and shouting.

Examples

1. Resident is alert and conversational and answers all questions during the BIMS interview, although not all answers are correct. Medical record documentation and staff report during the 7-day look-back period consistently noted that the resident was alert.

   Coding: C1300C would be **coded 0, behavior not present.**
   Rationale: All evidence indicates that the resident is alert during conversation, interview(s) and activities.

2. The resident is lying in bed. He arouses to soft touch but is only able to converse for a short time before his eyes close, and he appears to be sleeping. Again, he arouses to voice or touch but only for short periods during the interview. Information from other sources indicates that this was his condition throughout the look-back period.

   Coding: C1300C would be **coded 1, behavior continuously present, does not fluctuate.**
   Rationale: The resident's lethargy was consistent throughout the interview, and there is consistent documentation of lethargy in the medical record during the look-back period.

C1300: Signs and Symptoms of Delirium (cont.)

3. Resident is usually alert, oriented to time, place, and person. Today, at the time of the BIMS interview, resident is conversant at the beginning of the interview but becomes lethargic and difficult to arouse.

> **Coding:** C1300C would be **coded 2, behavior present, fluctuates.**
>
> **Rationale:** The level of consciousness fluctuated during the interview. If as few as one source notes fluctuation, then the behavior should be **coded 2, fluctuating**.

Coding Instructions for C1300D, Psychomotor Retardation

- **Code 0, behavior not present:** if the resident's movements and responses were noted to be appropriate during BIMS and across all information sources.

- **Code 1, behavior continuously present, did not fluctuate:** if, during the interview and according to other sources, the resident consistently had an unusually decreased level of activity such as being sluggish, staring into space, staying in one position, or moving or speaking very slowly.

- **Code 2, behavior present, fluctuates:** if, during the BIMS interview or according to other sources, the resident showed slowness or decreased movement and activity which varied during the interview(s) or during the look-back period.

> **DEFINITIONS**
>
> **PSYCHOMOTOR RETARDATION** Greatly reduced or slowed level of activity or mental processing. Psychomotor retardation differs from altered level of consciousness. Resident need not be lethargic (altered level of consciousness) to have slowness of response. Psychomotor retardation may be present with normal level of consciousness; also residents with lethargy or stupor do not necessarily have psychomotor retardation.

Examples

1. Resident answers questions promptly during interview and staff and medical record note similar behavior.

> **Coding:** Item C1300D would be **coded 0, behavior not present.**
>
> **Rationale:** There is no evidence of psychomotor retardation from any source.

2. The resident is alert, but has a prolonged delay before answering the interviewer's question. Staff reports that the resident has always been very slow in answering questions.

> **Coding:** C1300D would be **coded 1, behavior continuously present, does not fluctuate.**
>
> **Rationale:** The psychomotor retardation was continuously present according to sources that described the resident's response speed to questions.

3. Resident moves body very slowly (i.e., to pick up a glass). Staff reports that they have not noticed any slowness.

> **Coding:** C1300D would be **coded 2, behavior present, fluctuates.**
>
> **Rationale:** There is evidence that psychomotor retardation comes and goes.

C1600: Acute Onset of Mental Status Change

C1600. Acute Onset Mental Status Change	

Enter Code
☐
	Is there evidence of an acute change in mental status from the resident's baseline?
	   0. No
	   1. Yes

Item Rationale

Health-related Quality of Life

- Acute onset mental status change may indicate delirium or other serious medical complications, which may be reversible if detected and treated in a timely fashion.

Planning for Care

- Prompt detection of acute mental status change is essential in order to identify and treat or eliminate the cause.

Coding Instructions

- **Code 0, no:** if there is no evidence of acute mental status change from the resident's baseline.
- **Code 1, yes:** if resident has an alteration in mental status observed in the past 7 days or in the BIMS that represents a change from baseline.

Coding Tips

- Interview resident's family or significant others.
- Review medical record prior to 7-day look-back.

Examples

1. Resident was admitted to the nursing home 4 days ago. Her family reports that she was alert and oriented prior to admission. During the BIMS interview, she is lethargic and incoherent.

   Coding: Item C1600 would be **coded 1, yes.**

   Rationale: There is an acute change of the resident's behavior from alert and oriented (family report) to lethargic and incoherent during interview.

2. Nurse reports that a resident with poor short-term memory and disorientation to time suddenly becomes agitated, calling out to her dead husband, tearing off her clothes, and being completely disoriented to time, person, and place.

   Coding: Item C1600 would be **coded 1, yes.**

   Rationale: The new behaviors represent an acute change in mental status.

C1600: Acute Onset of Mental Status Change (cont.)

Other Examples of Acute Mental Status Changes

- A resident who is usually noisy or belligerent becomes quiet, lethargic, or inattentive.
- A resident who is normally quiet and content suddenly becomes restless or noisy.
- A resident who is usually able to find his or her way around the unit begins to get lost.

SECTION D: MOOD

Intent: The items in this section address mood distress, a serious condition that is underdiagnosed and undertreated in the nursing home and is associated with significant morbidity. It is particularly important to identify signs and symptoms of mood distress among nursing home residents because these signs and symptoms can be treatable.

It is important to note that coding the presence of indicators in Section D does not automatically mean that the resident has a diagnosis of depression or other mood disorder. Assessors do not make or assign a diagnosis in Section D, they simply record the presence or absence of specific clinical mood indicators. Facility staff should recognize these indicators and consider them when developing the resident's individualized care plan.

- Depression can be associated with:
  - psychological and physical distress (e.g., poor adjustment to the nursing home, loss of independence, chronic illness, increased sensitivity to pain),
  - decreased participation in therapy and activities (e.g., caused by isolation),
  - decreased functional status (e.g., resistance to daily care, decreased desire to participate in activities of daily living [ADLs]), and
  - poorer outcomes (e.g., decreased appetite, decreased cognitive status).
- Findings suggesting mood distress should lead to:
  - identifying causes and contributing factors for symptoms,
  - identifying interventions (treatment, personal support, or environmental modifications) that could address symptoms, and
  - ensuring resident safety.

D0100: Should Resident Mood Interview Be Conducted?

D0100. Should Resident Mood Interview be Conducted? - Attempt to conduct interview with all residents
Enter Code ☐	0. **No** (resident is rarely/never understood) → Skip to and complete D0500-D0600, Staff Assessment of Resident Mood (PHQ-9-OV) 1. **Yes** → Continue to D0200, Resident Mood Interview (PHQ-9©)

Item Rationale

This item helps to determine whether or not a resident or staff mood interview should be conducted.

Health-related Quality of Life

- Most residents who are capable of communicating can answer questions about how they feel.
- Obtaining information about mood directly from the resident, sometimes called "hearing the resident's voice," is more reliable and accurate than observation alone for identifying a mood disorder.

77

D0100: Should Resident Mood Interview Be Conducted? (cont.)

Planning for Care

- Symptom-specific information from direct resident interviews will allow for the incorporation of the resident's voice in the individualized care plan.

- If a resident cannot communicate, then **Staff Mood Interview** (D0500 A-J) should be conducted.

Steps for Assessment

1. Determine if the resident is rarely/never understood. If rarely/never understood, skip to D0500, Staff Assessment of Resident Mood (PHQ-9-OV©).

2. Review **Language** item (A1100) to determine if the resident needs or wants an interpreter to communicate with doctors or health care staff (A1100 = 1).

   - If the resident needs or wants an interpreter, complete the interview with an interpreter.

Coding Instructions

- **Code 0, no:** if the interview should not be conducted. This option should be selected for residents who are rarely/never understood, or who need an interpreter (A1100 = 1) but one was not available. Skip to item D0500, Staff Assessment of Resident Mood (PHQ-9-OV©).

- **Code 1, yes:** if the resident interview should be conducted. This option should be selected for residents who are able to be understood, and for whom an interpreter is not needed or is present. Continue to item D0200, Resident Mood Interview (PHQ-9©).

Coding Tips and Special Populations

- If the resident needs an interpreter, every effort should be made to have an interpreter present for the PHQ-9© interview. If it is absolutely not possible for a needed interpreter to be present on the day of the interview, code D0100 = 0 to indicate that an interview was not attempted and complete items D0500-D0650.

D0200: Resident Mood Interview (PHQ-9©)

D0200. Resident Mood Interview (PHQ-9©)

Say to resident: *"Over the last 2 weeks, have you been bothered by any of the following problems?"*

If symptom is present, enter 1 (yes) in column 1, Symptom Presence.
If yes in column 1, then ask the resident: *"About **how often** have you been bothered by this?"*
Read and show the resident a card with the symptom frequency choices. Indicate response in column 2, Symptom Frequency.

1. Symptom Presence	2. Symptom Frequency	1. Symptom Presence	2. Symptom Frequency
0. **No** (enter 0 in column 2)	0. **Never or 1 day**		
1. **Yes** (enter 0-3 in column 2)	1. **2-6 days** (several days)		
9. **No response** (leave column 2 blank)	2. **7-11 days** (half or more of the days)		
	3. **12-14 days** (nearly every day)	↓ Enter Scores in Boxes ↓	
A. *Little interest or pleasure in doing things*		☐	☐
B. *Feeling down, depressed, or hopeless*		☐	☐
C. *Trouble falling or staying asleep, or sleeping too much*		☐	☐
D. *Feeling tired or having little energy*		☐	☐
E. *Poor appetite or overeating*		☐	☐
F. *Feeling bad about yourself - or that you are a failure or have let yourself or your family down*		☐	☐
G. *Trouble concentrating on things, such as reading the newspaper or watching television*		☐	☐
H. *Moving or speaking so slowly that other people could have noticed. Or the opposite - being so fidgety or restless that you have been moving around a lot more than usual*		☐	☐
I. *Thoughts that you would be better off dead, or of hurting yourself in some way*		☐	☐

Item Rationale

Health-related Quality of Life

- Depression can be associated with:
  — psychological and physical distress,
  — decreased participation in therapy and activities,
  — decreased functional status, and
  — poorer outcomes.
- Mood disorders are common in nursing homes and are often underdiagnosed and undertreated.

Planning for Care

- Findings suggesting mood distress could lead to:
  — identifying causes and contributing factors for symptoms and
  — identifying interventions (treatment, personal support, or environmental modifications) that could address symptoms.

> **DEFINITIONS**
>
> **9-ITEM PATIENT HEALTH QUESTIONNAIRE (PHQ-9©)**
> A validated interview that screens for symptoms of depression. It provides a standardized severity score and a rating for evidence of a depressive disorder.

D0200: Resident Mood Interview (PHQ-9©) (cont.)

Steps for Assessment

Look-back period for this item is 14 days.

1. Conduct the interview preferably the day before or day of the ARD.
2. Interview any resident when D0100 = 1.
3. Conduct the interview in a private setting.
4. If an interpreter is used during resident interviews, the interpreter should not attempt to determine the intent behind what is being translated, the outcome of the interview, or the meaning or significance of the resident's responses. Interpreters are people who translate oral or written language from one language to another.
5. Sit so that the resident can see your face. Minimize glare by directing light sources away from the resident's face.
6. Be sure the resident can hear you.
   - Residents with a hearing impairment should be tested using their usual communication devices/techniques, as applicable.
   - Try an external assistive device (headphones or hearing amplifier) if you have any doubt about hearing ability.
   - Minimize background noise.
7. If you are administering the PHQ-9© in paper form, be sure that the resident can see the print. Provide large print or assistive device (e.g., page magnifier) if necessary.
8. Explain the reason for the interview before beginning.
   Suggested language: "I am going to ask you some questions about your mood and feelings over the past 2 weeks. I will also ask about some common problems that are known to go along with feeling down. Some of the questions might seem personal, but everyone is asked to answer them. This will help us provide you with better care."
9. Explain and /or show the interview response choices. A cue card with the response choices clearly written in large print might help the resident comprehend the response choices.
   Suggested language: "I am going to ask you how often you have been bothered by a particular problem over the last 2 weeks. I will give you the choices that you see on this card." (Say while pointing to cue card): "0-1 days—never or 1 day, 2-6 days—several days, 7-11 days—half or more of the days, or 12-14 days—nearly every day."
10. Interview the resident.
    Suggested language: "Over the last 2 weeks, have you been bothered by any of the following problems?"
    Then, for each question in **Resident Mood Interview** (D0200):
    - Read the item as it is written.
    - Do not provide definitions because the meaning **must be** based on the resident's interpretation. For example, the resident defines for himself what "tired" means; the item should be scored based on the resident's interpretation.
    - Each question **must be** asked in sequence to assess presence (column 1) and frequency (column 2) before proceeding to the next question.
    - Enter code 9 for any response that is unrelated, incomprehensible, or incoherent or if the resident's response is not informative with respect to the item being rated; this is considered a **nonsensical** response (e.g., when asked the question about "poor appetite or overeating," the resident answers, "I always win at poker.").

D0200: Resident Mood Interview (PHQ-9©) (cont.)

- For a **yes** response, ask the resident to tell you how often he or she was bothered by the symptom over the last 14 days. Use the response choices in D0200 Column 2, **Symptom Frequency**. Start by asking the resident the number of days that he or she was bothered by the symptom and read and show cue card with frequency categories/descriptions (0-1 days—never or 1 day, 2-6 days—several days, 7-11 days—half or more of the days, or 12-14 days—nearly every day).

Coding Instructions for Column 1. **Symptom Presence**

- **Code 0, no:** if resident indicates symptoms listed are not present enter 0. Enter 0 in Column 2 as well.
- **Code 1, yes:** if resident indicates symptoms listed are present enter 1. Enter 0, 1, 2, or 3 in Column 2, Symptom Frequency.
- **Code 9, no response:** if the resident was unable or chose not to complete the assessment, responded nonsensically and/or the facility was unable to complete the assessment. Leave Column 2, Symptom Frequency, blank.

Coding Instructions for Column 2. **Symptom Frequency**

Record the resident's responses as they are stated, regardless of whether the resident or the assessor attributes the symptom to something other than mood. Further evaluation of the clinical relevance of reported symptoms should be explored by the responsible clinician.

- **Code 0, never or 1 day:** if the resident indicates that he or she has never or has only experienced the symptom on 1 day.
- **Code 1, 2-6 days (several days):** if the resident indicates that he or she has experienced the symptom for 2-6 days.
- **Code 2, 7-11 days (half or more of the days):** if the resident indicates that he or she has experienced the symptom for 7-11 days.
- **Code 3, 12-14 days (nearly every day):** if the resident indicates that he or she has experienced the symptom for 12-14 days.

Coding Tips and Special Populations

- For question D0200I, **Thoughts That You Would Be Better Off Dead or of Hurting Yourself in Some Way:**
  - The checkbox in item D0350 reminds the assessor to notify a responsible clinician (psychologist, physician, etc). Follow facility protocol for evaluating possible self-harm.
  - Beginning interviewers may feel uncomfortable asking this item because they may fear upsetting the resident or may feel that the question is too personal. Others may worry that it will give the resident inappropriate ideas. However,
    - o Experienced interviewers have found that most residents who are having this feeling appreciate the opportunity to express it.

- o Asking about thoughts of self-harm does not give the person the idea. It does let the provider better understand what the resident is already feeling.
- o The best interviewing approach is to ask the question openly and without hesitation.
- If the resident uses his or her own words to describe a symptom, this should be briefly explored. If you determine that the resident is reporting the intended symptom but using his or her own words, ask him to tell you how often he or she was bothered by that symptom.
- Select only one frequency response per item.
- If the resident has difficulty selecting between two frequency responses, code for the higher frequency.
- Some items (e.g., item F) contain more than one phrase. If a resident gives different frequencies for the different parts of a single item, select the highest frequency as the score for that item.
- Residents may respond to questions:
  — verbally,
  — by pointing to their answers on the cue card, <u>OR</u>
  — by writing out their answers.

Interviewing Tips and Techniques

- Repeat a question if you think that it has been misunderstood or misinterpreted.
- Some residents may be eager to talk with you and will stray from the topic at hand. When a person strays, you should gently guide the conversation back to the topic.
  — **Example:** Say, "That's interesting, now I need to know…"; "Let's get back to…"; "I understand, can you tell me about…."
- Validate your understanding of what the resident is saying by asking for clarification.
  — **Example:** Say, "I think I hear you saying that…"; "Let's see if I understood you correctly."; "You said…. Is that right?"
- If the resident has difficulty selecting a frequency response, start by offering a single frequency response and follow with a sequence of more specific questions. This is known as unfolding.
  — **Example:** Say, "Would you say [name symptom] bothered you more than half the days in the past 2 weeks?"
    - o If the resident says "yes," show the cue card and ask whether it bothered him or her nearly every day (12-14 days) or on half or more of the days (7-11 days).
    - o If the resident says "no," show the cue card and ask whether it bothered him or her several days (2-6 days) or never or 1 day (0-1 day).

D0200: Resident Mood Interview (PHQ-9©) (cont.)

- Noncommittal responses such as "not really" should be explored. Residents may be reluctant to report symptoms and should be gently encouraged to tell you if the symptom bothered him or her, even if it was only some of the time. This is known as probing. Probe by asking neutral or nondirective questions such as:
  — "What do you mean?"
  — "Tell me what you have in mind."
  — "Tell me more about that."
  — "Please be more specific."
  — "Give me an example."

- Sometimes respondents give a long answer to interview items. To narrow the answer to the response choices available, it can be useful to summarize their longer answer and then ask them which response option best applies. This is known as echoing.
  — **Example:** Item D0200E, **Poor Appetite or Overeating**. The resident responds "the food is always cold and it just doesn't taste like it does at home. The doctor won't let me have any salt."
    o Possible interviewer response: "You're telling me the food isn't what you eat at home and you can't add salt. How often would you say that you were bothered by poor appetite or over-eating during the last 2 weeks?"
  — **Example:** Item D0200A, **Little Interest or Pleasure in Doing Things**. The resident, when asked how often he or she has been bothered by little interest or pleasure in doing things, responds, "There's nothing to do here, all you do is eat, bathe, and sleep. They don't do anything I like to do."
    o Possible interview response: "You're saying there isn't much to do here and I want to come back later to talk about some things you like to do. Thinking about how you've been feeling over the past 2 weeks, how often have you been bothered by little interest or pleasure in doing things."
  — **Example:** Item D0200B, **Feeling Down, Depressed, or Hopeless**. The resident, when asked how often he or she has been bothered by feeling down, depressed, or hopeless, responds: "How would you feel if you were here?"
    o Possible interview response: "You asked how I would feel, but it is important that I understand **your** feelings right now. How often would you say that you have been bothered by feeling down, depressed, or hopeless during the last 2 weeks?"

- If the resident has difficulty with longer items, separate the item into shorter parts, and provide a chance to respond after each part. This method, known as disentangling, is helpful if a resident has moderate cognitive impairment but can respond to simple, direct questions.
  — **Example**: Item D0200E, **Poor Appetite or Overeating**.
    o You can simplify this item by asking: "In the last 2 weeks, how often have you been bothered by poor appetite?" (pause for a response) "Or overeating?"

D0200: Resident Mood Interview (PHQ-9©) (cont.)

— **Example:** Item D0200C, **Trouble Falling or Staying Asleep, or Sleeping Too Much**.

  o You can break the item down as follows: "How often are you having problems falling asleep?" (pause for response) "How often are you having problems staying asleep?" (pause for response) "How often do you feel you are sleeping too much?"

— **Example:** Item D0200H, **Moving or Speaking So Slowly That Other People Could Have Noticed. Or the Opposite—Being So Fidgety or Restless That You Have Been Moving Around a Lot More than Usual**.

  o You can simplify this item by asking: "How often are you having problems with moving or speaking so slowly that other people could have noticed?" (pause for response) "How often have you felt so fidgety or restless that you move around a lot more than usual?"

D0300: Total Severity Score

D0300. Total Severity Score	
☐☐ **Enter Score**	**Add scores for all frequency responses in Column 2,** Symptom Frequency. Total score must be between 00 and 27. Enter 99 if unable to complete interview (i.e., Symptom Frequency is blank for 3 or more items).

Item Rationale

Health-related Quality of Life

- The score does not diagnose a mood disorder or depression but provides a standard score which can be communicated to the resident's physician, other clinicians and mental health specialists for appropriate follow up.

- The **Total Severity Score** is a summary of the frequency scores on the PHQ-9© that indicates the extent of potential depression symptoms and can be useful for knowing when to request additional assessment by providers or mental health specialists.

> **DEFINITIONS**
>
> **TOTAL SEVERITY SCORE**
> A summary of the frequency scores that indicates the extent of potential depression symptoms. The score does not diagnose a mood disorder, but provides a standard of communication with clinicians and mental health specialists.

Planning for Care

- The PHQ-9© **Total Severity Score** also provides a way for health care providers and clinicians to easily identify and track symptoms and how they are changing over time.

D0300: Total Severity Score (cont.)

Steps for Assessment

After completing D0200 A-I:

1. Add the numeric scores across all frequency items in **Resident Mood Interview** (D0200) Column 2.
2. Do not add up the score while you are interviewing the resident. Instead, focus your full attention on the interview.
3. The maximum resident score is 27 (3 x 9).

Coding Instructions

- The interview is successfully completed if the resident answered the frequency responses of at least 7 of the 9 items on the PHQ-9©.
- If symptom frequency is blank for 3 or more items, the interview is deemed **NOT** complete. **Total Severity Score** should be coded as "99" and the **Staff Assessment of Mood** should be conducted.
- Enter the total score as a two-digit number. The **Total Severity Score** will be between **00** and **27** (or "**99**" if symptom frequency is blank for 3 or more items).
- The software will calculate the Total Severity Score. For detailed instructions on manual calculations and examples, see Appendix E: PHQ-9© Total Severity Score Scoring Rules.

Coding Tips and Special Populations

- Responses to PHQ-9© can indicate possible depression. Responses can be interpreted as follows:
  - Major Depressive Syndrome is suggested if—of the 9 items—5 or more items are identified at a frequency of half or more of the days (7-11 days) during the look-back period and at least one of these, (1) little interest or pleasure in doing things, or (2) feeling down, depressed, or hopeless is identified at a frequency of half or more of the days (7-11 days) during the look-back period.
  - Minor Depressive Syndrome is suggested if, of the 9 items, (1) feeling down, depressed or hopeless, (2) trouble falling or staying asleep, or sleeping too much, or (3) feeling tired or having little energy are identified at a frequency of half or more of the days (7-11 days) during the look-back period and at least one of these, (1) little interest or pleasure in doing things, or (2) feeling down, depressed, or hopeless is identified at a frequency of half or more of the days (7-11 days).
  - In addition, PHQ-9© **Total Severity Score** can be used to track changes in severity over time. **Total Severity Score** can be interpreted as follows:

1-4:	minimal depression
5-9:	mild depression
10-14:	moderate depression
15-19:	moderately severe depression
20-27:	severe depression

D0350: Follow-up to D0200I

D0350. Safety Notification - Complete only if D0200I1 = 1 indicating possibility of resident self harm	
Enter Code ☐	**Was responsible staff or provider informed that there is a potential for resident self harm?** 0. **No** 1. **Yes**

Item Rationale

Health-related Quality of Life

- This item documents if appropriate clinical staff and/or mental health provider were informed that the resident expressed that he or she had thoughts of being better off dead, or hurting him or herself in some way.

- It is well-known that untreated depression can cause significant distress and increased mortality in the geriatric population beyond the effects of other risk factors.

- Although rates of suicide have historically been lower in nursing homes than for comparable individuals living in the community, indirect self-harm and life threatening behaviors, including poor nutrition and treatment refusal are common.

- Recognition and treatment of depression in the nursing home can be lifesaving, reducing the risk of mortality within the nursing home and also for those discharged to the community (available at http://www.agingcare.com/Featured-Stories/125788/Suicide-and-the-Elderly.htm).

Planning for Care

- Recognition and treatment of depression in the nursing home can be lifesaving, reducing the risk of mortality within the nursing home and also for those discharged to the community.

Steps for Assessment

- Complete item D0350 **only** if item D0200I1 **Thoughts That You Would Be Better Off Dead, or of Hurting Yourself in Some Way** = 1 indicating the possibility of resident self-harm.

Coding Tips and Special Populations

- **Code 0, no:** if responsible staff or provider was not informed that there is a potential for resident self-harm.

- **Code 1, yes:** if responsible staff or provider was informed that there is a potential for resident self-harm.

D0500: Staff Assessment of Resident Mood (PHQ-9-OV©)

D0500. Staff Assessment of Resident Mood (PHQ-9-OV®)		
Do not conduct if Resident Mood Interview (D0200-D0300) was completed		
Over the last 2 weeks, did the resident have any of the following problems or behaviors?		
If symptom is present, enter 1 (yes) in column 1, Symptom Presence. Then move to column 2, Symptom Frequency, and indicate symptom frequency.		
1. Symptom Presence 0. **No** (enter 0 in column 2) 1. **Yes** (enter 0-3 in column 2) **2. Symptom Frequency** 0. **Never or 1 day** 1. **2-6 days** (several days) 2. **7-11 days** (half or more of the days) 3. **12-14 days** (nearly every day)	**1.** Symptom Presence	**2.** Symptom Frequency
	↓ Enter Scores in Boxes ↓	
A. Little interest or pleasure in doing things	☐	☐
B. Feeling or appearing down, depressed, or hopeless	☐	☐
C. Trouble falling or staying asleep, or sleeping too much	☐	☐
D. Feeling tired or having little energy	☐	☐
E. Poor appetite or overeating	☐	☐
F. Indicating that s/he feels bad about self, is a failure, or has let self or family down	☐	☐
G. Trouble concentrating on things, such as reading the newspaper or watching television	☐	☐
H. Moving or speaking so slowly that other people have noticed. Or the opposite - being so fidgety or restless that s/he has been moving around a lot more than usual	☐	☐
I. States that life isn't worth living, wishes for death, or attempts to harm self	☐	☐
J. Being short-tempered, easily annoyed	☐	☐

Item Rationale

Health-related Quality of Life

- PHQ-9© **Resident Mood Interview** is preferred as it improves the detection of a possible mood disorder. However, a small percentage of patients are unable or unwilling to complete the PHQ-9© **Resident Mood Interview**. Therefore, staff should complete the PHQ-9-OV© **Staff Assessment of Mood** in these instances so that any behaviors, signs, or symptoms of mood distress are identified.

- Persons unable to complete the PHQ-9© **Resident Mood Interview** may still have a mood disorder.

- Even if a resident was unable to complete the **Resident Mood Interview**, important insights may be gained from the responses that were obtained during the interview, as well as observations of the resident's behaviors and affect during the interview.

- The identification of symptom presence and frequency as well as staff observations are important in the detection of mood distress, as they may inform need for and type of treatment.

- It is important to note that coding the presence of indicators in Section D does not automatically mean that the resident has a diagnosis of depression or other mood disorder. Assessors do not make or assign a diagnosis in Section D; they simply record the presence or absence of specific clinical mood indicators.

D0500: Staff Assessment of Resident Mood (PHQ-9-OV©) (cont.)

- Alternate means of assessing mood must be used for residents who cannot communicate or refuse or are unable to participate in the PHQ-9© **Resident Mood Interview**. This ensures that information about their mood is not overlooked.

Planning for Care

- When the resident is not able to complete the PHQ-9©, scripted interviews with staff who know the resident well should provide critical information for understanding mood and making care planning decisions.

Steps for Assessment

Look-back period for this item is 14 days.

1. Interview staff from all shifts who know the resident best. Conduct interview in a location that protects resident privacy.
2. The same administration techniques outlined above for the PHQ-9© **Resident Mood Interview** (pages D-4–D-6) and Interviewing Tips & Techniques (pages D-6–D-8) should also be followed when staff are interviewed.
3. Encourage staff to report symptom frequency, even if the staff believes the symptom to be unrelated to depression.
4. Explore unclear responses, focusing the discussion on the specific symptom listed on the assessment rather than expanding into a lengthy clinical evaluation.
5. If frequency cannot be coded because the resident has been in the facility for less than 14 days, talk to family or significant other and review transfer records to inform the selection of a frequency code.

Examples of Staff Responses That Indicate Need for Follow-up Questioning with the Staff Member

1. **D0500A, Little Interest or Pleasure in Doing Things**

   - The resident doesn't really do much here.
   - The resident spends most of the time in his or her room.

2. **D0500B, Feeling or Appearing Down, Depressed, or Hopeless**

   - She's 95- what can you expect?
   - How would you feel if you were here?

3. **D0500C, Trouble Falling or Staying Asleep, or Sleeping Too Much**

   - Her back hurts when she lies down.
   - He urinates a lot during the night.

4. **D0500D, Feeling Tired or Having Little Energy**

   - She's 95—she's always saying she's tired.
   - He's having a bad spell with his COPD right now.

5. **D0500E, Poor Appetite or Overeating**

   - She has not wanted to eat much of anything lately.
   - He has a voracious appetite, more so than last week.

6. **D0500F, Indicating That S/he Feels Bad about Self, Is a Failure, or Has Let Self or Family Down**

   - She does get upset when there's something she can't do now because of her stroke.
   - He gets embarrassed when he can't remember something he thinks he should be able to.

7. **D0500G, Trouble Concentrating on Things, Such as Reading the Newspaper or Watching Television**

   - She says there's nothing good on TV.
   - She never watches TV.
   - He can't see to read a newspaper.

8. **D0500H, Moving or Speaking So Slowly That Other People Have Noticed. Or the Opposite— Being So Fidgety or Restless That S/he Has Been Moving Around a Lot More than Usual**

   - His arthritis slows him down.
   - He's bored and always looking for something to do.

9. **D0500I, States That Life Isn't Worth Living, Wishes for Death, or Attempts to Harm Self**

   - She says God should take her already.
   - He complains that man was not meant to live like this.

10. **D0500J, Being Short-Tempered, Easily Annoyed**

    - She's OK if you know how to approach her.
    - He can snap but usually when his pain is bad.
    - Not with me.
    - He's irritable.

Coding Instructions for Column 1. Symptom Presence

- **Code 0, no:** if symptoms listed are not present. Enter 0 in Column 2, **Symptom Frequency**.
- **Code 1, yes:** if symptoms listed are present. Enter 0, 1, 2, or 3 in Column 2, **Symptom Frequency.**

D0500: Staff Assessment of Resident Mood (PHQ-9-OV©) (cont.)

Coding Instructions for Column 2. Symptom Frequency

- **Code 0, never or 1 day:** if staff indicate that the resident has never or has experienced the symptom on only 1 day.
- **Code 1, 2-6 days (several days):** if staff indicate that the resident has experienced the symptom for 2-6 days.
- **Code 2, 7-11 days (half or more of the days):** if staff indicate that the resident has experienced the symptom for 7-11 days.
- **Code 3, 12-14 days (nearly every day):** if staff indicate that the resident has experienced the symptom for 12-14 days.

Coding Tips and Special Populations

- Ask the staff member being interviewed to select how often over the past 2 weeks the symptom occurred. Use the descriptive and/or numeric categories on the form (e.g., "nearly every day" or 3 = 12-14 days) to select a frequency response.
- If you separated a longer item into its component parts, select the **highest** frequency rating that is reported.
- If the staff member has difficulty selecting between two frequency responses, code for the **higher** frequency.
- If the resident has been in the facility for less than 14 days, also talk to the family or significant other and review transfer records to inform selection of the frequency code.

D0600: Total Severity Score

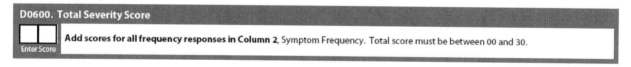

Item Rationale

Health-related Quality of Life

- Review Item Rationale for D0300, **Total Severity Score** (page D-10).
- The PHQ-9© Observational Version (PHQ-9-OV©) is adapted to allow the assessor to interview staff and identify a **Total Severity Score** for potential depressive symptoms.

Planning for Care

- The score can be communicated among health care providers and used to track symptoms and how they are changing over time.
- The score is useful for knowing when to request additional assessment by providers or mental health specialists for underlying depression.

D0600: Total Severity Score (cont.)

Steps for Assessment

After completing items D0500 A-J:

1. Add the numeric scores across all frequency items for **Staff Assessment of Mood, Symptom Frequency** (D0500) Column 2.

2. Maximum score is 30 (3×10).

Coding Instructions

The interview is successfully completed if the staff members were able to answer the frequency responses of at least 7 out of 10 items on the PHQ-9-OV$^©$.

- The software will calculate the Total Severity Score. For detailed instructions on manual calculations and examples, see Appendix E: PHQ-9-OV$^©$ Total Severity Score Scoring Rules.

Coding Tips and Special Populations

- Responses to PHQ-9-OV$^©$ can indicate possible depression. Responses can be interpreted as follows:

  — Major Depressive Syndrome is suggested if—of the 10 items, 5 or more items are identified at a frequency of half or more of the days (7-11 days) during the look-back period and at least one of these, (1) little interest or pleasure in doing things, or (2) feeling down, depressed, or hopeless is identified at a frequency of half or more of the days (7-11 days) during the look-back period.

  — Minor Depressive Syndrome is suggested if—of the 10 items, (1) feeling down, depressed or hopeless, (2) trouble falling or staying asleep, or sleeping too much, or (3) feeling tired or having little energy are identified at a frequency of half or more of the days (7-11 days) during the look-back period and at least one of these, (1) little interest or pleasure in doing things, or (2) feeling down, depressed, or hopeless is identified at a frequency of half or more of the days (7-11 days).

  — In addition, PHQ-9$^©$ **Total Severity Score** can be used to track changes in severity over time. **Total Severity Score** can be interpreted as follows:

    0-4: minimal depression
    5-9: mild depression
    10-14: moderate depression
    15-19: moderately severe depression
    20-30: severe depression

D0650: Follow-up to D0500I

D0650. Safety Notification - Complete only if D0500I1 = 1 indicating possibility of resident self harm	
Enter Code	Was responsible staff or provider informed that there is a potential for resident self harm?
[ ]	0. No
	1. Yes

Item Rationale

Health-related Quality of Life

- This item documents if appropriate clinical staff and/or mental health provider were informed that the resident expressed that they had thoughts of being better off dead, or hurting him or herself in some way.
- It is well known that untreated depression can cause significant distress and increased mortality in the geriatric population beyond the effects of other risk factors.
- Although rates of suicide have historically been lower in nursing homes than for comparable individuals living in the community, indirect self-harm and life-threatening behaviors, including poor nutrition and treatment refusal are common.

Planning for Care

- Recognition and treatment of depression in the nursing home can be lifesaving, reducing the risk of mortality within the nursing home and also for those discharged to the community (available at http://www.agingcare.com/Featured-Stories/125788/Suicide-and-the-Elderly.htm).

Steps for Assessment

1. Complete item D0650 only if item D0500I, **States That Life Isn't Worth Living, Wishes for Death, or Attempts to Harm Self** = 1 indicating the possibility of resident self-harm.

Coding Instructions

- **Code 0, no:** if responsible staff or provider was not informed that there is a potential for resident self-harm.
- **Code 1, yes:** if responsible staff or provider was informed that there is a potential for resident self-harm.

SECTION E: BEHAVIOR

Intent: The items in this section identify behavioral symptoms in the last seven days that may cause distress to the resident, or may be distressing or disruptive to facility residents, staff members or the care environment. These behaviors may place the resident at risk for injury, isolation, and inactivity and may also indicate unrecognized needs, preferences or illness. Behaviors include those that are potentially harmful to the resident himself or herself. The emphasis is identifying behaviors, which does not necessarily imply a medical diagnosis. Identification of the frequency and the impact of behavioral symptoms on the resident and on others is critical to distinguish behaviors that constitute problems from those that are not problematic. Once the frequency and impact of behavioral symptoms are accurately determined, follow-up evaluation and care plan interventions can be developed to improve the symptoms or reduce their impact.

This section focuses on the resident's actions, not the intent of his or her behavior. Because of their interactions with residents, staff may have become used to the behavior and may underreport or minimize the resident's behavior by presuming intent (e.g., "Mr. A. doesn't really mean to hurt anyone. He's just frightened."). Resident intent should **not** be taken into account when coding for items in this section.

E0100: Potential Indicators of Psychosis

E0100. Psychosis	
↓ Check all that apply	
☐	**A. Hallucinations** (perceptual experiences in the absence of real external sensory stimuli)
☐	**B. Delusions** (misconceptions or beliefs that are firmly held, contrary to reality)
☐	**Z. None of the above**

Item Rationale

Health-related Quality of Life

- Psychotic symptoms may be associated with
  — delirium,
  — dementia,
  — adverse drug effects,
  — psychiatric disorders, and
  — hearing or vision impairment.
- Hallucinations and delusions may
  — be distressing to residents and families,
  — cause disability,
  — interfere with delivery of medical, nursing, rehabilitative and personal care, and
  — lead to dangerous behavior or possible harm.

> **DEFINITIONS**
>
> **HALLUCINATION** The perception of the presence of something that is not actually there. It may be auditory or visual or involve smells, tastes or touch.
>
> **DELUSION** A fixed, false belief not shared by others that the resident holds even in the face of evidence to the contrary.

E0100: Potential Indicators of Psychosis (cont.)

Planning for Care

- Reversible and treatable causes should be identified and addressed promptly. When the cause is not reversible, the focus of management strategies should be to minimize the amount of disability and distress.

Steps for Assessment

1. Review the resident's medical record for the 7-day look-back period.
2. Interview staff members and others who have had the opportunity to observe the resident in a variety of situations during the 7-day look-back period.
3. Observe the resident during conversations and the structured interviews in other assessment sections and listen for statements indicating an experience of hallucinations, or the expression of false beliefs (delusions).
4. Clarify potentially false beliefs:

    - When a resident expresses a belief that is plausible but alleged by others to be false (e.g., history indicates that the resident's husband died 20 years ago, but the resident states her husband has been visiting her every day), try to verify the facts to determine whether there is reason to believe that it could have happened or whether it is likely that the belief is false.

    - When a resident expresses a clearly false belief, determine if it can be readily corrected by a simple explanation of verifiable (real) facts (which may only require a simple reminder or reorientation) or demonstration of evidence to the contrary. Do not, however, challenge the resident.

    - The resident's response to the offering of a potential alternative explanation is often helpful in determining whether the false belief is held strongly enough to be considered fixed.

Coding Instructions

Code based on behaviors observed and/or thoughts expressed in the last 7 days rather than the presence of a medical diagnosis. Check all that apply.

- **Check E0100A, hallucinations:** if hallucinations were present in the last 7 days. A hallucination is the perception of the presence of something that is not actually there. It may be auditory or visual or involve smells, tastes or touch.

- **Check E0100B, delusions:** if delusions were present in the last 7 days. A delusion is a fixed, false belief not shared by others that the resident holds true even in the face of evidence to the contrary.

- **Check E0100Z, none of the above:** if no hallucinations or delusions were present in the last 7 days.

E0100: Potential Indicators of Psychosis (cont.)

Coding Tips and Special Populations

- If a belief cannot be objectively shown to be false, or it is not possible to determine whether it is false, **do not** code it as a delusion.
- If a resident expresses a false belief but easily accepts a reasonable alternative explanation, **do not** code it as a delusion. If the resident continues to insist that the belief is correct despite an explanation or direct evidence to the contrary, **code as a delusion**.

Examples

1. A resident carries a doll which she believes is her baby and the resident appears upset. When asked about this, she reports she is distressed from hearing her baby crying and thinks she's hungry and wants to get her a bottle.

   Coding: E0100A would be **checked** and E0100B would be **checked.**
   Rationale: The resident believes the doll is a baby which is a delusion and she hears the doll crying which is an auditory hallucination.

2. A resident reports that he heard a gunshot. In fact, there was a loud knock on the door. When this is explained to him, he accepts the alternative interpretation of the loud noise.

   Coding: E0100Z would be **checked.**
   Rationale: He misinterpreted a real sound in the external environment. Because he is able to accept the alternative explanation for the cause of the sound, his report of a gunshot is not a fixed false belief and is therefore not a delusion.

3. A resident is found speaking aloud in her room. When asked about this, she states that she is answering a question posed to her by the gentleman in front of her. Staff note that no one is present and that no other voices can be heard in the environment.

   Coding: E0100A would be **checked.**
   Rationale: The resident reports an auditory sensation that occurs in the absence of any external stimulus. Therefore, this is a hallucination.

4. A resident announces that he must leave to go to work, because he is needed in his office right away. In fact, he has been retired for 15 years. When reminded of this, he continues to insist that he must get to his office.

   Coding: E0100B would be **checked.**
   Rationale: The resident adheres to the belief that he still works, even after being reminded about his retirement status. Because the belief is held firmly despite an explanation of the real situation, it is a delusion.

E0100: Potential Indicators of Psychosis (cont.)

5. A resident believes she must leave the facility immediately because her mother is waiting for her to return home. Staff know that, in reality, her mother is deceased and gently remind her that her mother is no longer living. In response to this reminder, the resident acknowledges, "Oh yes, I remember now. Mother passed away years ago."

> **Coding:** E0100Z would be **checked.**
>
> **Rationale:** The resident's initial false belief is readily altered with a simple reminder, suggesting that her mistaken belief is due to forgetfulness (i.e., memory loss) rather than psychosis. Because it is not a firmly held false belief, it does not fit the definition of a delusion.

E0200: Behavioral Symptom—Presence & Frequency

E0200. Behavioral Symptom - Presence & Frequency		
Note presence of symptoms and their frequency		
Coding: 0. **Behavior not exhibited** 1. **Behavior of this type occurred 1 to 3 days** 2. **Behavior of this type occurred 4 to 6 days, but less than daily** 3. **Behavior of this type occurred daily**	↓ Enter Codes in Boxes	
	☐	A. **Physical behavioral symptoms directed toward others** (e.g., hitting, kicking, pushing, scratching, grabbing, abusing others sexually)
	☐	B. **Verbal behavioral symptoms directed toward others** (e.g., threatening others, screaming at others, cursing at others)
	☐	C. **Other behavioral symptoms not directed toward others** (e.g., physical symptoms such as hitting or scratching self, pacing, rummaging, public sexual acts, disrobing in public, throwing or smearing food or bodily wastes, or verbal/vocal symptoms like screaming, disruptive sounds)

Item Rationale

Health-related Quality of Life

- New onset of behavioral symptoms warrants prompt evaluation, assurance of resident safety, relief of distressing symptoms, and compassionate response to the resident.

- Reversible and treatable causes should be identified and addressed promptly. When the cause is not reversible, the focus of management strategies should be to minimize the amount of disability and distress.

Planning for Care

- Identification of the frequency and the impact of behavioral symptoms on the resident and on others is critical to distinguish behaviors that constitute problems—and may therefore require treatment planning and intervention—from those that are not problematic.

- These behaviors may indicate unrecognized needs, preferences, or illness.

- Once the frequency and impact of behavioral symptoms are accurately determined, follow-up evaluation and interventions can be developed to improve the symptoms or reduce their impact.

- Subsequent assessments and documentation can be compared to baseline to identify changes in the resident's behavior, including response to interventions.

E0200: Behavioral Symptom-Presence & Frequency (cont.)

Steps for Assessment

1. Review the medical record for the 7-day look-back period.
2. Interview staff, across all shifts and disciplines, as well as others who had close interactions with the resident during the 7-day look-back period, including family or friends who visit frequently or have frequent contact with the resident.
3. Observe the resident in a variety of situations during the 7-day look-back period.

Coding Instructions

- **Code 0, behavior not exhibited:** if the behavioral symptoms were not present in the last 7 days. Use this code if the symptom has never been exhibited or if it previously has been exhibited but has been absent in the last 7 days.
- **Code 1, behavior of this type occurred 1-3 days:** if the behavior was exhibited 1-3 days of the last 7 days, regardless of the number or severity of episodes that occur on any one of those days.
- **Code 2, behavior of this type occurred 4-6 days, but less than daily:** if the behavior was exhibited 4-6 of the last 7 days, regardless of the number or severity of episodes that occur on any of those days.
- **Code 3, behavior of this type occurred daily:** if the behavior was exhibited daily, regardless of the number or severity of episodes that occur on any of those days.

Coding Tips and Special Populations

- Code based on whether the symptoms occurred and not based on an interpretation of the behavior's meaning, cause or the assessor's judgment that the behavior can be explained or should be tolerated.
- Code as present, even if staff have become used to the behavior or view it as typical or tolerable.
- Behaviors in these categories should be coded as present or not present, whether or not they might represent a rejection of care.
- Item E0200C does not include wandering.

Examples

1. Every morning, a nursing assistant tries to help a resident who is unable to dress himself. On the last 4 out of 6 mornings, the resident has hit or scratched the nursing assistant during attempts to dress him.

   Coding: E0200A would be **coded 2, behavior of this type occurred 4-6 days, but less than daily.**
   Rationale: Scratching the nursing assistant was a physical behavior directed toward others.

E0200: Behavioral Symptom-Presence & Frequency (cont.)

2. A resident has previously been found rummaging through the clothes in her roommate's dresser drawer. This behavior has not been observed by staff or reported by others in the last 7 days.

    Coding: E0200C would be **coded 0, behavior not exhibited.**
    Rationale: The behavior did not occur during the look-back period.

3. A resident throws his dinner tray at another resident who repeatedly spit food at him during dinner. This is a single, isolated incident.

    Coding: E0200A would be **coded 1, behavior of this type occurred 1-3 days of the last 7 days.**
    Rationale: Throwing a tray was a physical behavior directed toward others. Although a possible explanation exists, the behavior is noted as present because it occurred.

E0300: Overall Presence of Behavioral Symptoms

E0300. Overall Presence of Behavioral Symptoms	
Enter Code ☐	Were any behavioral symptoms in questions E0200 coded 1, 2, or 3? 0. **No** → Skip to E0800, Rejection of Care 1. **Yes** → Considering all of E0200, Behavioral Symptoms, answer E0500 and E0600 below

Item Rationale

To determine whether or not additional items E0500, **Impact on Resident**, and E0600, **Impact on Others,** are required to be completed.

Steps for Assessment

1. Review coding for item E0200 and follow these coding instructions:

Coding Instructions

*   **Code 0, no:** if E0200A, E0200B, and E0200C all are coded 0, not present. Skip to **Rejection of Care—Presence & Frequency** item (E0800).
*   **Code 1, yes:** if any of E0200A, E0200B, or E0200C were coded 1, 2, or 3. Proceed to complete **Impact on Resident** item (E0500), and **Impact on Others** item (E0600).

E0500: Impact on Resident

E0500. Impact on Resident	
	Did any of the identified symptom(s):
Enter Code ☐	**A. Put the resident at significant risk for physical illness or injury?** 0. No 1. Yes
Enter Code ☐	**B. Significantly interfere with the resident's care?** 0. No 1. Yes
Enter Code ☐	**C. Significantly interfere with the resident's participation in activities or social interactions?** 0. No 1. Yes

Item Rationale

Health-related Quality of Life

- Behaviors identified in item E0200 impact the resident's risk for significant injury, interfere with care or their participation in activities or social interactions.

Planning for Care

- Identification of the impact of the behaviors noted in E0200 may require treatment planning and intervention.
- Subsequent assessments and documentation can be compared to a baseline to identify changes in the resident's behavior, including response to interventions.

Steps for Assessment

1. Consider the previous review of the medical record, staff interviews across all shifts and disciplines, interviews with others who had close interactions with the resident and previous observations of the behaviors identified in E0200 for the 7-day look-back period.
2. Code E0500A, E0500B, and E0500C based on **all** of the behavioral symptoms coded in E0200.
3. Determine whether those behaviors put the resident at significant risk of physical illness or injury, whether the behaviors significantly interfered with the resident's care, and/or whether the behaviors significantly interfered with the resident's participation in activities or social interactions.

Coding Instructions for E0500A. Did Any of the Identified Symptom(s) Put the Resident at Significant Risk for Physical Illness or Injury?

- **Code 0, no:** if none of the identified behavioral symptom(s) placed the resident at clinically significant risk for a physical illness or injury.
- **Code 1, yes:** if any of the identified behavioral symptom(s) placed the resident at clinically significant risk for a physical illness or injury, even if no injury occurred.

E0500: Impact on Resident (cont.)

Coding Instructions for E0500B. Did Any of the Identified Symptom(s) Significantly Interfere with the Resident's Care?

- **Code 0, no:** if none of the identified behavioral symptom(s) significantly interfered with the resident's care.
- **Code 1, yes:** if any of the identified behavioral symptom(s) impeded the delivery of essential medical, nursing, rehabilitative or personal care, including but not limited to assistance with activities of daily living, such as bathing, dressing, feeding, or toileting.

Coding Instructions for E0500C. Did Any of the Identified Symptom(s) Significantly Interfere with the Resident's Participation in Activities or Social Interactions?

- **Code 0, no:** if none of the identified symptom(s) significantly interfered with the resident's participation in activities or social interactions.
- **Code 1, yes:** if any of the identified behavioral symptom(s) significantly interfered with or decreased the resident's participation or caused staff not to include residents in activities or social interactions.

Coding Tips and Special Populations

- For E0500A, code based on whether the risk for physical injury or illness is known to occur commonly under similar circumstances (i.e., with residents who exhibit similar behavior in a similar environment). Physical injury is trauma that results in pain or other distressing physical symptoms, impaired organ function, physical disability, or other adverse consequences, regardless of the need for medical, surgical, nursing, or rehabilitative intervention.
- For E0500B, code if the impact of the resident's behavior is impeding the delivery of care to such an extent that necessary or essential care (medical, nursing, rehabilitative or personal that is required to achieve the resident's goals for health and well-being) cannot be received safely, completely, or in a timely way without more than a minimal accommodation, such as simple change in care routines or environment.
- For E0500C, code if the impact of the resident's behavior is limiting or keeping the resident from engaging in solitary activities or hobbies, joining groups, or attending programmed activities or having positive social encounters with visitors, other residents, or staff.

Examples

1. A resident frequently grabs and scratches staff when they attempt to change her soiled brief, digging her nails into their skin. This makes it difficult to complete the care task.

   Coding: E0500B would be **coded 1, yes.**
   Rationale: This behavior interfered with delivery of essential personal care.

E0500: Impact on Resident (cont.)

2. During the last 7 days, a resident with vascular dementia and severe hypertension, hits staff during incontinent care making it very difficult to change her. Six out of the last seven days the resident refuses all her medication including her antihypertensive. The resident would close her mouth and shaking her head and will not take it even if re-approached multiple times.

    Coding: E0500A and E0500B would both be **coded 1, yes.**
    Rationale: The behavior interfered significantly with delivery of her medical and nursing care and put her at clinically significant risk for physical illness.

3. A resident paces incessantly. When staff encourage him to sit at the dinner table, he returns to pacing after less than a minute, even after cueing and reminders. He is so restless that he cannot sit still long enough to feed himself or receive assistance in obtaining adequate nutrition.

    Coding: E0500A and E0500B would both be **coded 1, yes.**
    Rationale: This behavior significantly interfered with personal care (i.e., feeding) and put the resident at risk for malnutrition and physical illness.

4. A resident repeatedly throws his markers and card on the floor during bingo.

    Coding: E0500C would be **coded 1, yes.**
    Rationale: This behavior interfered with his ability to participate in the activity.

5. A resident with severe dementia has continuous outbursts while awake despite all efforts made by staff to address the issue, including trying to involve the resident in prior activities of choice.

    Coding: E0500C would be **coded 1, yes.**
    Rationale: The staff determined the resident's behavior interfered with the ability to participate in any activities.

E0600: Impact on Others

	E0600. Impact on Others		
	Did any of the identified symptom(s):		
Enter Code	A. **Put others at significant risk for physical injury?**		
	0. No		
	1. Yes		
Enter Code	B. **Significantly intrude on the privacy or activity of others?**		
	0. No		
	1. Yes		
Enter Code	C. **Significantly disrupt care or living environment?**		
	0. No		
	1. Yes		

E0600: Impact on Others (cont.)

Item Rationale

Health-related Quality of Life

- Behaviors identified in item E0200 put others at risk for significant injury, intrude on their privacy or activities and/or disrupt their care or living environments. The impact on others is coded here in item E0600.

Planning for Care

- Identification of the behaviors noted in E0200 that have an impact on others may require treatment planning and intervention.
- Subsequent assessments and documentation can be compared with a baseline to identify changes in the resident's behavior, including response to interventions.

Steps for Assessment

1. Consider the previous review of the clinical record, staff interviews across all shifts and disciplines, interviews with others who had close interactions with the resident and previous observations of the behaviors identified in E0200 for the 7-day look-back period.
2. To code E0600, determine if the behaviors identified put others at significant risk of physical illness or injury, intruded on their privacy or activities, and/or interfered with their care or living environments.

Coding Instructions for E0600A. Did Any of the Identified Symptom(s) Put Others at Significant Risk for Physical Injury?

- **Code 0, no:** if none of the identified behavioral symptom(s) placed staff, visitors, or other residents at significant risk for physical injury.
- **Code 1, yes:** if any of the identified behavioral symptom(s) placed staff, visitors, or other residents at significant risk for physical injury.

Coding Instructions for E0600B. Did Any of the Identified Symptom(s) Significantly Intrude on the Privacy or Activity of Others?

- **Code 0, no:** if none of the identified behavioral symptom(s) significantly intruded on the privacy or activity of others.
- **Code 1, yes:** if any of the identified behavioral symptom(s) kept other residents from enjoying privacy or engaging in informal activities (not organized or run by staff). Includes coming in uninvited, invading, or forcing oneself on others' private activities.

E0600: Impact on Others (cont.)

Coding Instructions for E0600C. Did Any of the Identified Symptom(s) Significantly Disrupt Care or the Living Environment?

- **Code 0, no:** if none of the identified behavioral symptom(s) significantly disrupted delivery of care or the living environment.

- **Code 1, yes:** if any of the identified behavioral symptom(s) created a climate of excessive noise or interfered with the receipt of care or participation in organized activities by other residents.

Coding Tips and Special Populations

- For E0600A, code based on whether the behavior placed others at significant risk for physical injury. Physical injury is trauma that results in pain or other distressing physical symptoms, impaired organ function, physical disability or other adverse consequences, regardless of the need for medical, surgical, nursing, or rehabilitative intervention.

- For E0600B, code based on whether the behavior violates other residents' privacy or interrupts other residents' performance of activities of daily living or limits engagement in or enjoyment of informal social or recreational activities to such an extent that it causes the other residents to experience distress (e.g., displeasure or annoyance) or inconvenience, whether or not the other residents complain.

- For E600C, code based on whether the behavior interferes with staff ability to deliver care or conduct organized activities, interrupts receipt of care or participation in organized activities by other residents, and/or causes other residents to experience distress or adverse consequences.

Examples

1. A resident appears to intentionally stick his cane out when another resident walks by.

   Coding: E0600A would be **coded 1, yes**; E0600B and E0600C would be **coded 0, no.**
   Rationale: The behavior put the other resident at risk for falling and physical injury. You may also need to consider coding B and C depending on the specific situation in the environment or care setting.

2. A resident, when sitting in the hallway outside the community activity room, continually yells, repeating the same phrase. The yelling can be heard by other residents in hallways and activity/recreational areas but not in their private rooms.

   Coding: E0600A would be **coded 0, no**; E0600B and E0600C would be **coded 1, yes.**
   Rationale: The behavior does not put others at risk for significant injury. The behavior does create a climate of excessive noise, disrupting the living environment and the activity of others.

E0600: Impact on Others (cont.)

3. A resident repeatedly enters the rooms of other residents and rummages through their personal belongings. The other residents do not express annoyance.

   Coding: E0600A and E0600C would be **coded 0, no**; E0600B would be **coded 1, yes.**

   Rationale: This is an intrusion and violates other residents' privacy regardless of whether they complain or communicate their distress.

4. When eating in the dining room, a resident frequently grabs food off the plates of other residents. Although their food is replaced, so the behavior does not compromise their nutrition, other residents become anxious in anticipation of this recurring behavior.

   Coding: E0600A would be **coded 0, no**; E0600B and E0600C would be **coded 1, yes.**

   Rationale: This behavior violates other residents' privacy as it is an intrusion on the personal space and property (food tray) . In addition, the behavior is pervasive and disrupts the staff's ability to deliver nutritious meals in dining room (an organized activity).

5. A resident tries to seize the telephone out of the hand of another resident who is attempting to complete a private conversation. Despite being asked to stop, the resident persists in grabbing the telephone and insisting that he wants to use it.

   Coding: E0600A and E0600C would be **coded 0, no**; E0600B would be **coded 1, yes.**

   Rationale: This behavior is an intrusion on another resident's private telephone conversation.

6. A resident begins taunting two residents who are playing an informal card game, yelling that they will "burn in hell" if they don't stop "gambling."

   Coding: E0600A and E0600C would be **coded 0, no**; E0600B would be **coded 1, yes.**

   Rationale: The behavior is intruding on the other residents' game. The game is not an organized facility event and does not involve care. It is an activity in which the two residents wanted to engage.

7. A resident yells continuously during an exercise group, diverting staff attention so that others cannot participate in and enjoy the activity.

   Coding: E0600A and E0600B would be **coded 0, no**; E0600C would be **coded 1, yes.**

   Rationale: This behavior disrupts the delivery of physical care (exercise) to the group participants and creates an environment of excessive noise.

E0600: Impact on Others (cont.)

8. A resident becomes verbally threatening in a group discussion activity, frightening other residents. In response to this disruption, staff terminate the discussion group early to avoid eliciting the behavioral symptom.

    Coding: E0600A and E0600B would be **coded 0, no**; E0600C would be **coded 1, yes.**

    Rationale: This behavior does not put other residents at risk for significant injury. The behavior restricts full participation in the organized activity, and limits the enjoyment of other residents. It also causes fear, thereby disrupting the living environment.

E0800: Rejection of Care—Presence & Frequency

E0800. Rejection of Care - Presence & Frequency	
Enter Code [ ]	Did the resident **reject evaluation or care** (e.g., bloodwork, taking medications, ADL assistance) **that is necessary to achieve the resident's goals for health and well-being?** Do not include behaviors that have already been addressed (e.g., by discussion or care planning with the resident or family), and/or determined to be consistent with resident values, preferences, or goals. 0. **Behavior not exhibited** 1. **Behavior of this type occurred 1 to 3 days** 2. **Behavior of this type occurred 4 to 6 days,** but less than daily 3. **Behavior of this type occurred daily**

Item Rationale

Health-related Quality of Life

- Goals for health and well-being reflect the resident's wishes and objectives for health, function, and life satisfaction that define an acceptable quality of life for that individual.

- The resident's care preferences reflect desires, wishes, inclinations, or choices for care. Preferences do not have to appear logical or rational to the clinician. Similarly, preferences are not necessarily informed by facts or scientific knowledge and may not be consistent with "good judgment."

- It is really a matter of resident choice. When rejection/decline of care is first identified, the team then investigates and determines the rejection/decline of care is really a matter of resident's choice. Education is provided and the resident's choices become part of the plan of care. On future assessments, this behavior would not be coded in this item.

- A resident might reject/decline care because the care conflicts with his or her preferences and goals. In such cases, care rejection behavior is not considered a problem that warrants treatment to modify or eliminate the behavior.

- Care rejection may be manifested by verbally declining, statements of refusal, or through physical behaviors that convey aversion to, result in avoidance of, or interfere with the receipt of care.

- This type of behavior interrupts or interferes with the delivery or receipt of care by disrupting the usual routines or processes by which care is given, or by exceeding the level or intensity of resources that are usually available for the provision of care.

- A resident's rejection of care might be caused by an underlying neuropsychiatric, medical, or dental problem. This can interfere with needed care that is consistent with the resident's preferences or established care goals. In such cases, care rejection behavior may be a problem that requires assessment and intervention.

Planning for Care

- Evaluation of rejection of care assists the nursing home in honoring the resident's care preferences in order to meet his or her desired health care goals.

- Follow-up assessment should consider:
  - whether established care goals clearly reflect the resident's preferences and goals and
  - whether alternative approaches could be used to achieve the resident's care goals.

- Determine whether a previous discussion identified an objection to the type of care or the way in which the care was provided. If so, determine approaches to accommodate the resident's preferences.

> **DEFINITIONS**
>
> **REJECTION OF CARE**
> Behavior that interrupts or interferes with the delivery or receipt of care. Care rejection may be manifested by verbally declining or statements of refusal or through physical behaviors that convey aversion to or result in avoidance of or interfere with the receipt of care.
>
> **INTERFERENCE WITH CARE**
> Hindering the delivery or receipt of care by disrupting the usual routines or processes by which care is given, or by exceeding the level or intensity of resources that are usually available for the provision of care.

Steps for Assessment

1. Review the medical record.
2. Interview staff, across all shifts and disciplines, as well as others who had close interactions with the resident during the 7-day look-back period.
3. Review the record and consult staff to determine whether the rejected care is needed to achieve the resident's preferences and goals for health and well-being.
4. Review the medical record to find out whether the care rejection behavior was previously addressed and documented in discussions or in care planning with the resident, family, or significant other and determined to be an informed choice consistent with the resident's values, preferences, or goals; or whether that the behavior represents an objection to the way care is provided, but acceptable alternative care and/or approaches to care have been identified and employed.
5. If the resident exhibits behavior that appears to communicate a rejection of care (and that rejection behavior has not been previously determined to be consistent with the resident's values or goals), ask him or her directly whether the behavior is meant to decline or refuse care.

- If the resident indicates that the intention is to decline or refuse, then ask him or her about the reasons for rejecting care and about his or her goals for health care and well-being.

- If the resident is unable or unwilling to respond to questions about his or her rejection of care or goals for health care and well-being, then interview the family or significant other to ascertain the resident's health care preferences and goals.

Coding Instructions

- **Code 0, behavior not exhibited:** if rejection of care consistent with goals was not exhibited in the last 7 days.

- **Code 1, behavior of this type occurred 1-3 days:** if the resident rejected care consistent with goals 1-3 days during the 7-day look-back period, regardless of the number of episodes that occurred on any one of those days.

- **Code 2, behavior of this type occurred 4-6 days, but less than daily:** if the resident rejected care consistent with goals 4-6 days during the 7-day look-back period, regardless of the number of episodes that occurred on any one of those days.

- **Code 3, behavior of this type occurred daily:** if the resident rejected care consistent with goals daily in the 7-day look-back period, regardless of the number of episodes that occurred on any one of those days.

Coding Tips and Special Populations

- The intent of this item is to identify potential behavioral problems, not situations in which care has been rejected based on a choice that is consistent with the resident's preferences or goals for health and well-being or a choice made on behalf of the resident by a family member or other proxy decision maker.

- Do not include behaviors that have already been addressed (e.g., by discussion or care planning with the resident or family) and/or determined to be consistent with the resident's values, preferences, or goals.

Examples

1. A resident with heart failure who recently returned to the nursing home after surgical repair of a hip fracture is offered physical therapy and declines. She says that she gets too short of breath when she tries to walk even a short distance, making physical therapy intolerable. She does not expect to walk again and does not want to try. Her physician has discussed this with her and has indicated that her prognosis for regaining ambulatory function is poor.

   Coding: E0800 would be **coded 0, behavior not exhibited.**
   Rationale: This resident has communicated that she considers physical therapy to be both intolerable and futile. The resident discussed this with her physician. Her choice to not accept physical therapy treatment is consistent with her values and goals for health care. Therefore, this would **not** be coded as rejection of care.

2. A resident informs the staff that he would rather receive care at home, and the next day he calls for a taxi and exits the nursing facility. When staff try to persuade him to return, he firmly states, "Leave me alone. I always swore I'd never go to a nursing home. I'll get by with my visiting nurse service at home again." He is not exhibiting signs of disorientation, confusion, or psychosis and has never been judged incompetent.

   Coding: E0800 would be **coded 0, behavior not exhibited.**

   Rationale: His departure is consistent with his stated preferences and goals for health care. Therefore, this is **not** coded as care rejection.

3. A resident goes to bed at night without changing out of the clothes he wore during the day. When a nursing assistant offers to help him get undressed, he declines, stating that he prefers to sleep in his clothes tonight. The clothes are wet with urine. This has happened 2 of the past 5 days. The resident was previously fastidious, recently has expressed embarrassment at being incontinent, and has care goals that include maintaining personal hygiene and skin integrity.

   Coding: E0800 would be **coded 1, behavior of this type occurred 1-3 days.**

   Rationale: The resident's care rejection behavior is not consistent with his values and goals for health and well-being. Therefore, this is classified as care rejection that occurred twice.

4. A resident chooses not to eat supper one day, stating that the food causes her diarrhea. She says she knows she needs to eat and does not wish to compromise her nutrition, but she is more distressed by the diarrhea than by the prospect of losing weight.

   Coding: E0800 would be **coded 1, behavior of this type occurred 1-3 days.**

   Rationale: Although choosing not to eat is consistent with the resident's desire to avoid diarrhea, it is also in conflict with her stated goal to maintain adequate nutrition.

5. A resident is given his antibiotic medication prescribed for treatment of pneumonia and immediately spits the pills out on the floor. This resident's assessment indicates that he does not have any swallowing problems. This happened on each of the last 4 days. The resident's advance directive indicates that he would choose to take antibiotics to treat a potentially life-threatening infection.

   Coding: E0800 would be **coded 2, behavior of this type occurred 4-6 days, but less than daily.**

   Rationale: The behavioral rejection of antibiotics prevents the resident from achieving his stated goals for health care listed in his advance directives. Therefore, the behavior is coded as care rejection.

E0800: Rejection of Care—Presence & Frequency (cont.)

6. A resident who recently returned to the nursing home after surgery for a hip fracture is offered physical therapy and declines. She states that she wants to walk again but is afraid of falling. This occurred on 4 days during the look-back period.

    Coding: E0800 would be **coded 2, behavior of this type occurred 4-6 days.**

    Rationale: Even though the resident's health care goal is to regain her ambulatory status, her fear of falling results in rejection of physical therapy and interferes with her rehabilitation. This would be coded as rejection of care.

7. A resident who previously ate well and prided herself on following a healthy diet has been refusing to eat every day for the past 2 weeks. She complains that the food is boring and that she feels full after just a few bites. She says she wants to eat to maintain her weight and avoid getting sick, but she cannot push herself to eat anymore.

    Coding: E0800 would be **coded 3, behavior of this type occurred daily.**

    Rationale: The resident's choice not to eat is not consistent with her goal of weight maintenance and health. Choosing not to eat may be related to a medical condition such as a disturbance of taste sensation, gastrointestinal illness, endocrine condition, depressive disorder, or medication side effects.

E0900: Wandering—Presence & Frequency

E0900. Wandering - Presence & Frequency	
Enter Code	**Has the resident wandered?** 0. **Behavior not exhibited** → Skip to E1100, Change in Behavioral or Other Symptoms 1. **Behavior of this type occurred 1 to 3 days** 2. **Behavior of this type occurred 4 to 6 days,** but less than daily 3. **Behavior of this type occurred daily**

Item Rationale

Health-related Quality of Life

- Wandering may be a pursuit of exercise or a pleasurable leisure activity, or it may be related to tension, anxiety, agitation, or searching.

Planning for Care

- It is important to assess for reason for wandering. Determine the frequency of its occurrence, and any factors that trigger the behavior or that decrease the episodes.
- Assess for underlying tension, anxiety, psychosis, drug-induced psychomotor restlessness, agitation, or unmet need (e.g., for food, fluids, toileting, exercise, pain relief, sensory or cognitive stimulation, sense of security, companionship) that may be contributing to wandering.

E0900: Wandering—Presence & Frequency (cont.)

Steps for Assessment

1. Review the medical record and interview staff to determine whether wandering occurred during the 7-day look-back period.

   - Wandering is the act of moving (walking or locomotion in a wheelchair) from place to place with or without a specified course or known direction. Wandering may or may not be aimless. The wandering resident may be oblivious to his or her physical or safety needs. The resident may have a purpose such as searching to find something, but he or she persists without knowing the exact direction or location of the object, person or place. The behavior may or may not be driven by confused thoughts or delusional ideas (e.g., when a resident believes she must find her mother, who staff know is deceased).

2. If wandering occurred, determine the frequency of the wandering during the 7-day look-back period.

Coding Instructions for E0900

   - **Code 0, behavior not exhibited:** if wandering was not exhibited during the 7-day look-back period. Skip to **Change in Behavioral or Other Symptoms** item (E1100).

   - **Code 1, behavior of this type occurred 1-3 days:** if the resident wandered on 1-3 days during the 7-day look-back period, regardless of the number of episodes that occurred on any one of those days. Proceed to answer **Wandering—Impact** item (E1000).

   - **Code 2, behavior of this type occurred 4-6 days, but less than daily:** if the resident wandered on 4-6 days during the 7-day look-back period, regardless of the number of episodes that occurred on any one of those days. Proceed to answer **Wandering—Impact** item (E1000).

   - **Code 3, behavior of this type occurred daily:** if the resident wandered daily during the 7-day look-back period, regardless of the number of episodes that occurred on any one of those days. Proceed to answer **Wandering—Impact** item (E1000).

Coding Tips and Special Populations

   - Pacing (repetitive walking with a driven/pressured quality) within a constrained space is not included in wandering.
   - Wandering may occur even if resident is in a locked unit.
   - Traveling via a planned course to another specific place (such as going to the dining room to eat a meal or to an activity) is not considered wandering.

E1000: Wandering—Impact

Answer this item only if E0900, Wandering—Presence & Frequency, was coded 1 (behavior of this type occurred 1-3 days), 2 (behavior of this type occurred 4-6 days, but less than daily), or 3 (behavior of this type occurred daily).

E1000. Wandering - Impact	
Enter Code ☐	**A. Does the wandering place the resident at significant risk of getting to a potentially dangerous place** (e.g., stairs, outside of the facility)? 0. No 1. Yes
Enter Code ☐	**B. Does the wandering significantly intrude on the privacy or activities of others?** 0. No 1. Yes

Item Rationale

Health-related Quality of Life

- Not all wandering is harmful.
- Some residents who wander are at potentially higher risk for entering an unsafe situation.
- Some residents who wander can cause significant disruption to other residents.

Planning for Care

- Care plans should consider the impact of wandering on resident safety and disruption to others.
- Care planning should be focused on minimizing these issues.
- Determine the need for environmental modifications (door alarms, door barriers, etc.) that enhance resident safety if wandering places the resident at risk.
- Determine when wandering requires interventions to reduce unwanted intrusions on other residents or disruption of the living environment.

Steps for Assessment

1. Consider the previous review of the resident's wandering behaviors identified in E0900 for the 7-day look-back period.
2. Determine whether those behaviors put the resident at significant risk of getting into potentially dangerous places and/or whether wandering significantly intrudes on the privacy or activities of others based on clinical judgement for the individual resident.

Coding Instructions for E1000A. Does the Wandering Place the Resident at Significant Risk of Getting to a Potentially Dangerous Place?

- **Code 0, no:** if wandering does not place the resident at significant risk.
- **Code 1, yes:** if the wandering places the resident at significant risk of getting to a dangerous place (e.g., wandering outside the facility where there is heavy traffic) or encountering a dangerous situation (e.g., wandering into the room of another resident with dementia who is known to become physically aggressive toward intruders).

E1000: Wandering-Impact (cont.)

Coding Instructions for E1000B. Does the Wandering Significantly Intrude on the Privacy or Activities of Others?

- **Code 0, no:** if the wandering does not intrude on the privacy or activity of others.
- **Code 1, yes:** if the wandering intrudes on the privacy or activities of others (i.e., if the wandering violates other residents' privacy or interrupts other residents' performance of activities of daily living or limits engagement in or enjoyment of social or recreational activities), whether or not the other resident complains or communicates displeasure or annoyance.

Examples

1. A resident wanders away from the nursing home in his pajamas at 3 a.m. When staff members talk to him, he insists he is looking for his wife. This elopement behavior had occurred when he was living at home, and on one occasion he became lost and was missing for 3 days, leading his family to choose nursing home admission for his personal safety.

    Coding: E1000A would be **coded 1, yes.**

    Rationale: Wandering that results in elopement from the nursing home places the resident at significant risk of getting into a dangerous situation.

2. A resident wanders away from the nursing facility at 7 a.m. Staff find him crossing a busy street against a red light. When staff try to persuade him to return, he becomes angry and says, "My boss called, and I have to get to the office." When staff remind him that he has been retired for many years, he continues to insist that he must get to work.

    Coding: E1000A would be **coded 1, yes.**

    Rationale: This resident's wandering is associated with elopement from the nursing home and into a dangerous traffic situation. Therefore, this is coded as placing the resident at significant risk of getting to a place that poses a danger. In addition, delusions would be checked in item E0100.

3. A resident propels himself in his wheelchair into the room of another resident, blocking the door to the other resident's bathroom.

    Coding: E1000B would be **coded 1, yes.**

    Rationale: Moving about in this manner with the use of a wheelchair meets the definition of wandering, and the resident has intruded on the privacy of another resident and has interfered with that resident's ability to use the bathroom.

E1100: Change in Behavioral or Other Symptoms

E1100. Change in Behavior or Other Symptoms	
Consider all of the symptoms assessed in items E0100 through E1000	
Enter Code ☐	How does resident's current behavior status, care rejection, or wandering **compare to prior assessment (OBRA or PPS)?** 0. **Same** 1. **Improved** 2. **Worse** 3. **N/A** because no prior MDS assessment

E1100: Change in Behavioral or Other Symptoms (cont.)

Item Rationale

Health-related Quality of Life

- Change in behavior may be an important indicator of
  — a change in health status or a change in environmental stimuli,
  — positive response to treatment, and
  — adverse effects of treatment.

Planning for Care

- If behavior is worsening, assessment should consider whether it is related to
  — new health problems, psychosis, or delirium;
  — worsening of pre-existing health problems;
  — a change in environmental stimuli or caregivers that influences behavior; and
  — adverse effects of treatment.
- If behaviors are improved, assessment should consider what interventions should be continued or modified (e.g., to minimize risk of relapse or adverse effects of treatment).

Steps for Assessment

1. Review responses provided to items E0100-E1000 on the current MDS assessment.
2. Compare with responses provided on prior MDS assessment.
3. Taking all of these MDS items into consideration, make a global assessment of the change in behavior from the most recent to the current MDS.
4. Rate the overall behavior as same, improved, or worse.

Coding Instructions

- **Code 0, same:** if overall behavior is the same (unchanged).
- **Code 1, improved:** if overall behavior is improved.
- **Code 2, worse:** if overall behavior is worse.
- **Code 9, N/A:** if there was no prior MDS assessment of this resident.

Coding Tips

- For residents with multiple behavioral symptoms, it is possible that different behaviors will vary in different directions over time. That is, one behavior may improve while another worsens or remains the same. Using clinical judgment, this item should be rated to reflect the **overall** direction of behavior change, estimating the net effects of multiple behaviors.

E1100: Change in Behavioral or Other Symptoms (cont.)

Examples

1. On the prior assessment, the resident was reported to wander on 4 out of 5 days. Because of elopement, the behavior placed the resident at significant risk of getting to a dangerous place. On the current assessment, the resident was found to wander on 2 of the last 5 days. Because a door alarm system is now in use, the resident was not at risk for elopement and getting to a dangerous place. However, the resident is now wandering into the rooms of other residents, intruding on their privacy. This requires occasional redirection by staff.

    Coding: E1100 would be **coded 1, improved.**

    Rationale: Although one component of this resident's wandering behavior is worse because it has begun to intrude on the privacy of others, it is less frequent and less dangerous (without recent elopement) and is therefore improved overall since the last assessment. The fact that the behavior requires less intense surveillance or intervention by staff also supports the decision to rate the overall behavior as improved.

2. At the time of the last assessment, the resident was ambulatory and would threaten and hit other residents daily. He recently suffered a hip fracture and is not ambulatory. He is not approaching, threatening, or assaulting other residents. However, the resident is now combative when staff try to assist with dressing and bathing, and is hitting staff members daily.

    Coding: E1100 would be **coded 0, same.**

    Rationale: Although the resident is no longer assaulting other residents, he has begun to assault staff. Because the danger to others and the frequency of these behaviors is the same as before, the overall behavior is rated as unchanged.

3. On the prior assessment, a resident with Alzheimer's disease was reported to wander on 2 out of 7 days and has responded well to redirection. On the most recent assessment, it was noted that the resident has been wandering more frequently for 5 out of 7 days and has also attempted to elope from the building on two occasions.

    This behavior places the resident at significant risk of personal harm. The resident has been placed on more frequent location checks and has required additional redirection from staff. He was also provided with an elopement bracelet so that staff will be alerted if the resident attempts to leave the building. The intensity required of staff surveillance because of the dangerousness and frequency of the wandering behavior has significantly increased.

    Coding: E1100 would be **coded 2, worse.**

    Rationale: Because the danger and the frequency of the resident's wandering behavior have increased and there were two elopement attempts, the overall behavior is rated as worse.

SECTION F: PREFERENCES FOR CUSTOMARY ROUTINE AND ACTIVITIES

Intent: The intent of items in this section is to obtain information regarding the resident's preferences for his or her daily routine and activities. This is best accomplished when the information is obtained directly from the resident or through family or significant other, or staff interviews if the resident cannot report preferences. The information obtained during this interview is just a portion of the assessment. Nursing homes should use this as a guide to create an individualized plan based on the resident's preferences, and is not meant to be all-inclusive.

F0300: Should Interview for Daily and Activity Preferences Be Conducted?

F0300. Should Interview for Daily and Activity Preferences be Conducted? - Attempt to interview all residents able to communicate. If resident is unable to complete, attempt to complete interview with family member or significant other
Enter Code [ ]	0. **No** (resident is rarely/never understood <u>and</u> family/significant other not available) → Skip to and complete F0800, Staff Assessment of Daily and Activity Preferences 1. **Yes** → Continue to F0400, Interview for Daily Preferences

Item Rationale

Health-related Quality of Life

- Most residents capable of communicating can answer questions about what they like.
- Obtaining information about preferences directly from the resident, sometimes called "hearing the resident's voice," is the most reliable and accurate way of identifying preferences.
- If a resident cannot communicate, then family or significant other who knows the resident well may be able to provide useful information about preferences.

Planning for Care

- Quality of life can be greatly enhanced when care respects the resident's choice regarding anything that is important to the resident.
- Interviews allow the resident's voice to be reflected in the care plan.
- Information about preferences that comes directly from the resident provides specific information for individualized daily care and activity planning.

Steps for Assessment

1. Determine whether or not resident is rarely/never understood and if family/significant other is available. If resident is rarely/never understood and family is not available, skip to item F0800, Staff Assessment of Daily and Activity Preferences.
2. Review **Language** item (A1100) to determine whether or not the resident needs or wants an interpreter.
   - If the resident needs or wants an interpreter, complete the interview with an interpreter.
3. The resident interview should be conducted if the resident can respond:
   - verbally,
   - by pointing to their answers on the cue card, <u>OR</u>
   - by writing out their answers.

F0300: Should Interview for Daily and Activity Preferences Be Conducted? (cont.)

Coding Instructions

Record whether the resident preference interview should be attempted.

- **Code 0, no:** if the interview should not be attempted with the resident. This option should be selected for residents who are rarely/never understood, who need an interpreter but one was not available, and who do not have a family member or significant other available for interview. Skip to F0800, (Staff Assessment of Daily and Activity Preferences).

- **Code 1, yes:** if the resident interview should be attempted. This option should be selected for residents who are able to be understood, for whom an interpreter is not needed or is present, or who have a family member or significant other available for interview. Continue to F0400 (Interview for Daily Preferences) and F0500 (Interview for Activity Preferences).

Coding Tips and Special Populations

- If the resident needs an interpreter, every effort should be made to have an interpreter present for the MDS clinical interview. If it is not possible for a needed interpreter to be present on the day of the interview, **and** a family member or significant other is not available for interview, **code F0300 = 0** to indicate interview not attempted, and complete the Staff Assessment of Daily and Activity Preferences (F0800) instead of the interview with the resident (F0400 and F0500).

F0400: Interview for Daily Preferences

F0400. Interview for Daily Preferences		
Show resident the response options and say: **"While you are in this facility..."**		
	↓ **Enter Codes in Boxes**	
Coding: 1. **Very important** 2. **Somewhat important** 3. **Not very important** 4. **Not important at all** 5. **Important, but can't do or no choice** 9. **No response or non-responsive**	☐	A. how important is it to you to **choose what clothes to wear?**
	☐	B. how important is it to you to **take care of your personal belongings or things?**
	☐	C. how important is it to you to **choose between a tub bath, shower, bed bath, or sponge bath?**
	☐	D. how important is it to you to **have snacks available between meals?**
	☐	E. how important is it to you to **choose your own bedtime?**
	☐	F. how important is it to you to **have your family or a close friend involved in discussions about your care?**
	☐	G. how important is it to you to **be able to use the phone in private?**
	☐	H. how important is it to you to **have a place to lock your things to keep them safe?**

Item Rationale

Health-related Quality of Life

- Individuals who live in nursing homes continue to have distinct lifestyle preferences.

- A lack of attention to lifestyle preferences can contribute to depressed mood and increased behavior symptoms.

- Resident responses that something is important but that they can't do it or have no choice can provide clues for understanding pain, perceived functional limitations, and perceived environmental barriers.

Planning for Care

- Care planning should be individualized and based on the resident's preferences.

- Care planning and care practices that are based on resident preferences can lead to
  — improved mood,
  — enhanced dignity, and
  — increased involvement in daily routines and activities.

- Incorporating resident preferences into care planning is a dynamic, collaborative process. Because residents may adjust their preferences in response to events and changes in status, the preference assessment tool is intended as a first step in an ongoing dialogue between care providers and the residents. Care plans should be updated as residents' preferences change, paying special attention to preferences that residents state are important.

Steps for Assessment: Interview Instructions

1. Interview any resident not screened out by the **Should Interview for Daily and Activity Preferences Be Conducted?** item (F0300).
2. Conduct the interview in a private setting.
3. Sit so that the resident can see your face. Minimize glare by directing light sources away from the resident's face.
4. Be sure the resident can hear you.

    - Residents with hearing impairment should be interviewed using their usual communication devices/techniques, as applicable.

    - Try an external assistive device (headphones or hearing amplifier) if you have any doubt about hearing ability.

    - Minimize background noise.

5. Explain the reason for the interview before beginning.

    Suggested language: "I'd like to ask you a few questions about your daily routines. The reason I'm asking you these questions is that the staff here would like to know what's important to you. This helps us plan your care around your preferences so that you can have a comfortable stay with us. Even if you're only going to be here for a few days, we want to make your stay as personal as possible."

6. Explain the interview response choices. While explaining, also show the resident a clearly written list of the response options, for example a cue card.

Suggested language: "I am going to ask you how important various activities and routines are to you **while you are in this home.** I will ask you to answer using the choices you see on this card [read the answers while pointing to cue card]: 'Very Important,' 'Somewhat important,' 'Not very important,' 'Not important at all,' or 'Important, but can't do or no choice.'"

Explain the "Important, but can't do or no choice" response option.

Suggested language: "Let me explain the 'Important, but can't do or no choice' answer. You can select this answer if something would be important to you, but because of your health or because of what's available in this nursing home, you might not be able to do it. So, if I ask you about something that is important to you, but you don't think you're able to do it now, answer 'Important, but can't do or no choice.' If you choose this option, it will help us to think about ways we might be able to help you do those things."

7. Residents may respond to questions

- verbally,

- by pointing to their answers on the cue card, <u>OR</u>

- by writing out their answers.

8. If resident cannot report preferences, then interview family or significant others.

Coding Instructions

- **Code 1, very important:** if resident, family, or significant other indicates that the topic is "very important."

- **Code 2, somewhat important:** if resident, family, or significant other indicates that the topic is "somewhat important."

- **Code 3, not very important:** if resident, family, or significant other indicates that the topic is "not very important."

- **Code 4, not important at all:** if resident, family, or significant other indicates that the topic is "not important at all."

- **Code 5, important, but can't do or no choice:** if resident, family, or significant other indicates that the topic is "important," but that he or she is physically unable to participate, or has no choice about participating while staying in nursing home because of nursing home resources or scheduling.

> **DEFINITIONS**
>
> **NONSENSICAL RESPONSE**
> Any unrelated, incomprehensible, or incoherent response that is not informative with respect to the item being rated.

- **Code 9, no response or non-responsive:**
  — If resident, family, or significant other refuses to answer or says he or she does not know.
  — If resident does not give an answer to the question for several seconds and does not appear to be formulating an answer.
  — If resident provides an incoherent or nonsensical answer that does not correspond to the question.

Coding Tips and Special Populations

- Stop the interview and skip to Item F0700 if
  — the resident has given 3 nonsensical responses to 3 questions, OR
  — the resident has not responded to 3 of the questions.
- No look-back is provided for resident; he or she is being asked about current preferences while in the nursing home, therefore these questions can be completed anytime within the 7-day look-back period. Family or significant others are also responding to current preferences, but may have to consider past preferences if the resident is unable to communicate.

Interviewing Tips and Techniques

- Sometimes respondents give long or indirect answers to interview items. To narrow the answer to the response choices available, it can be useful to summarize their longer answer and then ask them which response option best applies. This is known as echoing.
- For these questions, it is appropriate to explore residents' answers and try to understand the reason.

Examples for F0400A, How Important Is It to You to Choose What Clothes to Wear (including hospital gowns or other garments provided by the facility)?

1. Resident answers, "It's very important. I've always paid attention to my appearance."

   Coding: F0400A would be **coded 1, very important**.

2. Resident replies, "I leave that up to the nurse. You have to wear what you can handle if you have a stiff leg."

   Interviewer echoes, "You leave it up to the nurses. Would you say that, while you are here, choosing what clothes to wear is [pointing to cue card] very important, somewhat important, not very important, not important at all, or that it's important, but you can't do it because of your leg?"

   Resident responds, "Well, it would be important to me, but I just can't do it."

   Coding: F0400A would be **coded 5, important, but can't do or no choice.**

F0400: Interview for Daily Preferences (cont.)

Examples for F0400B, How Important Is It to You to Take Care of Your Personal Belongings or Things?

1. Resident answers, "It's somewhat important. I'm not a perfectionist, but I don't want to have to look for things."

    Coding: F0400B would be **coded 2, somewhat important**.

DEFINITIONS

PERSONAL BELONGINGS OR THINGS Possessions such as eyeglasses, hearing aids, clothing, jewelry, books, toiletries, knickknacks, pictures.

2. Resident answers, "All my important things are at home."

    Interviewer clarifies, "Your most important things are at home. Do you have any other things while you're here that you think are important to take care of yourself?"

    Resident responds, "Well, my son brought me this CD player so that I can listen to music. It is very important to me to take care of that."

    Coding: F0400B would be **coded 1, very important.**

Examples for F0400C, How Important Is It to You to Choose between a Tub Bath, Shower, Bed Bath, or Sponge Bath?

1. Resident answers, "I like showers."

    Interviewer clarifies, "You like showers. Would you say that choosing a shower instead of other types of bathing is very important, somewhat important, not very important, not important at all, or that it's important, but you can't do it or have no choice?"

    The resident responds, "It's very important."

    Coding: F0400C would be **coded 1, very important.**

2. Resident answers, "I don't have a choice. I like only sponge baths, but I have to take shower two times a week."

    The interviewer says, "So how important is it to you to be able to choose to have a sponge bath while you're here?"

    The resident responds, "Well, it is very important, but I don't always have a choice because that's the rule."

    Coding: F0400C would be **coded 5, important, but can't do or no choice.**

Example for F0400D, How Important Is It to You to Have Snacks Available between Meals?

1. Resident answers, "I'm a diabetic, so it's very important that I get snacks."

    > **Coding:** F0400D would be **coded 1, very important.**

Example for F0400E, How Important Is It to You to Choose Your Own Bedtime?

1. Resident answers, "At home I used to stay up and watch TV. But here I'm usually in bed by 8. That's because they get me up so early."

    Interviewer echoes and clarifies, "You used to stay up later, but now you go to bed before 8 because you get up so early. Would you say it's [pointing to cue card] very important, somewhat important, not very important, not important at all, or that it's important, but you don't have a choice about your bedtime?"

    Resident responds, "I guess it would be important, but I can't do it because they wake me up so early in the morning for therapy and by 8 o'clock at night, I'm tired."

    > **Coding:** F0400E would be **coded 5, important, but can't do or no choice**.

Example for F0400F, How Important Is It to You to Have Your Family or a Close Friend Involved in Discussions about Your Care?

1. Resident responds, "They're not involved. They live in the city. They've got to take care of their own families."

    Interviewer replies, "You said that your family and close friends aren't involved right now. When you think about what you would prefer, would you say that it's very important, somewhat important, not very important, not important at all, or that it is important but you have no choice or can't have them involved in decisions about your care?"

    Resident responds, "It's somewhat important."

    > **Coding:** F0400F would be **coded 2, somewhat important**.

DEFINITIONS

BED BATH
Bath taken in bed using washcloths and water basin or other method in bed.

SHOWER
Bath taken standing or using gurney or shower chair in a shower room or stall.

SPONGE BATH
Bath taken sitting or standing at sink.

TUB BATH
Bath taken in bathtub.

SNACK
Food available between meals, including between dinner and breakfast.

Example for F0400G, How Important Is It to You to Be Able to Use the Phone in Private?

1. Resident answers "That's not a problem for me, because I have my own room. If I want to make a phone call, I just shut the door."

   Interviewer echoes and clarifies, "So, you can shut your door to make a phone call. If you had to rate how important it is to be able to use the phone in private, would you say it's very important, somewhat important, not very important, or not important at all?"

   Resident responds, "Oh, it's very important."

   Coding: F0400G would be **coded 1, very important**.

> **DEFINITIONS**
>
> **PRIVATE TELEPHONE CONVERSATION**
> A telephone conversation on which no one can listen in, other than the resident.

Example for F0400H, How Important Is It to You to Have a Place to Lock Your Things to Keep Them Safe?

1. Resident answers, "I have a safe deposit box at my bank, and that's where I keep family heirlooms and personal documents."

   Interviewer says, "That sounds like a good service. While you are staying here, how important is it to you to have a drawer or locker here?"

   Resident responds, "It's not very important. I'm fine with keeping all my valuables at the bank."

   Coding: F0400H would be **coded 3, not very important.**

F0500: Interview for Activity Preferences

F0500. Interview for Activity Preferences		
Show resident the response options and say: *"While you are in this facility..."*		
Coding: 1. **Very important** 2. **Somewhat important** 3. **Not very important** 4. **Not important at all** 5. **Important, but can't do or no choice** 9. **No response or non-responsive**	↓ Enter Codes in Boxes	
	☐	A. how important is it to you to **have books, newspapers, and magazines to read?**
	☐	B. how important is it to you to **listen to music you like?**
	☐	C. how important is it to you to **be around animals such as pets?**
	☐	D. how important is it to you to **keep up with the news?**
	☐	E. how important is it to you to **do things with groups of people?**
	☐	F. how important is it to you to **do your favorite activities?**
	☐	G. how important is it to you to **go outside to get fresh air when the weather is good?**
	☐	H. how important is it to you to **participate in religious services or practices?**

F0500: Interview for Activity Preferences (cont.)

Item Rationale

Health-related Quality of Life

- Activities are a way for individuals to establish meaning in their lives, and the need for enjoyable activities and pastimes does not change on admission to a nursing home.
- A lack of opportunity to engage in meaningful and enjoyable activities can result in boredom, depression, and behavior disturbances.
- Individuals vary in the activities they prefer, reflecting unique personalities, past interests, perceived environmental constraints, religious and cultural background, and changing physical and mental abilities.

Planning for Care

- These questions will be useful for designing individualized care plans that facilitate residents' participation in activities they find meaningful.
- Preferences may change over time and extend beyond those included here. Therefore, the assessment of activity preferences is intended as a first step in an ongoing informal dialogue between the care provider and resident.
- As with daily routines, responses may provide insights into perceived functional, emotional, and sensory support needs.

Coding Instructions

- **See Coding Instructions on page F-5.**
  Coding approach is identical to that for daily preferences.

Coding Tips and Special Populations

- **See Coding Tips on page F-5.**
  Coding tips include those for daily preferences.

- Include Braille and or audio recorded material when coding items in F0500A.

Interviewing Tips and Techniques

- **See Interview Tips and Techniques on page F-5.**
  Coding tips and techniques are identical to those for daily preferences.

DEFINITIONS

READ
Script, Braille, or audio recorded written material.

NEWS
News about local, state, national, or international current events.

KEEP UP WITH THE NEWS
Stay informed by reading, watching, or listening.

NEWSPAPERS AND MAGAZINES
Any type, such as journalistic, professional, and trade publications in script, Braille, or audio recorded format.

F0500: Interview for Activity Preferences (cont.)

Examples for F0500A, How Important Is It to You to Have Books (Including Braille and Audio-recorded Format), Newspapers, and Magazines to Read?

1. Resident answers, "Reading is very important to me."

    Coding: F0500A would be **coded 1, very important**.

2. Resident answers, "They make the print so small these days. I guess they are just trying to save money."

    Interviewer replies, "The print is small. Would you say that having books, newspapers, and magazines to read is very important, somewhat important, not very important, not important at all, or that it is important but you can't do it because the print is so small?"

    Resident answers: "It would be important, but I can't do it because of the print."

    Coding: F0500A would be **coded 5, important, but can't do or no choice.**

Example for F0500B, How Important Is It to You to Listen to Music You Like?

1. Resident answers, "It's not important, because all we have in here is TV. They keep it blaring all day long."

    Interviewer echoes, "You've told me it's not important because all you have is a TV. Would you say it's not very important or not important at all to you to listen to music you like while you are here? Or are you saying that it's important, but you can't do it because you don't have a radio or CD player?"

    Resident responds, "Yeah. I'd enjoy listening to some jazz if I could get a radio."

    Coding: F0500B would be **coded 5, important, but can't do or no choice.**

Examples for F0500C, How Important Is It to You to Be Around Animals Such as Pets?

1. Resident answers, "It's very important for me NOT to be around animals. You get hair all around and I might inhale it."

    Coding: F0500C would be **coded 4, not important at all.**

2. Resident answers, "I'd love to go home and be around my own animals. I've taken care of them for years and they really need me."

    Interviewer probes, "You said you'd love to be at home with your own animals. How important is it to you to be around pets while you're staying here? Would you say it is [points to card] very important, somewhat important, not very important, not important at all, or is it important, but you can't do it or don't have a choice about it."

    Resident responds, "Well, it's important to me to be around my own dogs, but I can't be around them. I'd say important but can't do."

    Coding: F0500C would be **coded 5, Important, but can't do or no choice.**

    Rationale: Although the resident has access to therapeutic dogs brought to the nursing home, he does not have access to the type of pet that is important to him.

F0500: Interview for Activity Preferences (cont.)

Example for F0500D, How Important Is It to You to Keep Up with the News?

1. Resident answers, "Well, they are all so liberal these days, but it's important to hear what they are up to."

   Interviewer clarifies, "You think it is important to hear the news. Would you say it is [points to card] very important, somewhat important, or it's important but you can't do it or have no choice?"

   Resident responds, "I guess you can mark me somewhat important on that one."

   Coding: F0500D would be **coded 2, somewhat important.**

Example for F0500E, How Important Is It to You to Do Things with Groups of People?

1. Resident answers, "I've never really liked groups of people. They make me nervous."

   Interviewer echoes and clarifies, "You've never liked groups. To help us plan your activities, would you say that while you're here, doing things with groups of people is very important, somewhat important, not very important, not important at all, or would it be important to you but you can't do it because you feel nervous about it?"

   Resident responds, "At this point I'd say it's not very important."

   Coding: F0500E would be **coded 3, not very important.**

Examples for F0500F, How Important Is It to You to Do Your Favorite Activities?

1. Resident answers, "Well, it's very important, but I can't really do my favorite activities while I'm here. At home, I used to like to play board games, but you need people to play and make it interesting. I also like to sketch, but I don't have the supplies I need to do that here. I'd say important but no choice."

   Coding: F0500F would be **coded 5, important, but can't do or no choice.**

2. Resident answers, "I like to play bridge with my bridge club."

   Interviewer probes, "Oh, you like to play bridge with your bridge club. How important is it to you to play bridge while you are here in the nursing home?"

   Resident responds, "Well, I'm just here for a few weeks to finish my rehabilitation. It's not very important."

   Coding: F0500F would be **coded 3, not very important**.
   Coding: F0500G would be **coded 1, very important.**

F0500: Interview for Activity Preferences (cont.)

Example for F0500G, How Important Is It to You to Go Outside to Get Fresh Air When the Weather Is Good (Includes Less Temperate Weather if Resident Has Appropriate Clothing)?

1. Resident answers, "They have such a nice garden here. It's very important to me to go out there."

Examples for F0500H, How Important Is It to You to Participate in Religious Services or Practices?

1. Resident answers, "I'm Jewish. I'm Orthodox, but they have Reform services here. So I guess it's not important."

   Interviewer clarifies, "You're Orthodox, but the services offered here are Reform. While you are here, how important would it be to you to be able to participate in religious services? Would you say it is very important, somewhat important, not very important, not important at all, or would it be important to you but you can't or have no choice because they don't offer Orthodox services."

   Resident responds, "It's important for me to go to Orthodox services if they were offered, but they aren't. So, can't do or no choice."

   > **Coding:** F0500I would be **coded 5, important, but can't do or no choice.**

2. Resident answers "My pastor sends taped services to me that I listen to in my room on Sundays. I don't participate in the services here."

   Interviewer probes, "You said your pastor sends you taped services. Would you say that it is very important, somewhat important, not very important, or not important at all, to you that you are able to listen to those tapes from your pastor?"

   Resident responds, "Oh, that's very important."

   > **Coding:** F0500I would be **coded 1, very important**.

DEFINITIONS

OUTSIDE
Any outdoor area in the proximity of the facility, including patio, porch, balcony, sidewalk, courtyard, or garden.

PARTICIPATE IN RELIGIOUS SERVICES
Any means of taking part in religious services or practices, such as listening to services on the radio or television, attending services in the facility or in the community, or private prayer or religious study.

RELIGIOUS PRACTICES
Rituals associated with various religious traditions or faiths, such as washing rituals in preparation for prayer, following kosher dietary laws, honoring holidays and religious festivals, and participating in communion or confession.

F0600: Daily and Activity Preferences Primary Respondent

F0600. Daily and Activity Preferences Primary Respondent	
Enter Code ☐	**Indicate primary respondent** for Daily and Activity Preferences (F0400 and F0500) 1. **Resident** 2. **Family or significant other** (close friend or other representative) 9. **Interview could not be completed** by resident or family/significant other ("No response" to 3 or more items")

Item Rationale

- This item establishes the source of the information regarding the resident's preferences.

Coding Instructions

- **Code 1, resident:** if resident was the primary source for the preference questions in F0400 and F0500.
- **Code 2, family or significant other:** if a family member or significant other was the primary source of information for F0400 and F0500.
- **Code 9, interview could not be completed:** if F0400 and F0500 could not be completed by the resident, a family member, or a representative of the resident.

F0700: Should the Staff Assessment of Daily and Activity Preferences Be Conducted?

F0700. Should the Staff Assessment of Daily and Activity Preferences be Conducted?	
Enter Code ☐	0. **No** (because Interview for Daily and Activity Preferences (F0400 and F0500) was completed by resident or family/significant other) → Skip to and complete G0110, Activities of Daily Living (ADL) Assistance 1. **Yes** (because 3 or more items in Interview for Daily and Activity Preferences (F0400 and F0500) were not completed by resident or family/significant other) → Continue to F0800, Staff Assessment of Daily and Activity Preferences

Item Rationale

Health-related Quality of Life

- Resident interview is preferred as it most accurately reflects what the resident views as important. However, a small percentage of residents are unable or unwilling to complete the interview for Daily and Activity Preferences.
- Persons unable to complete the preference interview should still have preferences evaluated and considered.

Planning for Care

- Even though the resident was unable to complete the interview, important insights may be gained from the responses that were obtained, observing behaviors, and observing the resident's affect during the interview.

Steps for Assessment

- Review resident, family, or significant other responses to F0400A-H and F0500A-H.

F0700: Should the Staff Assessment of Daily and Activity Preferences Be Conducted? (cont.)

Coding Instructions

- **Code 0, no:** if **Interview for Daily and Activity Preferences** items (F0400 and F0500) was completed by resident, family or significant other. Skip to Section G, Functional Status.
- **Code 1, yes:** if **Interview for Daily and Activity Preferences** items (F0400 through F0500) were not completed because the resident, family, or significant other was unable to answer 3 or more items (i.e. 3 or more items in F0400 through F0500 were coded as **9 or "-"**).

Coding Tips and Special Populations

- If the total number of unanswered questions in F0400 through F0500 is equal to 3 or more, the interview is considered incomplete.

F0800: Staff Assessment of Daily and Activity Preferences

F0800. Staff Assessment of Daily and Activity Preferences	
Do not conduct if Interview for Daily and Activity Preferences (F0400-F0500) was completed	
Resident Prefers:	
↓ Check all that apply	
☐	A. Choosing clothes to wear
☐	B. Caring for personal belongings
☐	C. Receiving tub bath
☐	D. Receiving shower
☐	E. Receiving bed bath
☐	F. Receiving sponge bath
☐	G. Snacks between meals
☐	H. Staying up past 8:00 p.m.
☐	I. Family or significant other involvement in care discussions
☐	J. Use of phone in private
☐	K. Place to lock personal belongings
☐	L. Reading books, newspapers, or magazines
☐	M. Listening to music
☐	N. Being around animals such as pets
☐	O. Keeping up with the news
☐	P. Doing things with groups of people
☐	Q. Participating in favorite activities
☐	R. Spending time away from the nursing home
☐	S. Spending time outdoors
☐	T. Participating in religious activities or practices
☐	Z. None of the above

F0800: Staff Assessment of Daily and Activity Preferences (cont.)

Item Rationale

Health-related Quality of Life

- Alternate means of assessing daily and preferences must be used for residents who cannot communicate. This ensures that information about their preferences is not overlooked.
- Activities allow residents to establish meaning in their lives. A lack of meaningful and enjoyable activities can result in boredom, depression, and behavioral symptoms.

Planning for Care

- Caregiving staff should use observations of resident behaviors to understand resident likes and dislikes in cases where the resident, family, or significant other cannot report the resident's preferences. This allows care plans to be individualized to each resident.

Steps for Assessment

1. Observe the resident when the care, routines, and activities specified in these items are made available to the resident.
2. Observations should be made by staff across all shifts and departments and others with close contact with the resident.
3. If the resident appears happy or content (e.g., is involved, pays attention, smiles) during an activity listed in **Staff Assessment of Daily and Activity Preferences** item (F0800), then that item should be checked.

   If the resident seems to resist or withdraw when these are made available, then do not check that item.

Coding Instructions

Check all that apply in the last 7 days based on staff observation of resident preferences.

- **F0800A.** Choosing clothes to wear
- **F0800B.** Caring for personal belongings
- **F0800C.** Receiving tub bath
- **F0800D.** Receiving shower
- **F0800E.** Receiving bed bath
- **F0800F.** Receiving sponge bath
- **F0800G.** Snacks between meals
- **F0800H.** Staying up past 8:00 p.m.
- **F0800I.** Family or significant other involvement in care discussions
- **F0800J.** Use of phone in private
- **F0800K.** Place to lock personal belongings

- **F0800L.** Reading books, newspapers, or magazines
- **F0800M.** Listening to music
- **F0800N.** Being around animals such as pets
- **F0800O.** Keeping up with the news
- **F0800P.** Doing things with groups of people
- **F0800Q.** Participating in favorite activities
- **F0800R.** Spending time away from the nursing home
- **F0800S.** Spending time outdoors
- **F0800T.** Participating in religious activities or practices
- **F0800Z.** None of the above

SECTION G: FUNCTIONAL STATUS

Intent: Items in this section assess the need for assistance with activities of daily living (ADLs), altered gait and balance, and decreased range of motion. In addition, on admission, resident and staff opinions regarding functional rehabilitation potential are noted.

G0110: Activities of Daily Living (ADL) Assistance

G0110. Activities of Daily Living (ADL) Assistance
Refer to the ADL flow chart in the RAI manual to facilitate accurate coding

Instructions for Rule of 3
- When an activity occurs three times at any one given level, code that level.
- When an activity occurs three times at multiple levels, code the most dependent, exceptions are total dependence (4), activity must require full assist every time, and activity did not occur (8), activity must not have occurred at all. Example, three times extensive assistance (3) and three times limited assistance (2), code extensive assistance (3).
- When an activity occurs at various levels, but not three times at any given level, apply the following:
  - When there is a combination of full staff performance, and extensive assistance, code extensive assistance.
  - When there is a combination of full staff performance, weight bearing assistance and/or non-weight bearing assistance code limited assistance (2).

If none of the above are met, code supervision.

1. ADL Self-Performance
Code for **resident's performance** over all shifts - not including setup. If the ADL activity occurred 3 or more times at various levels of assistance, code the most dependent - except for total dependence, which requires full staff performance every time

Coding:
Activity Occurred 3 or More Times
0. **Independent** - no help or staff oversight at any time
1. **Supervision** - oversight, encouragement or cueing
2. **Limited assistance** - resident highly involved in activity; staff provide guided maneuvering of limbs or other non-weight-bearing assistance
3. **Extensive assistance** - resident involved in activity, staff provide weight-bearing support
4. **Total dependence** - full staff performance every time during entire 7-day period
Activity Occurred 2 or Fewer Times
7. **Activity occurred only once or twice** - activity did occur but only once or twice
8. **Activity did not occur** - activity (or any part of the ADL) was not performed by resident or staff at all over the entire 7-day period

2. ADL Support Provided
Code for **most support provided** over all shifts; code regardless of resident's self-performance classification

Coding:
0. **No** setup or physical help from staff
1. **Setup** help only
2. **One** person physical assist
3. **Two+** persons physical assist
8. ADL activity itself **did not occur** during entire period

	1. Self-Performance	2. Support
	↓ Enter Codes in Boxes ↓	
A. Bed mobility - how resident moves to and from lying position, turns side to side, and positions body while in bed or alternate sleep furniture	☐	☐
B. Transfer - how resident moves between surfaces including to or from: bed, chair, wheelchair, standing position (**excludes** to/from bath/toilet)	☐	☐
C. Walk in room - how resident walks between locations in his/her room	☐	☐
D. Walk in corridor - how resident walks in corridor on unit	☐	☐
E. Locomotion on unit - how resident moves between locations in his/her room and adjacent corridor on same floor. If in wheelchair, self-sufficiency once in chair	☐	☐
F. Locomotion off unit - how resident moves to and returns from off-unit locations (e.g., areas set aside for dining, activities or treatments). **If facility has only one floor,** how resident moves to and from distant areas on the floor. If in wheelchair, self-sufficiency once in chair	☐	☐
G. Dressing - how resident puts on, fastens and takes off all items of clothing, including donning/removing a prosthesis or TED hose. Dressing includes putting on and changing pajamas and housedresses	☐	☐
H. Eating - how resident eats and drinks, regardless of skill. Do not include eating/drinking during medication pass. Includes intake of nourishment by other means (e.g., tube feeding, total parenteral nutrition, IV fluids administered for nutrition or hydration)	☐	☐
I. Toilet use - how resident uses the toilet room, commode, bedpan, or urinal; transfers on/off toilet; cleanses self after elimination; changes pad; manages ostomy or catheter; and adjusts clothes. Do not include emptying of bedpan, urinal, bedside commode, catheter bag or ostomy bag	☐	☐
J. Personal hygiene - how resident maintains personal hygiene, including combing hair, brushing teeth, shaving, applying makeup, washing/drying face and hands (**excludes** baths and showers)	☐	☐

G0110: Activities of Daily Living (ADL) Assistance (cont.)

Item Rationale

Health-related Quality of Life

- Almost all nursing home residents need some physical assistance. In addition, most are at risk of further physical decline. The amount of assistance needed and the risk of decline vary from resident to resident.

- A wide range of physical, neurological, and psychological conditions and cognitive factors can adversely affect physical function.

- Dependence on others for ADL assistance can lead to feelings of helplessness, isolation, diminished self-worth, and loss of control over one's destiny.

- As inactivity increases, complications such as pressure ulcers, falls, contractures, depression, and muscle wasting may occur.

Planning for Care

- Individualized care plans should address strengths and weakness, possible reversible causes such as de-conditioning, and adverse side effects of medications or other treatments. These may contribute to needless loss of self-sufficiency. In addition, some neurologic injuries such as stroke may continue to improve for months after an acute event.

- For some residents, cognitive deficits can limit ability or willingness to initiate or participate in self-care or restrict understanding of the tasks required to complete ADLs.

> **DEFINITIONS**
>
> **ADL**
> Tasks related to personal care; any of the tasks listed in items G0110A-J and G0120.
>
> **ADL ASPECTS**
> Components of an ADL activity. These are listed next to the activity in the item set. For example, the components of G0110H (Eating) are eating, drinking, and intake of nourishment or hydration by other means, including tube feeding, total parenteral nutrition and IV fluids for hydration.
>
> **ADL SELF-PERFORMANCE**
> Measures what the resident **actually did** (not what he or she might be capable of doing) within each ADL category over the last 7 days according to a performance-based scale.

- A resident's potential for maximum function is often underestimated by family, staff, and the resident. Individualized care plans should be based on an accurate assessment of the resident's self-performance and the amount and type of support being provided to the resident.

- Many residents might require lower levels of assistance if they are provided with appropriate devices and aids, assisted with segmenting tasks, or are given adequate time to complete the task while being provided graduated prompting and assistance. This type of supervision requires skill, time, and patience.

G0110: Activities of Daily Living (ADL) Assistance (cont.)

- Most residents are candidates for nursing-based rehabilitative care that focuses on maintaining and expanding self-involvement in ADLs.

- Graduated prompting/task segmentation (helping the resident break tasks down into smaller components) and allowing the resident time to complete an activity can often increase functional independence.

> **DEFINITIONS**
>
> **ADL SUPPORT PROVIDED**
> Measures the highest level of support **provided by staff** over the last 7 days, even if that level of support only occurred once.

Steps for Assessment

1. Review the documentation in the medical record for the 7-day look-back period.

2. Talk with direct care staff from each shift that has cared for the resident to learn what the resident does for himself during each episode of each ADL activity definition as well as the type and level of staff assistance provided. Remind staff that the focus is on the 7-day look-back period only.

3. When reviewing records, interviewing staff, and observing the resident, be specific in evaluating each component as listed in the ADL activity definition. For example, when evaluating Bed Mobility, determine the level of assistance required for moving the resident to and from a lying position, for turning the resident from side to side, and/or for positioning the resident in bed.

   To clarify your own understanding and observations about a resident's performance of an ADL activity (bed mobility, locomotion, transfer, etc.), ask probing questions, beginning with the general and proceeding to the more specific. See page G-9 for an example of using probes when talking to staff.

Coding Instructions

For each ADL activity:

- To assist in coding ADL self performance items, please use the algorithm on page G-6.

- Consider each episode of the activity that occurred during the 7-day look-back period.

- In order to be able to promote the highest level of functioning among residents, clinical staff must first identify what the resident actually does for himself or herself, noting when assistance is received and clarifying the types of assistance provided (verbal cueing, physical support, etc.).

- Code based on the resident's level of assistance when using special adaptive devices such as a walker, device to assist with donning socks, dressing stick, long-handle reacher, or adaptive eating utensils.

G0110: Activities of Daily Living (ADL) Assistance (cont.)

- A resident's ADL self-performance may vary from day to day, shift to shift, or within shifts. There are many possible reasons for these variations, including mood, medical condition, relationship issues (e.g., willing to perform for a nursing assistant that he or she likes), and medications. The responsibility of the person completing the assessment, therefore, is to capture the total picture of the resident's ADL self-performance over the 7-day period, 24 hours a day (i.e., not only how the evaluating clinician sees the resident, but how the resident performs on other shifts as well).

- The ADL self-performance coding options are intended to reflect real world situations where slight variations in self-performance are common. Refer to the algorithm on page G-6 for assistance in determining the most appropriate self-performance code.

- Although it is not necessary to know the actual number of times the activity occurred, it is necessary to know whether or not the activity occurred three or more times within the last 7 days.

- Because this section involves a two-part evaluation (ADL Self-Performance and ADL Support), each using its own scale, it is recommended that the Self-Performance evaluation be completed for all ADL activities before beginning the ADL Support evaluation.

- **Instructions for the Rule of Three:**

  — When an activity occurs three times at any one given level, code that level.

  — When an activity occurs three times at multiple levels, **code the most dependent**.

    o Example, three times extensive assistance (3) and three times limited assistance (2)—code extensive assistance (3).

    Exceptions are as follows:

    o Total dependence (4)—activity must require full assist every time, and

    o Activity did not occur (8)—activity must not have occurred at all.

  — When an activity occurs at more than one level, but not three times at any one level, apply the following:

    o Episodes of full staff performance are considered to be weight-bearing assistance (when every episode is full staff performance—this is total dependence).

    o When there are three or more episodes of a combination of full staff performance and weight-bearing assistance—code extensive assistance (3).

    o When there are three or more episodes of a combination of full staff performance, weight-bearing assistance, and non-weight-bearing assistance—code limited assistance (2).

- **If none of the above are met, code supervision.**

G0110: Activities of Daily Living (ADL) Assistance (cont.)

Coding Instructions for G0110, Column 1, **ADL-Self Performance**

- **Code 0, independent:** if resident completed activity with no help or oversight every time during the 7-day look-back period.

- **Code 1, supervision:** if oversight, encouragement, or cueing was provided **three** or more times during the last 7 days.

- **Code 2, limited assistance:** if resident was highly involved in activity and received physical help in guided maneuvering of limb(s) or other non-weight-bearing assistance on **three** or more times during the last 7 days.

- **Code 3, extensive assistance:** if resident performed part of the activity over the last 7 days, help of the following type(s) was provided three or more times:
  — Weight-bearing support provided three or more times.
  — Full staff performance of activity during part but not all of the last 7 days.

- **Code 4, total dependence:** if there was full staff performance of an activity with no participation by resident for any aspect of the ADL activity. The resident must be unwilling or unable to perform any part of the activity over the entire 7-day look-back period.

- **Code 7, activity occurred only once or twice:** if the activity occurred but **not** three times or more.

- **Code 8, activity did not occur:** if, over the 7-day look-back period, the ADL activity (or any part of the ADL) was not performed by the resident or staff at all.

Coding Instructions for G0110, Column 2, **ADL Support**

*Code for the **most** support provided over all shifts; code regardless of resident's self-performance classification.*

- **Code 0, no setup or physical help from staff:** if resident completed activity with no help or oversight.

- **Code 1, setup help only:** if resident is provided with materials or devices necessary to perform the ADL independently. This can include giving or holding out an item that the resident takes from the caregiver.

- **Code 2, one person physical assist:** if the resident was assisted by one staff person.

- **Code 3, two+ person physical assist:** if the resident was assisted by two or more staff persons.

- **Code 8, ADL activity itself did not occur during the entire period:** if, over the 7-day look-back period, the ADL activity did not occur.

G0110: Activities of Daily Living (ADL) Assistance (cont.)

ADL Self Performance Algorithm

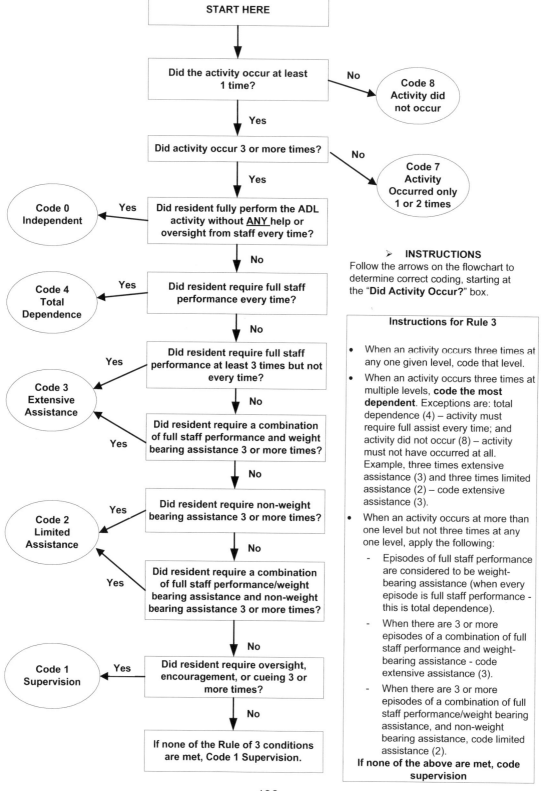

> ➤ **INSTRUCTIONS**
> Follow the arrows on the flowchart to determine correct coding, starting at the "**Did Activity Occur?**" box.

Instructions for Rule 3

- When an activity occurs three times at any one given level, code that level.
- When an activity occurs three times at multiple levels, **code the most dependent**. Exceptions are: total dependence (4) – activity must require full assist every time; and activity did not occur (8) – activity must not have occurred at all. Example, three times extensive assistance (3) and three times limited assistance (2) – code extensive assistance (3).
- When an activity occurs at more than one level but not three times at any one level, apply the following:
  - Episodes of full staff performance are considered to be weight-bearing assistance (when every episode is full staff performance - this is total dependence).
  - When there are 3 or more episodes of a combination of full staff performance and weight-bearing assistance - code extensive assistance (3).
  - When there are 3 or more episodes of a combination of full staff performance/weight bearing assistance, and non-weight bearing assistance, code limited assistance (2).

If none of the above are met, code supervision

G0110: Activities of Daily Living (ADL) Assistance (cont.)

Coding Tips and Special Populations

- Some residents sleep on furniture other than a bed (for example, a recliner). Consider assistance received in this alternative bed when coding bed mobility.
- Do **NOT** include the emptying of bedpan, urinal, bedside commode, catheter bag or ostomy bag in G0110 I.
- **Differentiating between guided maneuvering and weight-bearing assistance:** determine **who** is supporting the weight of the resident's extremity or body. For example, if the staff member supports some of the weight of the resident's hand while helping the resident to eat (e.g., lifting a spoon or a cup to mouth), or performs part of the activity for the resident, this is "weight-bearing" assistance for this activity. If the resident can lift the utensil or cup, but staff assistance is needed to guide the resident's hand to his or her mouth, this is guided maneuvering.
- Do **NOT** record the staff's assessment of the resident's potential capability to perform the ADL activity. The assessment of potential capability is covered in **ADL Functional Rehabilitation Potential** Item (G0900).
- Do **NOT** record the type and level of assistance that the resident "should" be receiving according to the written plan of care. The level of assistance actually provided might be very different from what is indicated in the plan. Record what actually happened.
- Do **NOT** include assistance provided by family or other visitors.
- **Some examples for coding for ADL Support Setup Help when the activity involves the following:**
  - Bed Mobility—handing the resident the bar on a trapeze, staff raises the ½ rails for the resident's use and then provides no further help.
  - Transfer—giving the resident a transfer board or locking the wheels on a wheelchair for safe transfer.
  - Locomotion
    - o Walking—handing the resident a walker or cane.
    - o Wheeling—unlocking the brakes on the wheelchair or adjusting foot pedals to facilitate foot motion while wheeling.
  - Dressing—retrieving clothes from the closet and laying out on the resident's bed; handing the resident a shirt.
  - Eating—cutting meat and opening containers at meals; giving one food item at a time.
  - Toilet Use—handing the resident a bedpan or placing articles necessary for changing an ostomy appliance within reach.
  - Personal Hygiene—providing a washbasin and grooming articles.
- **Supervision**
  - **Code Supervision** for residents seated together or in close proximity of one another during a meal who receive individual supervision with eating.
  - General supervision of a dining room is not the same as individual supervision of a resident and **is not** captured in the coding for Eating.

- **Coding activity did not occur, 8:**
  - **Toileting** would be **coded 8, activity did not occur**: only if elimination did not occur during the entire look-back period.
  - **Locomotion** would be **coded 8, activity did not occur**: if the resident was on bed rest and did not get out of bed, and there was no locomotion via bed, wheelchair, or other means during the look-back period.
  - **Eating** would be **coded 8, activity did not occur**: only if the resident received no nourishment by any route (oral, IV, TPN, enteral) during the 7-day look-back period.
- **Coding activity occurred only once or twice, 7:**
  - Walk in corridor would be **coded 7, activity occurred only once or twice**: if the resident came out of the room and ambulated in the hallway for a weekly tub bath but otherwise stayed in the room during the 7-day look-back period.
  - Locomotion off unit would be **coded 7, activity occurred only once or twice**: if the resident left the vicinity of his or her room only one or two times to attend an activity in another part of the building.
- **Residents with tube feeding, TPN, or IV fluids**
  - **Code extensive assistance (1 or 2 persons):** if the resident with tube feeding, TPN, or IV fluids did not participate in management of this nutrition but did participate in receiving oral nutrition. This is the correct code because the staff completed a portion of the ADL activity for the resident (managing the tube feeding, TPN, or IV fluids).
  - **Code totally dependent in eating:** only if resident was assisted in eating all food items and liquids at all meals and snacks (including tube feeding delivered totally by staff) and did not participate in any aspect of eating (e.g., did not pick up finger foods, did not give self tube feeding or assist with swallow or eating procedure).

Example of a Probing Conversation with Staff

1. Example of a probing conversation between the RN Assessment Coordinator and a nursing assistant (NA) regarding a resident's bed mobility assessment:

   RN: "Describe to me how Mrs. L. moves herself in bed. By that I mean once she is in bed, how does she move from sitting up to lying down, lying down to sitting up, turning side to side and positioning herself?"

   NA: "She can lay down and sit up by herself, but I help her turn on her side."

   RN: "She lays down and sits up without any verbal instructions or physical help?"

   NA: "No, I have to remind her to use her trapeze every time. But once I tell her how to do things, she can do it herself."

   RN: "How do you help her turn side to side?"

   NA: "She can help turn herself by grabbing onto her side rail. I tell her what to do. But she needs me to lift her bottom and guide her legs into a good position."

   RN: "Do you lift her by yourself or does someone help you?"

   NA: "I do it by myself."

   RN: "How many times during the last 7 days did you give this type of help?"

   NA: "Every day, probably 3 times each day."

G0110: Activities of Daily Living (ADL) Assistance (cont.)

In this example, the assessor inquired specifically how Mrs. L. moves to and from a lying position, how she turns from side to side, and how the resident positions herself while in bed. A resident can be independent in one aspect of bed mobility, yet require extensive assistance in another aspect. If the RN did not probe further, he or she would not have received enough information to make an accurate assessment of actual assistance Mrs. L. received. Because accurate coding is important as a basis for reporting on the type and amount of care provided, be sure to consider each activity definition fully.

Coding: Bed Mobility ADL assistance would be **coded 3 (self-performance) and 2 (support provided), extensive assistance with a one person assist.**

Examples for G0110A, Bed Mobility

1. Mrs. D. can easily turn and position herself in bed and is able to sit up and lie down without any staff assistance at any time during the 7-day look-back period. She requires use of a single side rail that staff place in the up position when she is in bed.

   Coding: G0110A1 would be **coded 0, independent**.
   G0110A2 would be **coded 1, setup help only**.
   Rationale: Resident is independent at all times in bed mobility during the 7-day look-back period and needs only setup help.

2. Resident favors lying on her right side. Because she has had a history of skin breakdown, staff must verbally remind her to reposition off her right side daily during the 7-day look-back period.

   Coding: G0110A1 would be **coded 1, supervision**.
   G0110A2 would be **coded 0, no setup or physical help from staff**.
   Rationale: Resident requires staff supervision, cueing, and reminders for repositioning more than three times during the look-back period.

3. Resident favors lying on her right side. Because she has had a history of skin breakdown, staff must sometimes cue the resident and guide (non-weight-bearing assistance) the resident to place her hands on the side rail and encourage her to change her position when in bed daily over the 7-day look-back period.

   Coding: G0110A1 would be **coded 2, limited assistance**.
   G0110A2 would be **coded 2, one person physical assist**.
   Rationale: Resident requires cueing and encouragement with setup and non-weight-bearing physical help daily during the 7-day look-back period.

4. Mr. Q. has slid to the foot of the bed four times during the 7-day look-back period. Two staff members had to physically lift and reposition him toward the head of the bed. Mr. Q. was able to assist by bending his knees and pushing with legs when reminded by staff.

   Coding: G0110A1 would be **coded 3, extensive assistance**.
   G0110A2 would be **coded 3, two+ persons physical assist**.
   Rationale: Resident required weight-bearing assistance of two staff members on four occasions during the 7-day look-back period with bed mobility.

G0110: Activities of Daily Living (ADL) Assistance (cont.)

5. Mrs. S. is unable to physically turn, sit up, or lie down in bed. Two staff members must physically turn her every 2 hours without any participation at any time from her at any time during the 7-day look-back period. She must be physically assisted to a seated position in bed when reading.

> **Coding:** G0110A1 would be **coded 4, total dependence**.
>
> G0110A2 would be **coded 3, two+ persons physical assist**.
>
> **Rationale:** Resident did not participate at any time during the 7-day look-back period and required two staff to position her in bed.

Examples for G0110B, Transfer

1. When transferring from bed to chair or chair back to bed, the resident is able to stand up from a seated position (without requiring any physical or verbal help) and walk from the bed to chair and chair back to the bed every day during the 7-day look back period.

> **Coding**: G0110B1 would be **coded 0, independent**.
>
> G0110B2 would be **coded 0, no setup or physical help from staff**.
>
> **Rationale:** Resident is independent each and every time she transferred during the 7-day look-back period and required no setup or physical help from staff.

2. Staff must supervise the resident as she transfers from her bed to wheelchair daily. Staff must bring the chair next to the bed and then remind her to hold on to the chair and position her body slowly.

> **Coding:** G0110B1 would be **coded 1, supervision**.
>
> G0110B2 would be **coded 1, setup help only**.
>
> **Rationale:** Resident requires staff supervision, cueing, and reminders for safe transfer. This activity happened daily over the 7-day look-back period.

3. Mrs. H. is able to transfer from the bed to chair when she uses her walker. Staff place the walker near her bed and then assist the resident with guided maneuvering as she transfers. The resident was noted to transfer from bed to chair six times during the 7-day look-back period.

> **Coding:** G0110B1 would be **coded 2, limited assistance**.
>
> G0110B2 would be **coded 2, one person physical assist**.
>
> **Rationale:** Resident requires staff to set up her walker and provide non-weight-bearing assistance when she is ready to transfer. The activity happened six times during the 7-day look-back period.

4. Mrs. B. requires weight-bearing assistance of one staff member to partially lift and support her when being transferred. The resident was noted to have been transferred 14 times in the 7-day look-back period and each time required weight-bearing assistance.

> **Coding:** G0110B1 would be **coded 3, extensive assistance**.
>
> G0110B2 would be **coded 2, one person physical assist**.
>
> **Rationale:** Resident partially participates in the task of transferring. The resident was noted to have transferred 14 times during the 7-day look-back period, each time requiring weight-bearing assistance of one staff member.

G0110: Activities of Daily Living (ADL) Assistance (cont.)

5. Mr. T. is in a physically debilitated state due to surgery. Two staff members must physically lift and transfer him to a reclining chair daily using a mechanical lift. Mr. T. is unable to assist or participate in any way.

> **Coding:** G0110B1 would be **coded 4, total dependence**.
> G0110B2 would be **coded 3, two+ persons physical assist**.
> **Rationale:** Resident did not participate and required two staff to transfer him out of his bed. The resident was transferred out of bed to the chair daily during the 7-day look-back period.

6. Mrs. D. is post-operative for extensive surgical procedures. Because of her ventilator dependent status in addition to multiple surgical sites, her physician has determined that she must remain on total bed rest. During the 7-day look-back period the resident was not moved from the bed.

> **Coding:** G0110B1 would be **coded 8, activity did not occur**.
> G0110B2 would be **coded 8, ADL activity itself did not occur during entire period**.
> **Rationale:** Activity did not occur.

7. Mr. M. has Parkinson's disease and needs weight-bearing assistance of two staff to transfer from his bed to his wheelchair. During the 7-day look-back period, Mr. M. was transferred once from the bed to the wheelchair and once from wheelchair to bed.

> **Coding:** G0110B1 would be **coded 7, activity occurred only once or twice**.
> G0110B2 would be **coded 3, two+ persons physical assist**.
> **Rationale:** The activity happened only twice during the look-back period, with the support of two staff members.

Examples for G0110C, **Walk in Room**

1. Mr. R. is able to walk freely in his room (obtaining clothes from closet, turning on TV) without any cueing or physical assistance from staff at all during the entire 7-day look-back period.

> **Coding:** G0110C1 would be **coded 0, independent**.
> G0110C2 would be **coded 0, no setup or physical help from staff**.
> **Rationale:** Resident is independent.

2. Mr. B. was able to walk in his room daily, but a staff member needed to cue and stand by during ambulation because the resident has had a history of an unsteady gait.

> **Coding:** G0110C1 would be **coded 1, supervision**.
> G0110C2 would be **coded 0, no setup or physical help from staff**.
> **Rationale:** Resident requires staff supervision, cueing, and reminders daily while walking in his room, but did not need setup or physical help from staff.

3. Mr. K. is able to walk in his room, and, with hand-held assist from one staff member, the resident was noted to ambulate daily during the 7-day look-back period.

   Coding: G0110C1 would be **coded 2, limited assistance**.
   G0110C2 would be **coded 2, one person physical assist**.
   Rationale: Resident requires hand-held (non-weight-bearing) assistance of one staff member daily for ambulation in his room.

4. Mr. A. has a bone spur on his heel and has difficulty ambulating in his room. He requires staff to help support him when he selects clothing from his closet. During the 7-day look-back period the resident was able to ambulate with weight-bearing assistance from one staff member in his room four times.

   Coding: G0110C1 would be **coded 3, extensive assistance**.
   G0110C2 would be **coded 2, one person physical assist**.
   Rationale: The resident was able to ambulate in his room four times during the 7-day look-back period with weight-bearing assistance of one staff member.

5. Mr. J. is attending physical therapy for transfer and gait training. He does not ambulate on the unit or in his room at this time. He calls for assistance to stand pivot to a commode next to his bed.

   Coding: G0110C1 would be **coded 8, activity did not occur**.
   G0110C2 would be **coded 8, ADL activity itself did not occur during entire period**.
   Rationale: Activity did not occur.

Examples for G0110D, Walk in Corridor

1. Mr. X. ambulated daily up and down the hallway on his unit with a cane and did not require any setup or physical help from staff at any time during the 7-day look-back period.

   Coding: G0110D1 would be **coded 0, independent**.
   G0110D2 would be **coded 0, no setup or physical help from staff**.
   Rationale: Resident requires no setup or help from the staff at any time during the entire 7-day look-back period.

2. Staff members provided verbal cueing while resident was walking in the hallway every day during the 7-day look-back period to ensure that the resident walked slowly and safely.

   Coding: G0110D1 would be **coded 1, supervision**.
   G0110D2 would be **coded 0, no setup or physical help from staff**.
   Rationale: Resident requires staff supervision, cueing, and reminders daily while ambulating in the hallway during the 7-day look-back period.

G0110: Activities of Daily Living (ADL) Assistance (cont.)

3. Mrs. Q. requires verbal cueing and physical guiding of her hand placement on the walker when walking down the unit hallway. She needs frequent verbal reminders of how to use her walker, where to place her hands, and to pick up her feet. Mrs. Q. needs to be physically guided to the day room. During the 7-day look-back period the resident was noted to ambulate in the hallway daily and required the above-mentioned support from one staff member.

   Coding: G0110D1 would be **coded 2, limited assistance**.
   G0110D2 would be **coded 2, one person physical assist**.
   Rationale: Resident requires non-weight-bearing assistance of one staff member for safe ambulation daily during the 7-day look-back period.

4. A resident had back surgery 2 months ago. Two staff members must physically support the resident as he is walking down the hallway because of his unsteady gait and balance problem. During the 7-day look-back period the resident was ambulated in the hallway three times with physical assist of two staff members.

   Coding: G0110D1 would be **coded 3, extensive assistance**.
   G0110D2 would be **coded 3, two+ persons physical assist**.
   Rationale: The resident was ambulated three times during the 7-day look-back period, with the resident partially participating in the task. Two staff members were required to physically support the resident so he could ambulate.

5. Mrs. J. ambulated in the corridor once with supervision and once with non-weight-bearing assistance of one staff member during the 7-day look-back period.

   Coding: G0110D1 would be **coded 7, activity occurred only once or twice**.
   G0110D2 would be **coded 2, one person physical assist**.
   Rationale: The activity occurred only twice during the look-back period. It does not matter that the level of assistance provided by staff was at different levels. During ambulation, the most support provided was physical help by one staff member.

Examples for G0110E, Locomotion on Unit

1. Mrs. L. is on complete bed rest. During the 7-day look-back period she did not get out of bed or leave the room.

   Coding: G0110E1 would be **coded 8, activity did not occur**.
   G0110E2 would be **coded 8, ADL activity itself did not occur during entire period**.
   Rationale: The resident was on bed rest during the look-back period and never left her room.

G0110: Activities of Daily Living (ADL) Assistance (cont.)

Examples for G0110F, Locomotion off Unit

1. Mr. R. does not like to go off his nursing unit. He prefers to stay in his room or the day room on his unit. He has visitors on a regular basis, and they visit with him in the day room on the unit. During the 7-day look-back period the resident did not leave the unit for any reason.

   Coding: G0110F1 would be **coded 8, activity did not occur**.
   G0110F2 would be **coded 8, ADL activity itself did not occur during entire period**.
   Rationale: Activity did not occur at all.

2. Mr. Q. is a wheelchair-bound and is able to self-propel on the unit. On two occasions during the 7-day look-back period, he self-propelled off the unit into the courtyard.

   Coding: G0110E1 would be **coded 7, activity occurred only once or twice**.
   G0110E2 would be **coded 0, independent**.
   Rationale: The activity of going off the unit happened only twice during the look-back period with no help or oversight from staff.

3. Mr. H. enjoyed walking in the nursing garden when weather permitted. Due to inclement weather during the assessment period, he required various levels of assistance on the days he walked through the garden. On two occasions, he required limited assistance for balance of one staff person and on another occasion he only required supervision. On one day he was able to walk through the garden completely by himself.

   Coding: G0100F1 would be **coded 1, supervision**.
   G0110F2 would be **coded 2, one person physical assist**.
   Rationale: Activity did not occur at any one level for three times and he did not require physical assistance for at least three times. The most support provided by staff was one person assist.

Examples for G0110G, Dressing

1. Mrs. C. did not feel well and chose to stay in her room. She requested to stay in night clothes and rest in bed for the entire 7-day look-back period. Each day, after washing up, Mrs. C. changed night clothes with staff assistance to guide her arms and assist in guiding her nightgown over her head and buttoning the front.

   Coding: G0110G1 would be **coded 2, limited assistance**.
   G0110G2 would be **coded 2, one person physical assist**.
   Rationale: Resident was highly involved in the activity and changed clothing daily with non-weight-bearing assistance from one staff member during the 7-day look-back period.

Examples for G0110H, Eating

1. After staff deliver Mr. K.'s meal tray, he consumes all food and fluids without any cueing or physical help during the entire 7-day look-back period.

   Coding: G0110H1 would be **coded 0, independent**.
   G0110H2 would be **coded 0, no setup or physical help from staff**.
   Rationale: Resident is completely independent in eating during the entire 7-day look-back period.

2. One staff member had to verbally cue the resident to eat slowly and drink throughout each meal during the 7-day look-back period.

   Coding: G0110H1 would be **coded 1, supervision**.
   G0110H2 would be **coded 0, no setup or physical help from staff**.
   Rationale: Resident required staff supervision, cueing, and reminders for safe meal completion daily during the 7-day look-back period.

3. Mr. V. is able to eat by himself. Staff must set up the tray, cut the meat, open containers, and hand him the utensils. Each day during the 7-day look-back period, Mr. V. required more help during the evening meal, as he was tired and less interested in completing his meal. In the evening, in addition to encouraging the resident to eat and handing him his utensils and cups, staff must also guide the resident's hand so he will get the utensil to his mouth.

   Coding: G0110H1 would be **coded 2, limited assistance**.
   G0110H2 would be **coded 2, one person physical assist**.
   Rationale: Resident is unable to complete the evening meal without staff providing him non-weight-bearing assistance daily.

4. Mr. F. begins eating each meal daily by himself. During the 7-day look-back period, after he had eaten only his bread, he stated he was tired and unable to complete the meal. One staff member physically supported his hand to bring the food to his mouth and provided verbal cues to swallow the food. The resident was then able to complete the meal.

   Coding: G0110H1 would be **coded 3, extensive assistance**.
   G0110H2 would be **coded 2, one person physical assist**.
   Rationale: Resident partially participated in the task daily at each meal, but one staff member provided weight-bearing assistance with some portion of each meal.

5. Mrs. U. is severely cognitively impaired. She is unable to feed herself. During the 7-day look-back period, one staff member had to assist her with eating every meal.

   Coding: G0110H1 would be **coded 4, total dependence**.
   G0110H2 would be **coded 2, one person physical assist**.
   Rationale: Resident did not participate and required one staff person to feed her all of her meal during the 7-day look-back period.

G0110: Activities of Daily Living (ADL) Assistance (cont.)

6. Mrs. D. receives all of her nourishment via a gastrostomy tube. She did not consume any food or fluid by mouth. During the 7-day look-back period, she did not participate in the gastrostomy nourishment process.

> **Coding:** G0110H1 would be **coded 4, total dependence**.
> G0110H2 would be **coded 2, one person physical assist**.
> **Rationale:** During the 7-day look-back period, she did not participate in eating and/or receiving of her tube feed during the entire period. She required full staff performance of these functions.

Examples for G0110I, Toilet Use

1. Mrs. L. transferred herself to the toilet, adjusted her clothing, and performed the necessary personal hygiene after using the toilet without any staff assistance daily during the entire 7-day look-back period.

> **Coding**: G0110I1 would be **coded 0, independent**.
> G0110I2 would be **coded 0, no setup or physical help from staff**.
> **Rationale:** Resident was independent in all her toileting tasks.

2. Staff member must remind resident to toilet frequently during the day and to unzip and zip pants and to wash his hands after using the toilet. During the 7-day look-back period, the resident required the above level of support multiple times each day.

> **Coding:** G0110I1 would be **coded 1, supervision**.
> G0110I2 would be **coded 0, no setup or physical help from staff**.
> **Rationale:** Resident required staff supervision, cueing and reminders daily.

3. Staff must assist Mr. P. to zip his pants, hand him a washcloth, and remind him to wash his hands after using the toilet daily. During the 7-day look-back period, the resident required the above level of support multiple times each day.

> **Coding:** G0110I1 would be **coded 2, limited assistance**.
> G0110I2 would be **coded 2, one person physical assist**.
> **Rationale:** Resident required staff to perform non-weight-bearing activities to complete the task multiple times each day during the 7-day look-back period.

4. Mrs. M. has had recent bouts of vertigo. During the 7-day look-back period, the resident required one staff member to assist and provide weight-bearing support to her as she transferred to the bedside commode four times.

> **Coding:** G0110I1 would be **coded 3, extensive assistance**.
> G0110I2 would be **coded 2, one person physical assist**.
> **Rationale:** During the 7-day look-back period, the resident required weight-bearing assistance with the support of one staff member to use the commode four times.

5. Miss W. is cognitively and physically impaired. During the 7-day look-back period, she was on strict bed rest. Staff were unable to physically transfer her to toilet during this time. Miss W. is incontinent of both bowel and bladder. One staff member was required to provide all the care for her elimination and personal hygiene needs several times each day.

    Coding: G0110I1 would be **coded 4, total dependence**.

    G0110I2 would be **coded 2, one person physical assist**.

    Rationale: Resident did not participate and required one staff person to provide total care for toileting and personal hygiene each time during the entire 7-day look-back period.

Examples for G0110J, Personal Hygiene

1. The nurse assistant takes Mr. L.'s comb, toothbrush, and toothpaste from the drawer and places them at the bathroom sink. Mr. L. combs his own hair and brushes his own teeth daily. During the 7-day look-back period, he required cueing to brush his teeth on three occasions.

    Coding: G0110J1 would be **coded 1, supervision**.

    G0110J2 would be **coded 1, setup help only**.

    Rationale: Staff placed grooming devices at sink for his use, and during the 7-day look-back period staff provided cueing three times.

2. Mrs. J. normally completes all hygiene tasks independently. Three mornings during the 7-day look-back period, however, she was unable to brush and style her hair because of elbow pain, so a staff member did it for her.

    Coding: G0110J1 would be **coded 2, limited assistance**.

    G0110J2 would be **coded 2, one person physical assist**.

    Rationale: A staff member had to complete part of the activity for the resident 3 days during the look-back period; the assistance was non-weight-bearing.

G0120: Bathing

G0120. Bathing	
How resident takes full-body bath/shower, sponge bath, and transfers in/out of tub/shower (**excludes** washing of back and hair). Code for **most dependent** in self-performance and support	
Enter Code	**A. Self-performance** 0. **Independent** - no help provided 1. **Supervision** - oversight help only 2. **Physical help limited to transfer only** 3. **Physical help in part of bathing activity** 4. **Total dependence** 8. **Activity itself did not occur** during the entire period
Enter Code	**B. Support provided** (Bathing support codes are as defined in item **G0110 column 2, ADL Support Provided**, above)

G0120: Bathing (cont.)

Item Rationale

Health-related Quality of Life

- The resident's choices regarding his or her bathing schedule should be accommodated when possible so that facility routine does not conflict with resident's desired routine.

DEFINITIONS

BATHING
How the resident takes a full body bath, shower or sponge bath, including transfers in and out of the tub or shower. It does not include the washing of back or hair.

Planning for Care

- The care plan should include interventions to address the resident's unique needs for bathing. These interventions should be periodically evaluated and, if objectives were not met, alternative approaches developed to encourage maintenance of bathing abilities.

Coding Instructions for G0120 A, Self Performance

Code for the maximum amount of assistance the resident received during the bathing episodes.

- **Code 0, independent:** if the resident required no help from staff.
- **Code 1, supervision:** if the resident required oversight help only.
- **Code 2, physical help limited to transfer only:** if the resident is able to perform the bathing activity, but required help with the transfer only.
- **Code 3, physical help in part of bathing activity:** if the resident required assistance with some aspect of bathing.
- **Code 4, total dependence:** if the resident is unable to participate in any of the bathing activity.
- **Code 8, activity itself did not occur:** if the resident was not bathed during the 7-day look-back period.

Coding Instructions for G0120B, Support Provided

- Bathing support codes are as defined **ADL Support Provided** item (G0110), Column 2.

Coding Tips

- Bathing is the only ADL activity for which the ADL Self-Performance codes in Item G0110, **Column 1 (Self-Performance),** do not apply. A unique set of self-performance codes is used in the bathing assessment given that bathing may not occur as frequently as the other ADL's in the 7-day look-back period.
- If a nursing home has a policy that all residents are supervised when bathing (i.e., they are never left alone while in the bathroom for a bath or shower, regardless of resident capability), it is appropriate to code the resident self-performance as supervision, even if the supervision is precautionary because the resident is still being individually supervised. Support for bathing in this instance would be coded according to whether or not the staff had to actually assist the resident during the bathing activity.

G0120: Bathing (cont.)

Examples

1. Resident received verbal cueing and encouragement to take twice-weekly showers. Once staff walked resident to bathroom, he bathed himself with periodic oversight.

   Coding: G0120A would be **coded 1, supervision**.

   G0120B would be **coded 0, no setup or physical help from staff**.

   Rationale: Resident needed only supervision to perform the bathing activity with no setup or physical help from staff.

2. For one bath, the resident received physical help of one person to position self in bathtub. However, because of her fluctuating moods, she received total help for her other bath from one staff member.

   Coding: G0120A would be **coded 4, total dependence**.

   G0120B would be **coded 2, one person physical assist**.

   Rationale: Coding directions for bathing state, "code for most dependent in self performance and support." Resident's most dependent episode during the 7-day look-back period was total help with the bathing activity with assist from one staff person.

3. On Monday, one staff member helped transfer resident to tub and washed his legs. On Thursday, the resident had physical help of one person to get into tub but washed himself completely.

   Coding: G0120A would be **coded 3, physical help in part of bathing activity**.

   G0120B would be **coded 2, one person physical assist**.

   Rationale: Resident's most dependent episode during the 7-day look-back period was assistance with part of the bathing activity from one staff person.

G0300: Balance During Transitions and Walking

G0300. Balance During Transitions and Walking		
After observing the resident, **code the following walking and transition items for most dependent**		
	↓ **Enter Codes in Boxes**	
Coding: 0. **Steady at all times** 1. **Not steady, but <u>able</u> to stabilize without human assistance** 2. **Not steady, <u>only able</u> to stabilize with human assistance** 8. **Activity did not occur**	☐	**A. Moving from seated to standing position**
	☐	**B. Walking** (with assistive device if used)
	☐	**C. Turning around** and facing the opposite direction while walking
	☐	**D. Moving on and off toilet**
	☐	**E. Surface-to-surface transfer** (transfer between bed and chair or wheelchair)

G0300: Balance During Transitions and Walking (cont.)

Item Rationale

Health-related Quality of Life

- Individuals with impaired balance and unsteadiness during transitions and walking
  - are at increased risk for falls;
  - often are afraid of falling;
  - may limit their physical and social activity, becoming socially isolated and depressed about limitations; and
  - can become increasingly immobile.

> **DEFINITIONS**
>
> **INTER-DISCIPLINARY TEAM**
> Refers to a team that includes staff from multiple disciplines such as nursing, therapy, physicians, and other advanced practitioners.

Planning for Care

- Individuals with impaired balance and unsteadiness should be evaluated for the need for
  - rehabilitation or assistive devices;
  - supervision or physical assistance for safety; and/or
  - environmental modification.
- Care planning should focus on preventing further decline of function, and/or on return of function, depending on resident-specific goals.
- Assessment should identify all related risk factors in order to develop effective care plans to maintain current abilities, slow decline, and/or promote improvement in the resident's functional ability.

Steps for Assessment

1. Complete this assessment for all residents.
2. Throughout the 7-day look-back period, interdisciplinary team members should carefully observe and document observations of the resident during transitions from sitting to standing, walking, turning, transferring on and off toilet, and transferring from wheelchair to bed and bed to wheelchair (for residents who use a wheelchair).
3. If staff have not systematically documented the resident's stability in these activities at least once during the 7-day look-back period, use the following process to code these items:
   a. Before beginning the activity, explain what the task is and what you are observing for.
   b. Have assistive devices the resident normally uses available.
   c. Start with the resident sitting up on the edge of his or her bed, in a chair or in a wheelchair (if he or she generally uses one).
   d. Ask the resident to stand up and stay still for 3-5 seconds. **Moving from seated to standing position (G0300A) should be rated at this time.**
   e. Ask the resident to walk approximately 15 feet using his or her usual **assistive device**. **Walking (G0300B) should be rated at this time.**

f. Ask the resident to turn around. **Turning around (G0300C) should be rated at this time.**
g. Ask the **resident to walk or wheel** from a starting point in his or her room into the bathroom, **prepare for toileting** as he or she normally does (including taking down pants or other clothes; underclothes can be kept on for this observation), and sit on the toilet. **Moving on and off toilet (G0300D) should be rated at this time.**
h. Ask residents who are not ambulatory and who use a wheelchair for mobility to transfer from a seated position in the wheelchair to a seated position on the bed. **Surface-to-surface transfer should be rated at this time (G0300E).**

Balance During Transitions and Walking Algorithm

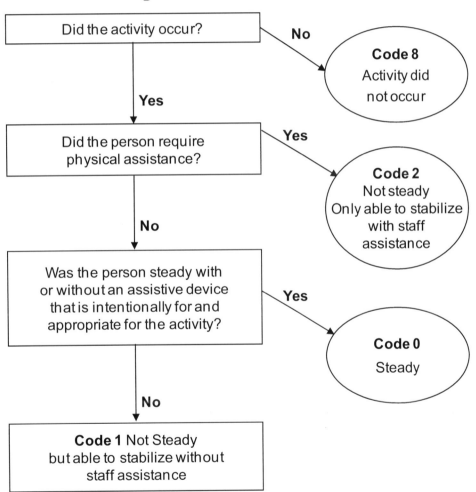

Coding Instructions G0300A, Moving from Seated to Standing Position

Code for the least steady episode, using assistive device if applicable.

- **Code 0, steady at all times:**
  - If all of the transitions from seated to standing position and from standing to seated position observed during the 7-day look-back period are steady.
  - If resident is stable when standing up using the arms of a chair or an assistive device identified for this purpose (such as a walker, locked wheelchair, or grab bar).
  - If an assistive device or equipment is used, the resident appropriately plans and integrates the use of the device into the transition activity.
  - If resident appears steady and not at risk of a fall when standing up.

- **Code 1, not steady, but able to stabilize without staff assistance:**
  - If any of transitions from seated to standing position or from standing to seated position during the 7-day look-back period are not steady, but the resident is able to stabilize without assistance from staff or object (e.g., a chair or table).
  - If the resident is unsteady using an assistive device but does not require staff assistance to stabilize.
  - If the resident attempts to stand, sits back down, then is able to stand up and stabilize without assistance from staff or object.
  - Residents coded in this category appear at increased risk for falling when standing up.

> **DEFINITIONS**
>
> **UNSTEADY** Residents may appear unbalanced or move with a sway or with uncoordinated or jerking movements that make them unsteady. They might exhibit unsteady gaits such as fast gaits with large, careless movements; abnormally slow gaits with small shuffling steps; or wide-based gaits with halting, tentative steps.

- **Code 2, not steady, only able to stabilize with staff assistance:**
  - If any of transitions from seated to standing or from standing to sitting are not steady, and the resident cannot stabilize without assistance from staff.
  - If the resident cannot stand but can transfer unassisted without staff assistance.
  - If the resident returned back to a seated position or was unable to move from a seated to standing or from standing to sitting position during the look-back period.
  - Residents coded in this category appear at high risk for falling during transitions.
  - If a lift device (a mechanical device operated by another person) is used because the resident requires staff assistance to stabilize, code as 2.

- **Code 8, activity did not occur:** if the resident did not move from seated to standing position during the 7-day look-back period.

G0300: Balance During Transitions and Walking (cont.)

Examples for G0300A, Moving from Seated to Standing Position

1. A resident sits up in bed, stands, and begins to sway, but steadies herself and sits down smoothly into her wheelchair.

    Coding: G0300A would be **coded 1, not steady, but able to stabilize without staff assistance**.

    Rationale: Resident was unsteady, but she was able to stabilize herself without assistance from staff.

2. A resident requires the use of a gait belt and physical assistance in order to stand.

    Coding: G0300A would be **coded 2, not steady, only able to stabilize with staff assistance**.

    Rationale: Resident required staff assistance to stand during the observation period.

3. A resident stands steadily by pushing himself up using the arms of a chair.

    Coding: G0300A would be **coded 0, steady at all times**.

    Rationale: Even though the resident used the arms of the chair to push himself up, he was steady at all times during the activity.

4. A resident locks his wheelchair and uses the arms of his wheelchair to attempt to stand. On the first attempt, he rises about halfway to a standing position then sits back down. On the second attempt, he is able to stand steadily.

    Coding: G0300A would be **coded 1, not steady, but able to stabilize without staff assistance**.

    Rationale: Even though the second attempt at standing was steady, the first attempt suggests he is unsteady and at risk for falling during this transition.

Coding Instructions G0300B, Walking (with Assistive Device if Used)

Code for the least steady episode, using assistive device if applicable.

*   **Code 0, steady at all times:**
    — If during the 7-day look-back period the resident's walking (with assistive devices if used) is steady at all times.
    — If an assistive device or equipment is used, the resident appropriately plans and integrates the use of the device and is steady while walking with it.
    — Residents in this category do not appear at risk for falls.
    — Residents who walk with an abnormal gait and/or with an assistive device can be steady, and if they are they should be coded in this category.

*   **Code 1, not steady, but able to stabilize without staff assistance:**
    — If during the 7-day look-back period the resident appears unsteady while walking (with assistive devices if used) but does not require staff assistance to stabilize.
    — Residents coded in this category appear at risk for falling while walking.

- **Code 2, not steady, only able to stabilize with staff assistance:**
  — If during the-7-day look-back period the resident at any time appeared unsteady and required staff assistance to be stable and safe while walking.
  — If the resident fell when walking during the look-back period.
  — Residents coded in this category appear at high risk for falling while walking.
- **Code 8, activity did not occur:**
  — If the resident did not walk during the 7-day look-back period.

Examples for G0300B, Walking (with Assistive Device if Used)

1. A resident with a recent stroke walks using a hemi-walker in her right hand because of left-sided weakness. Her gait is slow and short-stepped and slightly unsteady as she walks, she leans to the left and drags her left foot along the ground on most steps. She has not had to steady herself using any furniture or grab bars.

   Coding: G0300B would be **coded 1, not steady, but able to stabilize without staff assistance**.

   Rationale: Resident's gait is unsteady with or without an assistive device but does not require staff assistance.

2. A resident with Parkinson's disease ambulates with a walker. His posture is stooped, and he walks slowly with a short-stepped shuffling gait. On some occasions, his gait speeds up, and it appears he has difficulty slowing down. On multiple occasions during the 7-day observation period he has to steady himself using a handrail or a piece of furniture in addition to his walker.

   Coding: G0300B would be **coded 1, not steady, but able to stabilize without staff assistance**.

   Rationale: Resident has an unsteady gait but can stabilize himself using an object such as a handrail or piece of furniture.

3. A resident who had a recent total hip replacement ambulates with a walker. Although she is able to bear weight on her affected side, she is unable to advance her walker safely without staff assistance.

   Coding: G0300B would be **coded 2, not steady, only able to stabilize with staff assistance**.

   Rationale: Resident requires staff assistance to walk steadily and safely at any time during the observation period.

4. A resident with multi-infarct dementia walks with a short-stepped, shuffling-type gait. Despite the gait abnormality, she is steady.

   Coding: G0300B would be **coded 0, steady at all times**.

   Rationale: Resident walks steadily (with or without a normal gait and/or the use of an assistive device) at all times during the observation period.

G0300: Balance During Transitions and Walking (cont.)

Coding Instructions G0300C, Turning Around and Facing the Opposite Direction while Walking

Code for the least steady episode, using an assistive device if applicable.

- **Code 0, steady at all times:**
  - If all observed turns to face the opposite direction are steady without assistance of a staff during the 7-day look-back period.
  - If the resident is stable making these turns when using an assistive device.
  - If an assistive device or equipment is used, the resident appropriately plans and integrates the use of the device into the transition activity.
  - Residents coded as 0 should not appear to be at risk of a fall during a transition.

- **Code 1, not steady, but able to stabilize without staff assistance:**
  - If any transition that involves turning around to face the opposite direction is not steady, but the resident stabilizes without assistance from a staff.
  - If the resident is unstable with an assistive device but does not require staff assistance.
  - Residents coded in this category appear at increased risk for falling during transitions.

- **Code 2, not steady, only able to stabilize with staff assistance:**
  - If any transition that involves turning around to face the opposite direction is not steady, and the resident cannot stabilize without assistance from a staff.
  - If the resident fell when turning around to face the opposite direction during the look-back period.
  - Residents coded in this category appear at high risk for falling during transitions.

- **Code 8, activity did not occur:**
  - If the resident did not turn around to face the opposite direction while walking during the 7-day look-back period.

Examples for G0300C, Turning Around and Facing the Opposite Direction while Walking

1. A resident with Alzheimer's disease frequently wanders on the hallway. On one occasion, a nursing assistant noted that he was about to fall when turning around. However, by the time she got to him, he had steadied himself on the handrail.

    Coding: G0300C would be **coded 1, Not steady, but able to stabilize without staff assistance**.

    Rationale: The resident was unsteady when turning but able to steady himself on an object, in this instance, a handrail.

2. A resident with severe arthritis in her knee ambulates with a single-point cane. A nursing assistant observes her lose her balance while turning around to sit in a chair. The nursing assistant is able to get to her before she falls and lowers her gently into the chair.

    Coding: G0300C would be **coded 2, not steady, only able to stabilize with staff assistance**.

    Rationale: The resident was unsteady when turning around and would have fallen without staff assistance.

Coding for G0300D, Moving on and off Toilet

Code for the least steady episode of moving on and off a toilet or portable commode, using an assistive device if applicable. Include stability while manipulating clothing to allow toileting to occur in this rating.

- **Code 0, steady at all times:**
  — If all of the observed transitions on and off the toilet during the 7-day look-back period are steady without assistance of a staff.
  — If the resident is stable when transferring using an assistive device or object identified for this purpose.
  — If an assistive device is used (e.g., grab bar), the resident appropriately plans and integrates the use of the device into the transition activity.
  — Residents coded as 0 should not appear to be at risk of a fall during a transition.
- **Code 1, not steady, but able to stabilize without staff assistance:**
  — If any transitions on or off the toilet during the 7-day look-back period are not steady, **but** the resident stabilizes **without** assistance from a staff.
  — If resident is unstable with an assistive device but does not require staff assistance.
  — Residents coded in this category appear at increased risk for falling during transitions.
- **Code 2, not steady, only able to stabilize with staff assistance:**
  — If any transitions on or off the toilet during the 7-day look-back period are not steady, and the resident cannot stabilize without assistance from a staff.
  — If the resident fell when moving on or off the toilet during the look-back period.
  — Residents coded in this category appear at high risk for falling during transitions.
- **Code 8, activity did not occur:**
  — If the resident did not transition on and off the toilet during the 7-day look-back period.

Examples for G0300D, Moving on and off Toilet

1. A resident sits up in bed, stands up, pivots and grabs her walker. She then steadily walks to the bathroom where she pivots, pulls down her underwear, uses the grab bar and smoothly sits on the commode using the grab bar to guide her. After finishing, she stands and pivots using the grab bar and smoothly ambulates out of her room with her walker.

G0300: Balance During Transitions and Walking (cont.)

Coding: G0300D would be **coded 0, steady at all times**.

Rationale: This resident's use of the grab bar was not to prevent a fall after being unsteady, but to maintain steadiness during her transitions. The resident was able to smoothly and steadily transfer onto the toilet, using a grab bar.

2. A resident wheels her wheelchair into the bathroom, stands up, begins to lift her dress, sways, and grabs onto the grab bar to steady herself. When she sits down on the toilet, she leans to the side and must push herself away from the towel bar to sit upright steadily.

Coding: G0300D would be **coded 1, not steady, but able to stabilize without staff assistance**.

Rationale: The resident was unsteady when disrobing to toilet but was able to steady herself with a grab bar.

3. A resident wheels his wheelchair into the bathroom, stands, begins to pull his pants down, sways, and grabs onto the grab bar to steady himself. When he sits down on the toilet, he leans to the side and must push himself away from the sink to sit upright steadily. When finished, he stands, sways, and then is able to steady himself with the grab bar.

Coding: G0300D would be **coded 1, not steady, but able to stabilize without staff assistance**.

Rationale: The resident was unsteady when disrobing to toilet but was able to steady himself with a grab bar.

Coding Instructions G0300E, Surface-to-Surface Transfer (Transferring from Bed to Wheelchair or Wheelchair to Bed)

Code for the least steady episode.

- **Code 0, steady at all times:**
  - If all of the observed transfers during the 7-day look-back period are steady without assistance of a staff.
  - If the resident is stable when transferring using an assistive device identified for this purpose.
  - If an assistive device or equipment is used, the resident uses it independently and appropriately plans and integrates the use of the device into the transition activity.
  - Residents **coded 0** should not appear to be at risk of a fall during a transition.
- **Code 1, not steady, but able to stabilize without staff assistance:**
  - If any transfers during the look-back period are not steady, but the resident stabilizes without assistance from a staff.
  - If the resident is unstable with an assistive device but does not require staff assistance.
  - Residents coded in this category appear at increased risk for falling during transitions.

G0300: Balance During Transitions and Walking (cont.)

- **Code 2, not steady, only able to stabilize with staff assistance:**
  - If any transfers during the 7-day look-back period are not steady, and the resident can only stabilize with assistance from a staff.
  - If the resident fell during a surface-to-surface transfer during the look-back period.
  - Residents coded in this category appear at high risk for falling during transitions.
  - If a lift device (a mechanical device that is completely operated by another person) is used, and this mechanical device is being used because the resident requires staff assistance to stabilize, **code 2**.

- **Code 8, activity did not occur:**
  - If the resident did not transfer from bed to wheelchair/chair or wheelchair/chair to bed during the 7-day look-back period.

Examples for G0300E, Surface-to-Surface Transfer (Transferring from Bed to Wheelchair or Wheelchair to Bed)

1. A resident who uses her wheelchair for mobility stands up from the edge of her bed, pivots, and sits in her locked wheelchair in a steady fashion.

   Coding: G0300E would be **coded 0, steady at all times**.

   Rationale: The resident was steady when transferring from bed to wheelchair.

2. A resident who needs assistance ambulating transfers to his wheelchair from the bed. He is observed to stand halfway up and then sit back down on the bed. On a second attempt, a nursing assistant helps him stand up straight, pivot, and sit down in his wheelchair.

   Coding: G0300E would be **coded 2, not steady, only able to stabilize with staff assistance**.

   Rationale: The resident was unsteady when transferring from bed to wheelchair and required staff assistance to make a steady transfer.

3. A resident with an above-the-knee amputation sits on the edge of the bed and, using his locked wheelchair due to unsteadiness and the nightstand for leverage, stands and transfers to his wheelchair rapidly and almost misses the seat. He is able to steady himself using the nightstand and sit down into the wheelchair without falling to the floor.

   Coding: G0300E would be **coded 1, not steady, but able to stabilize without staff assistance**.

   Rationale: The resident was unsteady when transferring from bed to wheelchair but did not require staff assistance to complete the activity.

4. A resident who uses her wheelchair for mobility stands up from the edge of her bed, sways to the right, but then is quickly able to pivot and sits in her locked wheelchair in a steady fashion.

G0300: Balance During Transitions and Walking (cont.)

> **Coding:** G0300E would be **coded 1, not steady, but able to stabilize without staff assistance**.
>
> **Rationale:** The resident was unsteady when transferring from bed to wheelchair but was able to steady herself without staff assistance or an object.

Additional examples for G0300A-E, Balance during Transitions and Walking

1. A resident sits up in bed, stands up, pivots and sits in her locked wheelchair. She then wheels her chair to the bathroom where she stands, pivots, lifts gown and smoothly sits on the commode.

   > **Coding:** G0300A, G0300D, G0300E would be **coded 0, steady at all times**.
   >
   > **Rationale:** The resident was steady during each activity.

G0400: Functional Limitation in Range of Motion

G0400. Functional Limitation in Range of Motion		
Code for limitation that interfered with daily functions or placed resident at risk of injury		
Coding: 0. **No impairment** 1. **Impairment on one side** 2. **Impairment on both sides**	↓ Enter Codes in Boxes	
	☐	**A. Upper extremity** (shoulder, elbow, wrist, hand)
	☐	**B. Lower extremity** (hip, knee, ankle, foot)

Intent: The intent of G0400 is to determine whether functional limitation in range of motion (ROM) interferes with the resident's activities of daily living or places him or her at risk of injury. When completing this item, staff should refer back to item G0110 and view the limitation in ROM taking into account activities that the resident is able to perform.

> **DEFINITIONS**
>
> **FUNCTIONAL LIMITATION IN RANGE OF MOTION** Limited ability to move a joint that interferes with daily functioning (particularly with activities of daily living) or places the resident at risk of injury.

Item Rationale

Health-related Quality of Life

- Functional impairment could place the resident at risk of injury or interfere with performance of activities of daily living.

Planning for Care

- Individualized care plans should address possible reversible causes such as de-conditioning and adverse side effects of medications or other treatments.

Steps for Assessment

1. Review the medical record for references to functional range of motion limitation during the 7-day look-back period.
2. Talk with staff members who work with the resident as well as family/significant others about any impairment in functional ROM.

G0400: Functional Limitation in Range of Motion (cont.)

3. Coding for functional ROM limitations is a 3 step process:

   - Test the resident's upper and lower extremity ROM (See #6 below for examples).

   - If the resident is noted to have limitation of upper and/or lower extremity ROM, review G0110 and/or directly observe the resident to determine if the limitation interferes with function or places the resident at risk for injury.

   - Code G0400 A/B as appropriate based on the above assessment.

4. Assess the resident's ROM bilaterally at the shoulder, elbow, wrist, hand, hip, knee, ankle, foot, and other joints unless contraindicated (e.g., recent fracture, joint replacement or pain).

5. Staff observations of various activities, including ADLs, may be used to determine if any ROM limitations impact the resident's functional abilities.

6. Although this item codes for the presence or absence of functional limitation related to ROM; thorough assessment ought to be comprehensive and follow standards of practice for evaluating ROM impairment. Below are some suggested assessment strategies:

   - Ask the resident to follow your verbal instructions for each movement.

   - Demonstrate each movement (e.g., ask the resident to do what you are doing).

   - Actively assist the resident with the movements by supporting his or her extremity and guiding it through the joint ROM.

   Lower Extremity- includes hip, knee, ankle, and foot

   While resident is lying supine in a flat bed, instruct the resident to flex (pull toes up towards head) and extend (push toes down away from head) each foot. Then ask the resident to lift his or her leg one at a time, bending it at the knee to a right angle (90 degrees) Then ask the resident to slowly lower his or her leg and extend it flat on the mattress. If assessing lower extremity ROM by observing the resident, the flexion and extension of the food mimics the motion on the pedals of a bicycle. Extension might also be needed to don a shoe. If assessing bending at the knee, the motion would be similar to lifting of the leg when donning lower body clothing.

   Upper Extremity – includes shoulder, elbow, wrist, and fingers

   For each hand, instruct the resident to make a fist and then open the hand. With resident seated in a chair, instruct him or her to reach with both hands and touch palms to back of head. Then ask resident to touch each shoulder with the opposite hand. Alternatively, observe the resident donning or removing a shirt over the head. If assessing upper extremity ROM by observing the resident, making a fist mimics useful actions for grasping and letting go of utensils. When an individual reaches both hands to the back of the head, this mimics the action needed to comb hair.

Coding Tips

- Do not look at limited ROM in isolation. You must determine if the limited ROM impacts functional ability or places the resident at risk for injury.

G0400: Functional Limitation in Range of Motion (cont.)

Coding Instructions for G0400A, Upper Extremity (Shoulder, Elbow, Wrist, Hand); G0400B, Lower Extremity (Hip, Knee, Ankle, Foot)

- **Code 0, no impairment:** if resident has full functional range of motion on the right and left side of upper/lower extremities.
- **Code 1, impairment on one side:** if resident has an upper and/or lower extremity impairment on one side that interferes with daily functioning or places the resident at risk of injury.
- **Code 2, impairment on both sides:** if resident has an upper and/or lower extremity impairment on both sides that interferes with daily functioning or places the resident at risk of injury.

Examples for G0400A, Upper Extremity (Shoulder, Elbow, Wrist, Hand); G0400B, Lower Extremity (Hip, Knee, Ankle, Foot)

1. The resident can perform all arm, hand, and leg motions on the right side, with smooth coordinated movements. She is able to perform grooming activities (e.g. brush teeth, comb her hair) with her right upper extremity, and is also able to pivot to her wheelchair with the assist of one person. She is, however, unable to voluntarily move her left side (limited arm, hand and leg motion) as she has a flaccid left hemiparesis from a prior stroke.

   Coding: G0400A would be **coded 1, upper extremity impairment on one side**. G0400B would be **coded 1, lower extremity impairment on one side**.

   Rationale: Impairment due to left hemiparesis affects both upper and lower extremities on one side. Even though this resident has limited ROM that impairs function on the left side, as indicated above, the resident can perform ROM fully on the right side. Even though there is impairment on one side, the facility should always attempt to provide the resident with assistive devices or physical assistance that allows for the resident to be as independent as possible.

2. The resident had shoulder surgery and can't brush her hair or raise her right arm above her head. The resident has no impairment on the lower extremities.

   Coding: G0400A would be **coded 1, upper extremity impairment on one side**. G0400B would be **coded 0, no impairment**.

   Rationale: Impairment due to shoulder surgery affects only one side of her upper extremities.

G0400: Functional Limitation in Range of Motion (cont.)

3. The resident has a diagnosis of Parkinson's and ambulates with a shuffling gate. The resident has had 3 falls in the past quarter and often forgets his walker which he needs to ambulate. He has tremors of both upper extremities that make it very difficult to feed himself, brush his teeth or write.

> **Coding**: G0400A would be **coded 2, upper extremity impairment on both sides**.
>
> G0400B would be **coded 2, lower extremity impairment on both sides**.
>
> **Rationale:** Impairment due to Parkinson's disease affects the resident at the upper and lower extremities on both sides.

G0600: Mobility Devices

G0600. Mobility Devices	
↓ Check all that were normally used	
☐	A. Cane/crutch
☐	B. Walker
☐	C. Wheelchair (manual or electric)
☐	D. Limb prosthesis
☐	Z. None of the above were used

Item Rationale

Health-related Quality of Life

- Maintaining independence is important to an individual's feelings of autonomy and self-worth. The use of devices may assist the resident in maintaining that independence.

Planning for Care

- Resident ability to move about his or her room, unit or nursing home may be directly related to the use of devices. It is critical that nursing home staff assure that the resident's independence is optimized by making available mobility devices on a daily basis, if needed.

Steps for Assessment

1. Review the medical record for references to locomotion during the 7-day look-back period.

2. Talk with staff members who work with the resident as well as family/significant others about devices the resident used for mobility during the look-back period.

3. Observe the resident during locomotion.

G0600: Mobility Devices (cont.)

Coding Instructions

Record the type(s) of mobility devices the resident normally uses for locomotion (in room and in facility). Check all that apply:

- **Check G0600A, cane/crutch:** if the resident used a cane or crutch, including single prong, tripod, quad cane, etc.

- **Check G0600B, walker:** if the resident used a walker or hemi-walker, including an enclosed frame-wheeled walker with/without a posterior seat and lap cushion. Also check this item if the resident walks while pushing a wheelchair for support.

- **Check G0600C, wheelchair (manual or electric):** if the resident normally sits in wheelchair when moving about. Include hand-propelled, motorized, or pushed by another person.

- **Check G0600D, limb prosthesis:** if the resident used an artificial limb to replace a missing extremity.

- **Check G0600Z, none of the above:** if the resident used none of the mobility devices listed in G0600 or locomotion did not occur during the look-back period.

Examples

1. The resident uses a quad cane daily to walk in the room and on the unit. The resident uses a standard push wheelchair that she self-propels when leaving the unit due to her issues with endurance.

   Coding: G0600A, use of cane/crutch, and **G0600C, wheelchair,** would be checked.
   Rationale: The resident uses a quad cane in her room and on the unit and a wheelchair off the unit.

2. The resident has an artificial leg that is applied each morning and removed each evening. Once the prosthesis is applied the resident is able to ambulate independently.

   Coding: G0600D, limb prosthesis, would be checked.
   Rationale: The resident uses a leg prosthesis for ambulating.

G0900: Functional Rehabilitation Potential

Complete only on first assessment (OBRA or PPS) since most recent admission (A0310A = 1)

G0900. Functional Rehabilitation Potential
Complete only if A0310A = 01
Enter Code ☐	**A. Resident believes he or she is capable of increased independence** in at least some ADLs 0. **No** 1. **Yes** 2. **Unable to determine**
Enter Code ☐	**B. Direct care staff believe resident is capable of increased independence** in at least some ADLs 0. **No** 1. **Yes**

G0900: Functional Rehabilitation Potential (cont.)

Item Rationale

Health-related Quality of Life

- Attaining and maintaining independence is important to an individual's feelings of autonomy and self-worth.

- Independence is also important to health status, as decline in function can trigger all of the complications of immobility, depression, and social isolation.

Planning for Care

- Beliefs held by the resident and staff that the resident has the capacity for greater independence and involvement in self-care in at least some ADL areas may be important clues to assist in setting goals.

- Even if highly independent in an activity, the resident or staff may believe the resident can gain more independence (e.g., walk longer distances, shower independently).

- Disagreement between staff beliefs and resident beliefs should be explored by the interdisciplinary team.

Steps for Assessment: Interview Instructions for G0900A, Resident Believes He or She Is Capable of Increased Independence in at Least Some ADLs

1. Ask if the resident thinks he or she could be more self-sufficient given more time.
2. Listen to and record what the resident believes, even if it appears unrealistic.
   - It is sometimes helpful to have a conversation with the resident that helps him/her break down this question. For example, you might ask the resident what types of things staff assist him with and how much of those activities the staff do for the resident. Then ask the resident, "Do you think that you could get to a point where you do more or all of the activity yourself?"

Coding Instructions for G0900A, Resident Believes He or She Is Capable of Increased Independence in at Least Some ADLs

- **Code 0, no:** if the resident indicates that he or she believes he or she will probably stay the same and continue with his or her current needs for assistance.

- **Code 1, yes:** if the resident indicates that he or she thinks he or she can improve. Code even if the resident's expectation appears unrealistic.

- **Code 9, unable to determine:** if the resident cannot indicate any beliefs about his or her functional rehabilitation potential.

G0900: Functional Rehabilitation Potential (cont.)

Example for G0900A, Resident Believes He or She Is Capable of Increased Independence in at Least Some ADLs

1. Mr. N. is cognitively impaired and receives limited physical assistance in locomotion for safety purposes. However, he believes he is capable of walking alone and often gets up and walks by himself when staff are not looking.

   Coding: G0900A would be **coded 1, yes**.
   Rationale: The resident believes he is capable of increased independence.

Steps for Assessment for G0900B, Direct Care Staff Believe Resident Is Capable of Increased Independence in at Least Some ADLs

1. Discuss in interdisciplinary team meeting.

2. Ask staff who routinely care for or work with the resident if they think he or she is capable of greater independence in at least some ADLs.

Coding Instructions for G0900B, Direct Care Staff Believe Resident Is Capable of Increased Independence in at Least Some ADLs

- **Code 0, no:** if staff believe the resident probably will stay the same and continue with current needs for assistance. Also **code 0** if staff believe the resident is likely to experience a decrease in his or her capacity for ADL care performance.

- **Code 1, yes:** if staff believe the resident can gain greater independence in ADLs or if staff indicate they are not sure about the potential for improvement, because that indicates some potential for improvement.

Example for G0900B, Direct Care Staff Believe Resident Is Capable of Increased Independence in at Least Some ADLs

1. The nurse assistant who totally feeds Mrs. W. has noticed in the past week that Mrs. W. has made several attempts to pick up finger foods. She believes Mrs. W. could become more independent in eating if she received close supervision and cueing in a small group for restorative care in eating.

   Coding: G0900B would be **coded 1, yes**.
   Rationale: Based upon observation of the resident, the nurse assistant believes Mrs. W. is capable of increased independence.

SECTION H: BLADDER AND BOWEL

Intent: The intent of the items in this section is to gather information on the use of bowel and bladder appliances, the use of and response to urinary toileting programs, urinary and bowel continence, bowel training programs, and bowel patterns. Each resident who is incontinent or at risk of developing incontinence should be identified, assessed, and provided with individualized treatment (medications, non-medicinal treatments and/or devices) and services to achieve or maintain as normal elimination function as possible.

H0100: Appliances

H0100. Appliances	
↓ Check all that apply	
☐	A. **Indwelling catheter** (including suprapubic catheter and nephrostomy tube)
☐	B. **External catheter**
☐	C. **Ostomy** (including urostomy, ileostomy, and colostomy)
☐	D. **Intermittent catheterization**
☐	Z. **None of the above**

Item Rationale

Health-related Quality of Life

- It is important to know what appliances are in use and the history and rationale for such use.
- External catheters should fit well and be comfortable, minimize leakage, maintain skin integrity, and promote resident dignity.
- Indwelling catheters should not be used unless there is valid medical justification. Assessment should include consideration of the risk and benefits of an indwelling catheter, the anticipated duration of use, and consideration of complications resulting from the use of an indwelling catheter. Complications can include an increased risk of urinary tract infection, blockage of the catheter with associated bypassing of urine, expulsion of the catheter, pain, discomfort, and bleeding.
- Ostomies (and periostomal skin) should be free of redness, tenderness, excoriation, and breakdown. Appliances should fit well, be comfortable, and promote resident dignity.

Planning for Care

- Care planning should include interventions that are consistent with the resident's goals and minimize complications associated with appliance use.

> **DEFINITIONS**
>
> **INDWELLING CATHETER**
> A catheter that is maintained within the bladder for the purpose of continuous drainage of urine.
>
> **SUPRAPUBIC CATHETER**
> An indwelling catheter that is placed by a urologist directly into the bladder through the abdomen. This type of catheter is frequently used when there is an obstruction of urine flow through the urethra.
>
> **NEPHROSTOMY TUBE**
> A catheter inserted through the skin into the kidney in individuals with an abnormality of the ureter (the fibromuscular tube that carries urine from the kidney to the bladder) or the bladder.

H0100: Appliances (cont.)

- Care planning should be based on an assessment and evaluation of the resident's history, physical examination, physician orders, progress notes, nurses' notes and flow sheets, pharmacy and lab reports, voiding history, resident's overall condition, risk factors and information about the resident's continence status, catheter status, environmental factors related to continence programs, and the resident's response to catheter/continence services.

Steps for Assessment

Examine the resident to note the presence of any urinary or bowel appliances.

Review the medical record, including bladder and bowel records, for documentation of current or past use of urinary or bowel appliances.

Coding Instructions

*Check next to each appliance that was used at any time in the past 7 days. Select **none of the above** if none of the appliances A-D were used in the past 7 days.*

- **H0100A,** indwelling catheter (including suprapubic catheter and nephrostomy tube)
- **H0100B,** external catheter
- **H0100C,** ostomy (including urostomy, ileostomy, and colostomy)
- **H0100D,** intermittent catheterization
- **H0100Z,** none of the above

Coding Tips and Special Populations

- Suprapubic catheters and nephrostomy tubes should be coded as an indwelling catheter (H0100A) only and not as an ostomy (H0100C).
- In men, condom catheters, and in females, external urinary pouches, are commonly used intermittently or at night only. This use should be coded as external catheter.
- Do not code gastrostomies or other feeding ostomies in this section. Only appliances used for elimination are coded here.
- Do not include one time catheterization for urine specimen during look back period as intermittent catheterization.

DEFINITIONS

EXTERNAL CATHETER
Device attached to the shaft of the penis like a condom for males or a receptacle pouch that fits around the labia majoria for females and connected to a drainage bag.

OSTOMY
Any type of surgically created opening of the gastrointestinal or genitourinary tract for discharge of body waste.

UROSTOMY
A stoma for the urinary system used in cases where long-term drainage of urine through the bladder and urethra is not possible, e.g., after extensive surgery or in case of obstruction.

ILEOSTOMY
A stoma that has been constructed by bringing the end or loop of small intestine (the ileum) out onto the surface of the skin.

COLOSTOMY
A stoma that has been constructed by connecting a part of the colon onto the anterior abdominal wall.

INTERMITTENT CATHETERIZATION
Sterile insertion and removal of a catheter through the urethra for bladder drainage.

H0200: Urinary Toileting Program

	H0200. Urinary Toileting Program

Enter Code ☐	**A. Has a trial of a toileting program (e.g., scheduled toileting, prompted voiding, or bladder training)** been attempted on admission/reentry or since urinary incontinence was noted in this facility?
	  0. **No** → Skip to H0300, Urinary Continence
	  1. **Yes** → Continue to H0200B, Response
	  9. **Unable to determine** → Skip to H0200C, Current toileting program or trial

Enter Code ☐	**B. Response** - What was the resident's response to the trial program?
	  0. **No improvement**
	  1. **Decreased wetness**
	  2. **Completely dry** (continent)
	  9. **Unable to determine** or trial in progress

Enter Code ☐	**C. Current toileting program or trial** - Is a toileting program (e.g., scheduled toileting, prompted voiding, or bladder training) currently being used to manage the resident's urinary continence?
	  0. **No**
	  1. **Yes**

Item Rationale

Health-related Quality of Life

- An individualized, resident-centered toileting program may decrease or prevent urinary incontinence, minimizing or avoiding the negative consequences of incontinence.

- Determining the type of urinary incontinence can allow staff to provide more individualized programming or interventions to enhance the resident's quality of life and functional status.

- Many incontinent residents (including those with dementia) respond to a toileting program, especially during the day.

Planning for Care

- The steps toward ensuring that the resident receives appropriate treatment and services to restore as much bladder function as possible are

  — determining if the resident is currently experiencing some level of incontinence or is at risk of developing urinary incontinence;

  — completing an accurate, thorough assessment of factors that may predispose the resident to having urinary incontinence; and

  — implementing appropriate, individualized interventions and modifying them as appropriate.

- If the toileting program or bladder retraining leads to a decrease or resolution of incontinence, the program should be maintained.

- Research has shown that one quarter to one third of residents will have a decrease or resolution of incontinence in response to a toileting program.

- If incontinence is not decreased or resolved with a toileting trial, consider whether other reversible or treatable causes are present.

- Residents may need to be referred to practitioners who specialize in diagnosing and treating conditions that affect bladder function.

- Residents who do not respond to a toileting trial and for whom other reversible or treatable causes are not found should receive supportive management (such as checking the resident for incontinence and changing his or her brief if needed and providing good skin care).

H0200: Urinary Toileting Program (cont.)

Steps for Assessment: H0200A, Trial of a Toileting Program

The look-back period for this item is to the most recent admission/readmission assessment, the most recent prior assessment, or to when incontinence was first noted.

1. Review the medical record for evidence of a trial of an individualized, resident-centered toileting program. A toileting trial should include observations of at least 3 days of toileting patterns with prompting to toilet and of recording results in a bladder record or voiding diary. Toileting programs may have different names, e.g., habit training/scheduled voiding, bladder rehabilitation/bladder retraining.
2. Review records of voiding patterns (such as frequency, volume, duration, nighttime or daytime, quality of stream) over several days for those who are experiencing incontinence.
3. Voiding records help detect urinary patterns or intervals between incontinence episodes and facilitate providing care to avoid or reduce the frequency of episodes.
4. Simply tracking continence status using a bladder record or voiding diary should not be considered a trial of an individualized, resident-centered toileting program.
5. Residents should be reevaluated whenever there is a change in cognition, physical ability, or urinary tract function. Nursing home staff must use clinical judgment to determine when it is appropriate to reevaluate a resident's ability to participate in a toileting trial or, if the toileting trial was unsuccessful, the need for a trial of a different toileting program.

Steps for Assessment: H0200B, Response to Trial Toileting Program

1. Review the resident's responses as recorded during the toileting trial, noting any change in the number of incontinence episodes or degree of wetness the resident experiences.

DEFINITIONS

BLADDER REHABILITATION/ BLADDER RETRAINING
A behavioral technique that requires the resident to resist or inhibit the sensation of urgency (the strong desire to urinate), to postpone or delay voiding, and to urinate according to a timetable rather than to the urge to void.

PROMPTED VOIDING
Prompted voiding includes (1) regular monitoring with encouragement to report continence status, (2) using a schedule and prompting the resident to toilet, and (3) praise and positive feedback when the resident is continent and attempts to toilet.

HABIT TRAINING/ SCHEDULED VOIDING
A behavior technique that calls for scheduled toileting at regular intervals on a planned basis to match the resident's voiding habits or needs.

CHECK AND CHANGE
Involves checking the resident's dry/wet status at regular intervals and using incontinence devices and products.

H0200: Urinary Toileting Program (cont.)

Steps for Assessment: H0200C, Current Toileting Program or Trial

1. Review the medical record for evidence of a toileting program being used to manage incontinence during the 7-day look-back period. Note the number of days during the look-back period that the toileting program was implemented or carried out.

2. Look for documentation in the medical record showing that the following three requirements have been met:

   - implementation of an individualized, resident-specific toileting program that was based on an assessment of the resident's unique voiding pattern

   - evidence that the individualized program was communicated to staff and the resident (as appropriate) verbally and through a care plan, flow records, and a written report

   - notations of the resident's response to the toileting program and subsequent evaluations, as needed

3. Guidance for developing a toileting program may be obtained from sources found in Appendix C.

Coding Instructions H0200A, Toileting Program Trial

- **Code 0, no:** if for any reason the resident did not undergo a toileting trial. This includes residents who are continent of urine with or without toileting assistance, or who use a permanent catheter or ostomy, as well as residents who prefer not to participate in a trial. Skip to **Urinary Continence** item (H0300).

- **Code 1, yes:** for residents who underwent a trial of an individualized, resident-centered toileting program at least once since admission/readmission, **prior assessment**, or when urinary incontinence was first noted.

- **Code 9, unable to determine:** if records cannot be obtained to determine if a trial toileting program has been attempted. If code 9, skip H0200B and go to H0200C, **Current Toileting Program or Trial**.

Coding Instructions H0200B, Toileting Program Trial Response

- **Code 0, no improvement:** if the frequency of resident's urinary incontinence did not decrease during the toileting trial.

- **Code 1, decreased wetness:** if the resident's urinary incontinence frequency decreased, but the resident remained incontinent. There is no quantitative definition of improvement. However, the improvement should be clinically meaningful—for example, having at least one less incontinent void per day than before the toileting program was implemented.

- **Code 2, completely dry (continent):** if the resident becomes completely continent of urine, with no episodes of urinary incontinence during the toileting trial. (For residents who have undergone more than one toileting program trial during their stay, use the most recent trial to complete this item.)

- **Code 9, unable to determine or trial in progress:** if the response to the toileting trial cannot be determined because information cannot be found or because the trial is still in progress.

H0200: Urinary Toileting Program (cont.)

Coding Instructions H0200C, Current Toileting Program

- **Code 0, no:** if an individualized resident-centered toileting program (i.e., prompted voiding, scheduled toileting, or bladder training) is used less than 4 days of the 7-day look-back period to manage the resident's urinary continence.

- **Code 1, yes:** for residents who are being managed, during 4 or more days of the 7-day look-back period, with some type of systematic toileting program (i.e., bladder rehabilitation/bladder retraining, prompted voiding, habit training/scheduled voiding). Some residents prefer to not be awakened to toilet. If that resident, however, is on a toileting program during the day, code "yes."

Coding Tips for H0200A-C

- Toileting (or trial toileting) programs refer to a specific approach that is organized, planned, documented, monitored, and evaluated that is consistent with the nursing home's policies and procedures and current standards of practice. A toileting program does not refer to
  - — simply tracking continence status,
  - — changing pads or wet garments, and
  - — random assistance with toileting or hygiene.
- For a resident currently undergoing a trial of a toileting program,
  - — H0200A would be **coded 1, yes, a trial toileting program is attempted,**
  - — H0200B would be **coded 9, unable to determine or trial in progress,** and
  - — H0200C would be **coded 1, current toileting program**.

Example

1. Mrs. H. has a diagnosis of advanced Alzheimer's disease. She is dependent on the staff for her ADLs, does not have the cognitive ability to void in the toilet or other appropriate receptacle, and is totally incontinent. Her voiding assessment/diary indicates no pattern to her incontinence. Her care plan states that due to her total incontinence, staff should follow the facility standard policy for incontinence, which is to check and change every 2 hours while awake and apply a superabsorbent brief at bedtime so as not to disturb her sleep.

   Coding: H0200A would be **coded as 0, no** H0200B and H0200C would be skipped.
   Rationale: Based on this resident's voiding assessment/diary, there was no pattern to her incontinence. Therefore, H0200A would be coded as 0, no. Due to total incontinence a toileting program is not appropriate for this resident. Since H0200A is coded 0, no skip to H0300, Urinary Continence.

H0200: Urinary Toileting Program (cont.)

2. Mr. M., who has a diagnosis of congestive heart failure (CHF) and a history of left-sided hemiplegia from a previous stroke, has had an increase in urinary incontinence. The team has assessed him for a reversible cause of the incontinence and has evaluated his voiding pattern using a voiding assessment/diary. After completing the assessment, it was determined that incontinence episodes could be reduced. A plan was developed and implemented that called for toileting every hour for 4 hours after receiving his 8 a.m. diuretic, then every 3 hours until bedtime at 9 p.m. The team has communicated this approach to the resident and the care team and has placed these interventions in the care plan. The team will reevaluate the resident's response to the plan after 1 month and adjust as needed.

> **Coding**: H0200A would be **coded as 1, yes.**
>
> H0200B would be **coded as 9, unable to determine or trial in progress**
>
> H0200C would be **coded as 1, current toileting program or trial.**
>
> **Rationale:** Based on this resident's voiding assessment/diary, it was determined that this resident could benefit from a toileting program. Therefore H0200A is coded as 1, yes. Based on the assessment it was determined that incontinence episodes could be reduced, therefore H0200B is coded as 9, unable to determine or trial in progress. An individualized plan has been developed, implemented, and communicated to the resident and staff, therefore H0200C is coded as 1, current toileting program or trial.

H0300: Urinary Continence

H0300. Urinary Continence	
Enter Code ☐	**Urinary continence -** Select the one category that best describes the resident 0. **Always continent** 1. **Occasionally incontinent** (less than 7 episodes of incontinence) 2. **Frequently incontinent** (7 or more episodes of urinary incontinence, but at least one episode of continent voiding) 3. **Always incontinent** (no episodes of continent voiding) 9. **Not rated,** resident had a catheter (indwelling, condom), urinary ostomy, or no urine output for the entire 7 days

Item Rationale

Health-related Quality of Life

- Incontinence can
    - interfere with participation in activities,
    - be socially embarrassing and lead to increased feelings of dependency,
    - increase risk of long-term institutionalization,
    - increase risk of skin rashes and breakdown,
    - increased risk of repeated urinary tract infections, and
    - increase the risk of falls and injuries resulting from attempts to reach a toilet unassisted.

DEFINITIONS

URINARY INCONTINENCE
The involuntary loss of urine.

CONTINENCE
Any void into a commode, urinal, or bedpan that occurs voluntarily, or as the result of prompted toileting, assisted toileting, or scheduled toileting.

H0300: Urinary Continence (cont.)

Planning for Care

- For many residents, incontinence can be resolved or minimized by
  - identifying and treating underlying potentially reversible causes, including medication side effects, urinary tract infection, constipation and fecal impaction, and immobility (especially among those with the new or recent onset of incontinence);
  - eliminating environmental physical barriers to accessing commodes, bedpans, and urinals; and
  - bladder retraining, prompted voiding, or scheduled toileting.
- For residents whose incontinence does not have a reversible cause and who do not respond to retraining, prompted voiding, or scheduled toileting, the interdisciplinary team should establish a plan to maintain skin dryness and minimize exposure to urine.

Steps for Assessment

1. Review the medical record for bladder or incontinence records or flow sheets, nursing assessments and progress notes, physician history, and physical examination.
2. Interview the resident if he or she is capable of reliably reporting his or her continence. Speak with family members or significant others if the resident is not able to report on continence.
3. Ask direct care staff who routinely work with the resident on all shifts about incontinence episodes.

Coding Instructions

- **Code 0, always continent:** if throughout the 7-day look-back period the resident has been continent of urine, without any episodes of incontinence.
- **Code 1, occasionally incontinent:** if during the 7-day look-back period the resident was incontinent less than 7 episodes. This includes incontinence of any amount of urine sufficient to dampen undergarments, briefs, or pads during daytime or nighttime.
- **Code 2, frequently incontinent:** if during the 7-day look-back period, the resident was incontinent of urine during seven or more episodes but had at least one continent void. This includes incontinence of any amount of urine, daytime and nighttime.
- **Code 3, always incontinent:** if during the 7-day look-back period, the resident had no continent voids.
- **Code 9, not rated:** if during the 7-day look-back period the resident had an indwelling bladder catheter, condom catheter, ostomy, or no urine output (e.g., is on chronic dialysis with no urine output) for the entire 7 days.

Coding Tips and Special Populations

- If intermittent catheterization is used to drain the bladder, code continence level based on continence between catheterizations.

H0300: Urinary Continence (cont.)

Examples

1. An 86-year-old female resident has had longstanding stress-type incontinence for many years. When she has an upper respiratory infection and is coughing, she involuntarily loses urine. However, during the current 7-day look-back period, the resident has been free of respiratory symptoms and has not had an episode of incontinence.

    Coding: H0300 would be **coded 0, always continent.**

    Rationale: Even though the resident has known intermittent stress incontinence, she was continent during the current 7-day look-back period.

2. A resident with multi-infarct dementia is incontinent of urine on three occasions on day one of observation, continent of urine in response to toileting on days two and three, and has one urinary incontinence episode during each of the nights of days four, five, six, and seven of the look-back period.

    Coding: H0300 would be **coded as 2, frequently incontinent.**

    Rationale: The resident had seven documented episodes of urinary incontinence over the look-back period. The criterion for "frequent" incontinence has been set at seven or more episodes over the 7-day look-back period with at least one continent void.

3. A resident with Parkinson's disease is severely immobile, and cannot be transferred to a toilet. He is unable to use a urinal and is managed by adult briefs and bed pads that are regularly changed. He did not have a continent void during the 7-day look-back period.

    Coding: H0300 would be **coded as 3, always incontinent.**

    Rationale: The resident has no urinary continent episodes and cannot be toileted due to severe disability or discomfort. Incontinence is managed by a check and change in protocol.

4. A resident had one continent urinary void during the 7-day look-back period, after the nursing assistant assisted him to the toilet and helped with clothing. All other voids were incontinent.

    Coding: H0300 would be **coded as 2, frequently incontinent.**

    Rationale: The resident had at least one continent void during the look-back period. The reason for the continence does not enter into the coding decision.

H0400: Bowel Continence

H0400. Bowel Continence	
Enter Code	**Bowel continence** - Select the one category that best describes the resident 0. **Always continent** 1. **Occasionally incontinent** (one episode of bowel incontinence) 2. **Frequently incontinent** (2 or more episodes of bowel incontinence, but at least one continent bowel movement) 3. **Always incontinent** (no episodes of continent bowel movements) 9. **Not rated**, resident had an ostomy or did not have a bowel movement for the entire 7 days

H0400: Bowel Continence (cont.)

Item Rationale

Health-related Quality of Life
- Incontinence can
  — interfere with participation in activities,
  — be socially embarrassing and lead to increased feelings of dependency,
  — increase risk of long-term institutionalization,
  — increase risk of skin rashes and breakdown, and
  — increase the risk of falls and injuries resulting from attempts to reach a toilet unassisted.

Planning for Care
- For many residents, incontinence can be resolved or minimized by
  — identifying and managing underlying potentially reversible causes, including medication side effects, constipation and fecal impaction, and immobility (especially among those with the new or recent onset of incontinence); and
  — eliminating environmental physical barriers to accessing commodes, bedpans, and urinals.
- For residents whose incontinence does not have a reversible cause and who do not respond to retraining programs, the interdisciplinary team should establish a plan to maintain skin dryness and minimize exposure to stool.

Steps for Assessment

1. Review the medical record for bowel records and incontinence flow sheets, nursing assessments and progress notes, physician history and physical examination.
2. Interview the resident if he or she is capable of reliably reporting his or her bowel habits. Speak with family members or significant other if the resident is unable to report on continence.
3. Ask direct care staff who routinely work with the resident on all shifts about incontinence episodes.

Coding Instructions

- **Code 0, always continent:** if during the 7-day look-back period the resident has been continent of bowel on all occasions of bowel movements, without any episodes of incontinence.
- **Code 1, occasionally incontinent:** if during the 7-day look-back period the resident was incontinent of stool once. This includes incontinence of any amount of stool day or night.
- **Code 2, frequently incontinent:** if during the 7-day look-back period, the resident was incontinent of bowel more than once, but had at least one continent bowel movement. This includes incontinence of any amount of stool day or night.
- **Code 3, always incontinent:** if during the 7-day look-back period, the resident was incontinent of bowel for all bowel movements and had no continent bowel movements.

H0400: Bowel Continence (cont.)

- **Code 9, not rated:** if during the 7-day look-back period the resident had an ostomy or did not have a bowel movement for the entire 7 days. (Note that these residents should be checked for fecal impaction and evaluated for constipation.)

Coding Tips and Special Populations

- Bowel incontinence precipitated by loose stools or diarrhea from any cause (including laxatives) would count as incontinence.

H0500: Bowel Toileting Program

H0500. Bowel Toileting Program	
Enter Code ☐	**Is a toileting program currently being used to manage the resident's bowel continence?** 0. No 1. Yes

Item Rationale

Health-related Quality of Life

- A systematically implemented bowel toileting program may decrease or prevent bowel incontinence, minimizing or avoiding the negative consequences of incontinence.
- Many incontinent residents respond to a bowel toileting program, especially during the day.

Planning for Care

- If the bowel toileting program leads to a decrease or resolution of incontinence, the program should be maintained.
- If bowel incontinence is not decreased or resolved with a bowel toileting trial, consider whether other reversible or treatable causes are present.
- Residents who do not respond to a bowel toileting trial and for whom other reversible or treatable causes are not found should receive supportive management (such as a regular check and change program with good skin care).
- Residents with a colostomy or colectomy may need their diet monitored to promote healthy bowel elimination and careful monitoring of skin to prevent skin irritation and breakdown.
- When developing a toileting program the provider may want to consider assessing the resident for adequate fluid intake, adequate fiber in the diet, exercise, and scheduled times to attempt bowel movement (Newman, 2009).

H0500: Bowel Toileting Program (cont.)

Steps for Assessment

1. Review the medical record for evidence of a bowel toileting program being used to manage bowel incontinence during the 7-day look-back period.
2. Look for documentation in the medical record showing that the following three requirements have been met:

   - implementation of an individualized, resident-specific bowel toileting program based on an assessment of the resident's unique bowel pattern;
   - evidence that the individualized program was communicated to staff and the resident (as appropriate) verbally and through a care plan, flow records, verbal and a written report; and
   - notations of the resident's response to the toileting program and subsequent evaluations, as needed.

Coding Instructions

- **Code 0, no:** if the resident is not currently on a toileting program targeted specifically at managing bowel continence.
- **Code 1, yes:** if the resident is currently on a toileting program targeted specifically at managing bowel continence.

H0600: Bowel Patterns

H0600. Bowel Patterns	
Enter Code	**Constipation present?** 0. **No** 1. **Yes**

Item Rationale

Health-related Quality of Life

- Severe constipation can cause abdominal pain, anorexia, vomiting, bowel incontinence, and delirium.
- If unaddressed, constipation can lead to fecal impaction.

Planning for Care

- This item identifies residents who may need further evaluation of and intervention on bowel habits.
- Constipation may be a manifestation of serious conditions such as
  — dehydration due to a medical condition or inadequate access to and intake of fluid, and
  — side effect of medications.

> **DEFINITIONS**
>
> **CONSTIPATION**
> If the resident has two or fewer bowel movements during the 7-day look-back period or if for most bowel movements their stool is hard and difficult for them to pass (no matter what the frequency of bowel movements).

H0600: Bowel Patterns (cont.)

Steps for Assessment

1. Review the medical record for bowel records or flow sheets, nursing assessments and progress notes, physician history and physical examination to determine if the resident has had problems with constipation during the 7-day look-back period.
2. Residents who are capable of reliably reporting their continence and bowel habits should be interviewed. Speak with family members or significant others if the resident is unable to report on bowel habits.
3. Ask direct care staff who routinely work with the resident on all shifts about problems with constipation.

Coding Instructions

- **Code 0, no:** if the resident shows no signs of constipation during the 7-day look-back-period.

- **Code 1, yes:** if the resident shows signs of constipation during the 7-day look-back period.

Coding Tips and Special Populations

- Fecal impaction is constipation.

DEFINITIONS

FECAL IMPACTION
A large mass of dry, hard stool that can develop in the rectum due to chronic constipation. This mass may be so hard that the resident is unable to move it from the rectum. Watery stool from higher in the bowel or irritation from the impaction may move around the mass and leak out, causing soiling, often a sign of a fecal impaction.

SECTION I: ACTIVE DIAGNOSES

Intent: The items in this section are intended to code diseases that have a relationship to the resident's current functional status, cognitive status, mood or behavior status, medical treatments, nursing monitoring, or risk of death. One of the important functions of the MDS assessment is to generate an updated, accurate picture of the resident's health status.

Active Diagnoses in the Last 7 Days

Active Diagnoses in the last 7 days - Check all that apply Diagnoses listed in parentheses are provided as examples and should not be considered as all-inclusive lists	
Cancer	
☐	I0100. **Cancer** (with or without metastasis)
Heart/Circulation	
☐	I0200. **Anemia** (e.g., aplastic, iron deficiency, pernicious, and sickle cell)
☐	I0300. **Atrial Fibrillation or Other Dysrhythmias** (e.g., bradycardias and tachycardias)
☐	I0400. **Coronary Artery Disease (CAD)** (e.g., angina, myocardial infarction, and atherosclerotic heart disease (ASHD))
☐	I0500. **Deep Venous Thrombosis (DVT), Pulmonary Embolus (PE), or Pulmonary Thrombo-Embolism (PTE)**
☐	I0600. **Heart Failure** (e.g., congestive heart failure (CHF) and pulmonary edema)
☐	I0700. **Hypertension**
☐	I0800. **Orthostatic Hypotension**
☐	I0900. **Peripheral Vascular Disease (PVD) or Peripheral Arterial Disease (PAD)**
Gastrointestinal	
☐	I1100. **Cirrhosis**
☐	I1200. **Gastroesophageal Reflux Disease (GERD) or Ulcer** (e.g., esophageal, gastric, and peptic ulcers)
☐	I1300. **Ulcerative Colitis, Crohn's Disease, or Inflammatory Bowel Disease**
Genitourinary	
☐	I1400. **Benign Prostatic Hyperplasia (BPH)**
☐	I1500. **Renal Insufficiency, Renal Failure, or End-Stage Renal Disease (ESRD)**
☐	I1550. **Neurogenic Bladder**
☐	I1650. **Obstructive Uropathy**
Infections	
☐	I1700. **Multidrug-Resistant Organism (MDRO)**
☐	I2000. **Pneumonia**
☐	I2100. **Septicemia**
☐	I2200. **Tuberculosis**
☐	I2300. **Urinary Tract Infection (UTI) (LAST 30 DAYS)**
☐	I2400. **Viral Hepatitis** (e.g., Hepatitis A, B, C, D, and E)
☐	I2500. **Wound Infection** (other than foot)
Metabolic	
☐	I2900. **Diabetes Mellitus (DM)** (e.g., diabetic retinopathy, nephropathy, and neuropathy)
☐	I3100. **Hyponatremia**
☐	I3200. **Hyperkalemia**
☐	I3300. **Hyperlipidemia** (e.g., hypercholesterolemia)
☐	I3400. **Thyroid Disorder** (e.g., hypothyroidism, hyperthyroidism, and Hashimoto's thyroiditis)
Musculoskeletal	
☐	I3700. **Arthritis** (e.g., degenerative joint disease (DJD), osteoarthritis, and rheumatoid arthritis (RA))
☐	I3800. **Osteoporosis**
☐	I3900. **Hip Fracture** - any hip fracture that has a relationship to current status, treatments, monitoring (e.g., sub-capital fractures, and fractures of the trochanter and femoral neck)
☐	I4000. **Other Fracture**
Neurological	
☐	I4200. **Alzheimer's Disease**
☐	I4300. **Aphasia**
☐	I4400. **Cerebral Palsy**
☐	I4500. **Cerebrovascular Accident (CVA), Transient Ischemic Attack (TIA), or Stroke**
☐	I4800. **Dementia** (e.g. Non-Alzheimer's dementia such as vascular or multi-infarct dementia; mixed dementia; frontotemporal dementia such as Pick's disease; and dementia related to stroke, Parkinson's or Creutzfeldt-Jakob diseases)

I: Active Diagnoses in the Last 7 Days (cont.)

	Active Diagnoses in the last 7 days - Check all that apply
	Diagnoses listed in parentheses are provided as examples and should not be considered as all-inclusive lists

Neurological - Continued

- [ ] **I4900. Hemiplegia or Hemiparesis**
- [ ] **I5000. Paraplegia**
- [ ] **I5100. Quadriplegia**
- [ ] **I5200. Multiple Sclerosis (MS)**
- [ ] **I5250. Huntington's Disease**
- [ ] **I5300. Parkinson's Disease**
- [ ] **I5350. Tourette's Syndrome**
- [ ] **I5400. Seizure Disorder or Epilepsy**
- [ ] **I5500. Traumatic Brain Injury (TBI)**

Nutritional

- [ ] **I5600. Malnutrition** (protein or calorie) or at risk for malnutrition

Psychiatric/Mood Disorder

- [ ] **I5700. Anxiety Disorder**
- [ ] **I5800. Depression** (other than bipolar)
- [ ] **I5900. Manic Depression** (bipolar disease)
- [ ] **I5950. Psychotic Disorder** (other than schizophrenia)
- [ ] **I6000. Schizophrenia** (e.g., schizoaffective and schizophreniform disorders)
- [ ] **I6100. Post Traumatic Stress Disorder (PTSD)**

Pulmonary

- [ ] **I6200. Asthma, Chronic Obstructive Pulmonary Disease (COPD), or Chronic Lung Disease** (e.g., chronic bronchitis and restrictive lung diseases such as asbestosis)
- [ ] **I6300. Respiratory Failure**

Vision

- [ ] **I6500. Cataracts, Glaucoma, or Macular Degeneration**

None of Above

- [ ] **I7900. None of the above active diagnoses** within the last 7 days

Other

- [ ] **I8000. Additional active diagnoses**
  Enter diagnosis on line and ICD code in boxes. Include the decimal for the code in the appropriate box.

  A. _____

  B. _____

  C. _____

  D. _____

  E. _____

  F. _____

  G. _____

  H. _____

  I. _____

  J. _____

I: Active Diagnoses in the Last 7 Days (cont)

Item Rationale

Health-Related Quality of Life

- Disease processes can have a significant adverse affect on an individual's health status and quality of life.

Planning for Care

- This section identifies active diseases and infections that drive the current plan of care.

Steps for Assessment

There are two look-back periods for this section:

- Diagnosis identification (Step 1) is a 60-day look-back period.
- Diagnosis status: Active or Inactive (Step 2) is a 7-day look-back period (except for Item I2300 UTI, which does not use the active 7-day look-back period).

1. **Identify diagnoses:** The disease conditions in this section require a physician-documented diagnosis (or by a nurse practitioner, physician assistant, or clinical nurse specialist if allowable under state licensure laws) in the **last 60 days.**

   Medical record sources for physician diagnoses include progress notes, the most recent history and physical, transfer documents, discharge summaries, diagnosis/problem list, and other resources as available. If a diagnosis/problem list is used, only diagnoses confirmed by the physician should be entered.

   - Although open communication regarding diagnostic information between the physician and other members of the interdisciplinary team is important, it is also essential that diagnoses communicated verbally be documented in the medical record by the physician to ensure follow-up.
   - Diagnostic information, including past history obtained from family members and close contacts, must also be documented in the medical record by the physician to ensure validity and follow-up.

2. **Determine whether diagnoses are active:** Once a diagnosis is identified, it must be determined if the diagnosis is **active.** Do not include conditions that have been resolved or have no **longer** affected the resident's functioning or plan of care during the last 7 days. Item I2300 UTI, has specific coding criteria and does not use the active 7-day look-back. Please refer to Page I-8 for specific coding instructions for Item I2300 UTI.

DEFINITIONS

ACTIVE DIAGNOSES
Diagnoses that have a direct relationship to the resident's functional status, cognitive status, mood or behavior, medical treatments, nursing monitoring, or risk of death during the 7-day look-back period.

FUNCTIONAL LIMITATIONS
Loss of range of motion, contractures, muscle weakness, fatigue, decreased ability to perform ADLs, paresis, or paralysis.

I: Active Diagnoses in the Last 7 Days (cont)

- **Active** diagnoses have a direct relationship to the resident's functional status, cognitive status, mood or behavior, medical treatments, nursing monitoring, or risk of death during the look-back period.

- Check the following information sources in the medical record for the last 7 days to identify "active" diagnoses: transfer documents, physician progress notes, recent history and physical, recent discharge summaries, nursing assessments, nursing care plans, medication sheets, doctor's orders, consults and official diagnostic reports, and other sources as available.

Coding Instructions

Code diseases that have a documented diagnosis in the last 60 days and have a relationship to the resident's functional status, cognitive status, mood or behavior status, medical treatments, nursing monitoring, or risk of death during the 7-day look-back period (except Item I2300 UTI, which does not use the active diagnosis 7-day look-back. Please refer to Item I2300 UTI, Page I-8 for specific coding instructions).

- Document active diagnoses on the MDS as follows:

  — Diagnoses are listed by major disease category: Cancer; Heart/Circulation; Gastrointestinal; Genitourinary; Infections; Metabolic; Musculoskeletal; Neurological; Nutritional; Psychiatric/Mood Disorder; Pulmonary; and Vision.

  — Examples of diseases are included for some disease categories. Diseases to be coded in these categories are not meant to be limited to only those listed in the examples. For example, **I0200, Anemia,** includes anemia of any etiology, including those listed (e.g., aplastic, iron deficiency, pernicious, sickle cell).

- Check off each active disease. Check all that apply.

- If a disease or condition is **not** specifically listed, check the "Other" box (I8000) and write in the ICD code and name for that diagnosis.

- Computer specifications are written such that the ICD code should be automatically justified. The important element is to insure that the ICD code's decimal point is in it's own box and should be right justified (aligned with the right margin so that any unused boxes and on the left.)If a diagnosis is a V-code, another diagnosis for the related primary medical condition should be checked in items I0100-I7900 or entered in I8000.

Cancer

- **I0100,** cancer (with or without metastasis)

Heart/Circulation

- **I0200,** anemia (e.g., aplastic, iron deficiency, pernicious, sickle cell)

- **I0300,** atrial fibrillation or other dysrhythmias (e.g., bradycardias, tachycardias)

- **I0400,** coronary artery disease (CAD) (e.g., angina, myocardial infarction, atherosclerotic heart disease [ASHD])

I: Active Diagnoses in the Last 7 Days (cont.)

- **I0500,** deep venous thrombosis (DVT), pulmonary embolus (PE), or pulmonary thrombo-embolism (PTE)
- **I0600,** heart failure (e.g., congestive heart failure [CHF], pulmonary edema)
- **I0700,** hypertension
- **I0800,** orthostatic hypotension
- **I0900,** peripheral vascular disease or peripheral arterial disease

Gastrointestinal

- **I1100,** cirrhosis
- **I1200,** gastroesophageal reflux disease (GERD) or ulcer (e.g., esophageal, gastric, and peptic ulcers)
- **I1300,** ulcerative colitis or Crohn's disease or inflammatory bowel disease

Genitourinary

- **I1400,** benign prostatic hyperplasia (BPH)
- **I1500,** renal insufficiency, renal failure, or end-stage renal disease (ESRD)
- **I1550,** neurogenic bladder
- **I1650,** obstructive uropathy

Infections

- **I1700,** multidrug resistant organism (MDRO)
- **I2000,** pneumonia
- **I2100,** septicemia
- **I2200,** tuberculosis
- **I2300,** urinary tract infection (UTI) (last 30 days)
- **I2400,** viral hepatitis (e.g., hepatitis A, B, C, D, and E)
- **I2500,** wound infection (other than foot)

Metabolic

- **I2900,** diabetes mellitus (DM) (e.g., diabetic retinopathy, nephropathy, neuropathy)
- **I3100,** hyponatremia
- **I3200,** hyperkalemia
- **I3300,** hyperlipidemia (e.g., hypercholesterolemia)
- **I3400,** thyroid disorder (e.g., hypothyroidism, hyperthyroidism, Hashimoto's thyroiditis)

I: Active Diagnoses in the Last 7 Days (cont.)

Musculoskeletal

- **I3700,** arthritis (e.g., degenerative joint disease [DJD], osteoarthritis, rheumatoid arthritis [RA])
- **I3800,** osteoporosis
- **I3900,** hip fracture (any hip fracture that has a relationship to current status, treatments, monitoring (e.g., subcapital fractures and fractures of the trochanter and femoral neck)
- **I4000,** other fracture

Neurological

- **I4200,** Alzheimer's disease
- **I4300,** aphasia
- **I4400,** cerebral palsy
- **I4500,** cerebrovascular accident (CVA), transient ischemic attack (TIA), or stroke
- **I4800,** dementia (e.g., non-Alzheimer's dementia, including vascular or multi-infarct dementia; mixed dementia; frontotemporal dementia, such as Pick's disease; and dementia related to stroke, Parkinson's disease or Creutzfeldt-Jakob diseases)
- **I4900,** hemiplegia or hemiparesis
- **I5000,** paraplegia
- **I5100,** quadriplegia
- **I5200,** multiple sclerosis (MS)
- **I5250,** Huntington's disease
- **I5300,** Parkinson's disease
- **I5350,** Tourette's syndrome
- **I5400,** seizure disorder or epilepsy
- **I5500,** traumatic brain injury (TBI)

Nutritional

- **I5600,** malnutrition (protein or calorie) or at risk for malnutrition

Psychiatric/Mood Disorder

- **I5700,** anxiety disorder
- **I5800,** depression (other than bipolar)
- **I5900,** manic depression (bipolar disease)
- **I5950,** psychotic disorder (other than schizophrenia)
- **I6000,** schizophrenia (e.g., schizoaffective and schizophreniform disorders)
- **I6100,** post-traumatic stress disorder (PTSD)

I: Active Diagnoses in the Last 7 Days (cont.)

Pulmonary

- **I6200,** asthma, chronic obstructive pulmonary disease (COPD), or chronic lung disease (e.g., chronic bronchitis and restrictive lung diseases, such as asbestosis)
- **I6300,** respiratory failure

Vision

- **I6500,** cataracts, glaucoma, or macular degeneration

None of Above

- **I7900,** none of the above active diagnoses within the past 7 days

Other

- **I8000,** additional active diagnoses

Coding Tips

The following indicators may assist assessors in determining whether a diagnosis should be coded as active in the MDS.

- **There may be specific documentation in the medical record by a physician, nurse practitioner, physician assistant, or clinical nurse specialist of active diagnosis.**
  - The physician may specifically indicate that a condition is active. Specific documentation may be found in progress notes, most recent history and physical, transfer notes, hospital discharge summary, etc.
  - For example, the physician documents that the resident has inadequately controlled hypertension and will modify medications. This would be sufficient documentation of active disease and would require no additional confirmation.
- **In the absence of specific documentation that a disease is active, the following indicators may be used to confirm active disease:**
  - Recent onset or acute exacerbation of the disease or condition indicated by a positive study, test or procedure, hospitalization for acute symptoms and/or recent change in therapy in the last 7 days. Examples of a recent onset or acute exacerbation include the following: new diagnosis of pneumonia indicated by chest X-ray; hospitalization for fractured hip; or a blood transfusion for a hematocrit of 24. Sources may include radiological reports, hospital discharge summaries, doctor's orders, etc.
  - Symptoms and abnormal signs indicating ongoing or decompensated disease in the last 7 days. For example, intermittent claudication (lower extremity pain on exertion) in conjunction with a diagnosis of peripheral vascular disease would indicate active disease. Sometimes signs and symptoms can be nonspecific and could be caused by several disease processes. Therefore, a symptom must be specifically attributed to the disease. For example, a productive cough would confirm a diagnosis of pneumonia if specifically noted as such by a physician. Sources may include radiological reports, nursing assessments and care plans, progress notes, etc.

I: Active Diagnoses in the Last 7 Days (cont.)

— Listing a disease/diagnosis (e.g., arthritis) on the resident's medical record problem list is not sufficient for determining active or inactive status. To determine if arthritis, for example, is an "active" diagnosis, the reviewer would check progress notes (including the history and physical) during the 7-day look-back period for notation of treatment of symptoms of arthritis, doctor's orders for medications for arthritis, and documentation of physical or other therapy for functional limitations caused by arthritis.

— Ongoing therapy with medications or other interventions to manage a condition that requires monitoring for therapeutic efficacy or to monitor potentially severe side effects in the last 7 days. A medication indicates active disease if that medication is prescribed to manage an ongoing condition that requires monitoring or is prescribed to decrease active symptoms associated with a condition. This includes medications used to limit disease progression and complications. If a medication is prescribed for a condition that requires regular staff monitoring of the drug's effect on that condition (therapeutic efficacy), then the prescription of the medication would indicate active disease.

- **It is expected that nurses monitor all medications for adverse effects as part of usual nursing practice.** For coding purposes, this monitoring relates to management of pharmacotherapy and not to management or monitoring of the underlying disease.

- **Item I2300 Urinary tract infection (UTI):**

  — The UTI has a look-back period of 30 days for active disease instead of 7 days.

  — **Code only if all the following are met**

    1. Physician, nurse practitioner, physician assistant, or clinical nurse specialist or other authorized licensed staff as permitted by state law diagnosis of a UTI in last 30 days,

    2. Sign or symptom attributed to UTI, which may or may not include but not be limited to: fever, urinary symptoms (e.g., peri-urethral site burning sensation, frequent urination of small amounts), pain or tenderness in flank, confusion or change in mental status, change in character of urine (e.g. pyuria),

    3. "Significant laboratory findings" (The attending physician should determine the level of significant laboratory findings and whether or not a culture should be obtained), and

    4. Current medication or treatment for a UTI in the last 30 days.

In response to questions regarding the resident with colonized MRSA, we consulted with the Centers for Disease Control (CDC) who provided the following information:

A physician often prescribes empiric antimicrobial therapy for a suspected infection **after a culture is obtained, but prior to receiving the culture results**. The confirmed diagnosis of UTI will depend on the culture results and other clinical assessment to determine appropriateness and continuation of antimicrobial therapy. This should not be any different, even if the resident is known to be colonized with an antibiotic resistant organism. An appropriate culture will help to ensure the diagnosis of infection is correct, and the appropriate antimicrobial is prescribed to treat the infection. The CDC does not recommend routine antimicrobial treatment for the purposes of attempting to eradicate colonization of MRSA or any other antimicrobial resistant organism.

The CDC's Healthcare Infection Control Practices Advisory Committee (HICPAC) has released infection prevention and control guidelines that contain recommendations that should be applied in all healthcare settings. At this site you will find information related to UTI's and many other issues related to infections in LTC. http://www.cdc.gov/ncidod/dhqp/gl_longterm_care.html

Examples of Active Disease

1. A resident is prescribed hydrochlorothiazide for hypertension. The resident requires regular blood pressure monitoring to determine whether blood pressure goals are achieved by the current regimen. Physician progress note documents hypertension.

   Coding: Hypertension item (I0700), would be **checked**.
   Rationale: This would be considered an active diagnosis because of the need for ongoing monitoring to ensure treatment efficacy.

2. Warfarin is prescribed for a resident with atrial fibrillation to decrease the risk of embolic stroke. The resident requires monitoring for change in heart rhythm, for bleeding, and for anticoagulation.

   Coding: Atrial fibrillation item (I0300), would be **checked**.
   Rationale: This would be considered an active diagnosis because of the need for ongoing monitoring to ensure treatment efficacy as well as to monitor for side effects related to the medication.

3. A resident with a past history of healed peptic ulcer is prescribed a non-steroidal anti-inflammatory (NSAID) medication for arthritis. The physician also prescribes a proton-pump inhibitor to decrease the risk of peptic ulcer disease (PUD) from NSAID treatment.

   Coding: Arthritis item (I3700), would be **checked**.
   Rationale: Arthritis would be considered an active diagnosis because of the need for medical therapy. Given that the resident has a history of a healed peptic ulcer without current symptoms, the proton-pump inhibitor prescribed is preventive and therefore PUD would not be coded as an active disease.

4. The resident had a stroke 4 months ago and continues to have left-sided weakness, visual problems, and inappropriate behavior. The resident is on aspirin and has physical therapy and occupational therapy three times a week. The physician's note 25 days ago lists stroke.

   Coding: Cerebrovascular Vascular Accident (CVA), Transient Ischemic Attack (TIA), or Stroke item (I4500), would be **checked**.

I: Active Diagnoses in the Last 7 Days (cont.)

Rationale: The physician note within the last 30 days indicates stroke, and the resident is receiving medication and therapies to manage continued symptoms from stroke.

Examples of Inactive Diagnoses (do not code)

1. The admission history states that the resident had pneumonia 2 months prior to this admission. The resident has recovered completely, with no residual effects and no continued treatment during the 7-day look back period.

   Coding: Pneumonia item (I2000), would **not be checked.**

   Rationale: The pneumonia diagnosis would not be considered active because of the resident's complete recovery and the discontinuation of any treatment during the look-back period.

2. The problem list includes a diagnosis of coronary artery disease (CAD). The resident had an angioplasty 3 years ago, is not symptomatic, and is not taking any medication for CAD.

   Coding: CAD item (I0400), would **not be checked.**

   Rationale: The resident has had no symptoms and no treatment during the 7-day look-back period; thus, the CAD would be considered inactive.

3. Mr. J fell and fractured his hip 2 years ago. At the time of the injury, the fracture was surgically repaired. Following the surgery, the resident received several weeks of physical therapy in an attempt to restore him to his previous ambulation status, which had been independent without any devices. Although he received therapy services at that time, he now requires assistance to stand from the chair and uses a walker. He also needs help with lower body dressing because of difficulties standing and leaning over.

   Coding: Hip Fracture item (I3900), would **not be checked.**

   Rationale: Although the resident has mobility and self-care limitations in ambulation and ADLs due to the hip fracture, he has not received therapy services during the 7-day look-back period; thus, Hip Fracture would be considered inactive.

SECTION J: HEALTH CONDITIONS

Intent: The intent of the items in this section is to document a number of health conditions that impact the resident's functional status and quality of life. The items include an assessment of pain which uses an interview with the resident or staff if the resident is unable to participate. The pain items assess the presence of pain, pain frequency, effect on function, intensity, management and control. Other items in the section assess dyspnea, tobacco use, prognosis, problem conditions, and falls.

J0100: Pain Management (5-Day Look Back)

J0100. Pain Management - Complete for all residents, regardless of current pain level	
At any time in the last 5 days, has the resident:	
Enter Code [ ]	A. **Been on a scheduled pain medication regimen?** 0. No 1. Yes
Enter Code [ ]	B. **Received PRN pain medications?** 0. No 1. Yes
Enter Code [ ]	C. **Received non-medication intervention for pain?** 0. No 1. Yes

Item Rationale

Health-related Quality of Life

- Pain can cause suffering and is associated with inactivity, social withdrawal, depression, and functional decline.
- Pain can interfere with participation in rehabilitation.
- Effective pain management interventions can help to avoid these adverse outcomes.

Planning for Care

- Goals for pain management for most residents should be to achieve a consistent level of comfort while maintaining as much function as possible.
- Identification of pain management interventions facilitates review of the effectiveness of pain management and revision of the plan if goals are not met.
- Residents may have more than one source of pain and will need a comprehensive, individualized management regimen.
- Most residents with moderate to severe pain will require regularly dosed pain medication, and some will require additional PRN (as-needed) pain medications for breakthrough pain.
- Some residents with intermittent or mild pain may have orders for PRN dosing only.

> **DEFINITIONS**
>
> **PAIN MEDICATION REGIMEN**
> Pharmacological agent(s) prescribed to relieve or prevent the recurrence of pain. Include all medications used for pain management by any route and any frequency during the look-back period. Include oral, transcutaneous, subcutaneous, intramuscular, rectal, intravenous injections or intraspinal delivery. This item does not include medications that primarily target treatment of the underlying condition, such as chemotherapy or steroids, although such treatments may lead to pain reduction.

J0100: Pain Management (cont.)

- Non-medication pain (non-pharmacologic) interventions for pain can be important adjuncts to pain treatment regimens.

- Interventions must be included as part of a care plan that aims to prevent or relieve pain and includes monitoring for effectiveness and revision of care plan if stated goals are not met. There must be documentation that the intervention was received and its effectiveness was assessed. It does not have to have been successful to be counted.

Steps for Assessment

1. Review the medical record and interview staff and direct caregivers to determine what, if any, pain management interventions the resident received during the 5-day look-back period. Include information from all disciplines.

Coding Instructions for J0100A-C

Determine all interventions for pain provided to the resident during the 5-day look-back period. Answer these items even if the resident currently denies pain.

Coding Instructions for J0100A, Been on a Scheduled Pain Medication Regimen

- **Code 0, no:** if the medical record does not contain documentation that a scheduled pain medication was received.

- **Code 1, yes:** if the medical record contains documentation that a scheduled pain medication was received.

Coding Instructions for J0100B, Received PRN Pain Medication

- **Code 0, no:** if the medical record does not contain documentation that a PRN medication was received or offered.

- **Code 1, yes:** if the medical record contains documentation that a PRN medication was either received OR was offered but declined.

Coding Instructions for J0100C, Received Non-medication Intervention for Pain

- **Code 0, no:** if the medical record does not contain documentation that a non-medication pain intervention was received.

DEFINITIONS

SCHEDULED PAIN MEDICATION REGIMEN
Pain medication order that defines dose and specific time interval for pain medication administration. For example, "once a day," "every 12 hours."

PRN PAIN MEDICATIONS
Pain medication order that specifies dose and indicates that pain medication may be given on an as needed basis, including a time interval, such as "every 4 hours as needed for pain" or "every 6 hours as needed for pain."

NON-MEDICATION PAIN INTERVENTION
Scheduled and implemented non-pharmacological interventions include, but are not limited to: bio-feedback, application of heat/cold, massage, physical therapy, nerve block, stretching and strengthening exercises, chiropractic, electrical stimulation, radiotherapy, ultrasound and acupuncture. Herbal medications are not included in this category.

J0100: Pain Management (cont.)

- **Code 1, yes:** if the medical record contains documentation that a non-medication pain intervention was scheduled as part of the care plan and it is documented that the intervention was actually received and assessed for efficacy.

Coding Tips

- Code only pain medication regimens without PRN pain medications in J0100A. Code receipt of PRN pain medications in J0100B.
- For coding J0100B code only residents with PRN pain medication regimens here. If the resident has a scheduled pain medication J0100A should be coded.

Examples

1. The resident's medical record documents that she received the following pain management in the past 5 days:

   - Hydrocodone/acetaminophen 5/500 1 tab PO every 6 hours. Discontinued on day 1 of look-back period.
   - Acetaminophen 500mg PO every 4 hours. Started on day 2 of look-back period.
   - Cold pack to left shoulder applied by PT BID. PT notes that resident reports significant pain improvement after cold pack applied.

     Coding: J0100A would be **coded 1, yes**.
     Rationale: Medical record indicated that resident received a scheduled pain medication during the 5-day look-back period.
     Coding: J0100B would be **coded 0, no**.
     Rationale: No documentation was found in the medical record that resident received or was offered and declined any PRN medications during the 5-day look-back period.
     Coding: J0100C would be **coded 1, yes**.
     Rationale: The medical record indicates that the resident received scheduled non-medication pain intervention (cold pack to the left shoulder) during the 5-day look-back period.

2. The resident's medical record includes the following pain management documentation:

   - Morphine sulfate controlled-release 15 mg PO Q 12 hours: Resident refused every dose of medication during the 5-day look-back period. No other pain management interventions were documented.

     Coding: J0100A would be **coded 0, no.**
     Rationale: The medical record documented that the resident did not receive scheduled pain medication during the 5-day look-back period. Residents may refuse scheduled medications; however, medications are not considered "received" if the resident refuses the dose.

J0100: Pain Management (cont.)

Coding: J0100B would be **coded 0, no**.
Rationale: The medical record contained no documentation that the resident received or was offered and declined any PRN medications during the 5-day look-back period.
Coding: J0100C would be **coded 0, no**.
Rationale: The medical record contains no documentation that the resident received non-medication pain intervention during the 5-day look-back period.

J0200: Should Pain Assessment Interview Be Conducted?

J0200. Should Pain Assessment Interview be Conducted?
Attempt to conduct interview with all residents. If resident is comatose, skip to J1100, Shortness of Breath (dyspnea)
Enter Code [ ]   0. **No** (resident is rarely/never understood) → Skip to and complete J0800, Indicators of Pain or Possible Pain   1. **Yes** → Continue to J0300, Pain Presence

Item Rationale

Health-related Quality of Life

- Most residents who are capable of communicating can answer questions about how they feel.
- Obtaining information about pain directly from the resident, sometimes called "hearing the resident's voice," is more reliable and accurate than observation alone for identifying pain.
- If a resident cannot communicate (e.g., verbal, gesture, written), then staff observations for pain behavior (J0800 and J0850) will be used.

Planning for Care

- Interview allows the resident's voice to be reflected in the care plan.
- Information about pain that comes directly from the resident provides symptom-specific information for individualized care planning.

Steps for Assessment

1. Determine whether the resident is understood at least sometimes. Review **Language** item (A1100), to determine whether the resident needs or wants an interpreter.

- If an interpreter is needed or requested, every effort should be made to have an interpreter present for the MDS clinical interview.

J0200: Should Pain Assessment Interview Be Conducted? (cont.)

Coding Instructions

*Attempt to complete the interview if the resident is at least sometimes understood and an **interpreter is present** or not required.*

- **Code 0, no:** if the resident is rarely/never understood or an interpreter is required but not available. Skip to **Indicators of Pain or Possible Pain** item (J0800).
- **Code 1, yes:** if the resident is at least sometimes understood and an interpreter is present or not required. Continue to **Pain Presence** item (J0300).

Coding Tips and Special Populations

- If it is not possible for an interpreter to be present during the look-back period, code J0200 = 0 to indicate interview not attempted and complete **Staff Assessment of Pain** item (J0800), instead of the **Pain Interview** items (J0300-J0600).

J0300-J0600: Pain Assessment Interview

Pain Assessment Interview

J0300. Pain Presence
Enter Code ☐	Ask resident: **"Have you had pain or hurting at any time in the last 5 days?"** 0. **No** → Skip to J1100, Shortness of Breath 1. **Yes** → Continue to J0400, Pain Frequency 9. **Unable to answer** → Skip to J0800, Indicators of Pain or Possible Pain

J0400. Pain Frequency
Enter Code ☐	Ask resident: **"How much of the time have you experienced pain or hurting** over the last 5 days?" 1. **Almost constantly** 2. **Frequently** 3. **Occasionally** 4. **Rarely** 9. **Unable to answer**

J0500. Pain Effect on Function
Enter Code ☐	**A.** Ask resident: "*Over the past 5 days, has pain made it hard for you to sleep at night?*" 0. **No** 1. **Yes** 9. **Unable to answer**
Enter Code ☐	**B.** Ask resident: "*Over the past 5 days, have you limited your day-to-day activities because of pain?*" 0. **No** 1. **Yes** 9. **Unable to answer**

J0600. Pain Intensity - Administer **ONLY ONE** of the following pain intensity questions (A or B)
Enter Rating ☐☐	**A. Numeric Rating Scale (00-10)** Ask resident: "*Please rate your worst pain over the last 5 days on a zero to ten scale, with zero being no pain and ten as the worst pain you can imagine.*" (Show resident 00-10 pain scale) **Enter two-digit response. Enter 99 if unable to answer.**
Enter Code ☐	**B. Verbal Descriptor Scale** Ask resident: "*Please rate the intensity of your worst pain over the last 5 days.*" (Show resident verbal scale) 1. **Mild** 2. **Moderate** 3. **Severe** 4. **Very severe, horrible** 9. **Unable to answer**

J0300-J0600: Pain Assessment Interview (cont.)

Item Rationale

Health-related Quality of Life

- The effects of unrelieved pain impact the individual in terms of functional decline, complications of immobility, skin breakdown and infections.
- Pain significantly adversely affects a person's quality of life and is tightly linked to depression, diminished self-confidence and self-esteem, as well as an increase in behavior problems, particularly for cognitively-impaired residents.
- Some older adults limit their activities in order to avoid having pain. Their report of lower pain frequency may reflect their avoidance of activity more than it reflects adequate pain management.

Planning for Care

- Directly asking the resident about pain rather than relying on the resident to volunteer the information or relying on clinical observation significantly improves the detection of pain.
- Resident self-report is the most reliable means for assessing pain.
- Pain assessment provides a basis for evaluation treatment need and response to treatment.
- Assessing whether pain interferes with sleep or activities provides additional understanding of the functional impact of pain and potential care planning implications.
- Assessment of pain provides insight into the need to adjust the timing of pain interventions to better cover sleep or preferred activities.
- Pain assessment prompts discussion about factors that aggravate and alleviate pain.
- Similar pain stimuli can have varying impact on different individuals.
- Consistent use of a standardized pain intensity scale improves the validity and reliability of pain assessment. Using the same scale in different settings may improve continuity of care.
- Pain intensity scales allow providers to evaluate whether pain is responding to pain medication regime(s) and/or non-pharmacological intervention(s).

Steps for Assessment: Basic Interview Instructions for Pain Assessment Interview (J0300-J0600)

1. Interview any resident not screened out by the **Should Pain Assessment Interview be Conducted?** item (**J0200**).
2. The Pain Assessment Interview for residents consists of four items: the primary question **Pain Presence** item (J0300), and three follow-up questions **Pain Frequency** item (J0400); **Pain Effect on Function** item (J0500); and **Pain Intensity** item (J0600). If the resident is unable to answer the primary question on **Pain Presence** item J0300, skip to the **Staff Assessment for Pain** beginning with **Indicators of Pain or Possible Pain** item (J0800).

J0300-J0600: Pain Assessment Interview (cont.)

3. The look-back period on these items is 5 days. Because this item asks the resident to recall pain during the past 5 days, this assessment should be conducted close to the end of the 5-day look-back period; preferably on the day before, or the day of the ARD. This should more accurately capture pain episodes that occur during the 5-day look-back period.
4. Conduct the interview in a private setting.
5. Be sure the resident can hear you.

   • Residents with hearing impairment should be tested using their usual communication devices/techniques, as applicable.

   • Try an external assistive device (headphones or hearing amplifier) if you have any doubt about hearing ability.

   • Minimize background noise.

6. Sit so that the resident can see your face. Minimize glare by directing light sources away from the resident's face.
7. Give an introduction before starting the interview.
   Suggested language: "I'd like to ask you some questions about pain. The reason I am asking these questions is to understand how often you have pain, how severe it is, and how pain affects your daily activities. This will help us to develop the best plan of care to help manage your pain."
8. Directly ask the resident each item in J0300 through J0600 in the order provided.

   • Use other terms for pain or follow-up discussion if the resident seems unsure or hesitant. Some residents avoid use of the term "pain" but may report that they "hurt." Residents may use other terms such as "aching" or "burning" to describe pain.

9. If the resident chooses not to answer a particular item, accept their refusal and move on to the next item. **Code 9** and move to the next item.
10. If the resident is unsure about whether the pain occurred in the 5-day time interval, prompt the resident to think about the most recent episode of pain and try to determine whether it occurred within the look-back period.

> ### DEFINITIONS
>
> **PAIN** Any type of physical pain or discomfort in any part of the body. It may be localized to one area or may be more generalized. It may be acute or chronic, continuous or intermittent, or occur at rest or with movement. Pain is very subjective; pain is whatever the experiencing person says it is and exists whenever he or she says it does.

J0300: Pain Presence (5-Day Look Back)

Pain Assessment Interview
J0300. Pain Presence
Enter Code [ ] Ask resident: "***Have you had pain or hurting at any time* in the last 5 days?**" 0. **No** → Skip to J1100, Shortness of Breath 1. **Yes** → Continue to J0400, Pain Frequency 9. **Unable to answer** → Skip to J0800, Indicators of Pain or Possible Pain

J0300: Pain Presence (cont.)

Steps for Assessment

1. Ask the resident: "Have you had pain or hurting at any time in the last 5 days?"

Coding Instructions for J0300, **Pain Presence**

Code for the presence or absence of pain regardless of pain management efforts during the 5-day look-back period.

> **DEFINITIONS**
>
> **NONSENSICAL RESPONSE**
> Any unrelated, incomprehensible, or incoherent response that is not informative with respect to the item being coded.

- **Code 0, no:** if the resident responds "no" to any pain in the 5-day look-back period. **Code 0, no pain**, even if the reason for no pain is that the resident received pain management interventions. If coded 0, the pain interview is complete. Skip to **Shortness of Breath** item (J1100).

- **Code 1, yes:** if the resident responds "yes" to pain at any time during the look-back period. If coded 1, proceed to items J0400, J0500, J0600 AND J0700.

- **Code 9, unable to answer:** if the resident is unable to answer, does not respond, or gives a nonsensical response. If coded 9, skip to the Staff Assessment for Pain beginning with **Indicators of Pain or Possible Pain** item (J0800).

Coding Tips

- Rates of self-reported pain are higher than observed rates. Although some observers have expressed concern that residents may not complain and may deny pain, the regular and objective use of self-report pain scales enhances residents' willingness to report.

Examples

1. When asked about pain, Mrs. S. responds, "No. I have been taking the pain medication regularly, so fortunately I have had no pain."

    Coding: J0300 would be **coded 0, no**. The assessor would skip to **Shortness of Breath** item (J1100).
    Rationale: Mrs. S. reports having no pain during the look-back period. Even though she received pain management interventions during the look-back period, the item is coded "No," because there was no pain.

2. When asked about pain, Mr. T. responds, "No pain, but I have had a terrible burning sensation all down my leg."

    Coding: J0300 would be **coded 1, yes**. The assessor would proceed to **Pain Frequency** item (J0400).
    Rationale: Although Mr. T.'s initial response is "no," the comments indicate that he has experienced pain (burning sensation) during the look-back period.

J0300: Pain Presence (cont.)

3. When asked about pain, Ms. G. responds, "I was on a train in 1905."

> **Coding:** J0300 would be **coded 9, unable to respond.** The assessor would skip to **Indicators of Pain** item (J0800).
> **Rationale:** Ms. G. has provided a nonsensical answer to the question. The assessor will complete the **Staff Assessment for Pain** beginning with **Indicators of Pain** item (J0800).

J0400: Pain Frequency (5-Day Look Back)

J0400. Pain Frequency	
Enter Code ☐	Ask resident: *"How much of the time have you experienced pain or hurting over the last 5 days?"* 1. **Almost constantly** 2. **Frequently** 3. **Occasionally** 4. **Rarely** 9. **Unable to answer**

Steps for Assessment

1. Ask the resident: "How much of the time have you experienced pain or hurting over the last 5 days?" Staff may present response options on a written sheet or cue card. This can help the resident respond to the items.
2. If the resident provides a related response but does not use the provided response scale, help clarify the best response by echoing (repeating) the resident's own comment and providing related response options. This interview approach frequently helps the resident clarify which response option he or she prefers.
3. If the resident, despite clarifying statement and repeating response options, continues to have difficulty selecting between two of the provided responses, then select the more frequent of the two.

Coding Instructions

Code for pain frequency during the 5-day look-back period.

- **Code 1, almost constantly:** if the resident responds "almost constantly" to the question.
- **Code 2, frequently:** if the resident responds "frequently" to the question.
- **Code 3, occasionally:** if the resident responds "occasionally" to the question.
- **Code 4, rarely:** if the resident responds "rarely" to the question.
- **Code 9, unable to answer:** if the resident is unable to respond, does not respond, or gives a nonsensical response. Proceed to items J0500, J0600 AND J0700.

J0400: Pain Frequency (cont.)

Coding Tips

- No predetermined definitions are offered to the resident related to frequency of pain.
  - The response should be based on the resident's interpretation of the frequency options.
  - Facility policy should provide standardized tools to use throughout the facility in assessing pain to ensure consistency in interpretation and documentation of the resident's pain.

Examples

1. When asked about pain, Mrs. C. responds, "All the time. It has been a terrible week. I have not been able to get comfortable for more than 10 minutes at a time since I started physical therapy four days ago."

   Coding: J0400 would be **coded 1, almost constantly**.
   Rationale: Mrs. C. describes pain that has occurred "all the time."

2. When asked about pain, Mr. J. responds, "I don't know if it is frequent or occasional. My knee starts throbbing every time they move me from the bed or the wheelchair."

   The interviewer says: "Your knee throbs every time they move you. If you had to choose an answer, would you say that you have pain frequently or occasionally?"

   Mr. J. is still unable to choose between frequently and occasionally.

   Coding: J0400 would be **coded 2, frequently**.
   Rationale: The interviewer appropriately echoed Mr. J.'s comment and provided related response options to help him clarify which response he preferred. Mr. J. remained unable to decide between frequently and occasionally. The interviewer therefore coded for the higher frequency of pain.

3. When asked about pain, Miss K. responds: "I can't remember. I think I had a headache a few times in the past couple of days, but they gave me Tylenol and the headaches went away."

   The interviewer clarifies by echoing what Miss K. said: "You've had a headache a few times in the past couple of days and the headaches went away when you were given Tylenol. If you had to choose from the answers, would you say you had pain occasionally or rarely?"

   Miss K. replies "Occasionally."

   Coding: J0400 would be **coded 3, occasionally**.
   Rationale: After the interviewer clarified the resident's choice using echoing, the resident selected a response option.

198

J0400: Pain Frequency (cont.)

4. When asked about pain, Ms. M. responds, "I would say rarely. Since I started using the patch, I don't have much pain at all, but four days ago the pain came back. I think they were a bit overdue in putting on the new patch, so I had some pain for a little while that day."

> **Coding:** J0400 would be **coded 4, rarely**.
> **Rationale:** Ms. M. selected the "rarely" response option.

J0500: Pain Effect on Function (5-Day Look Back)

J0500.	Pain Effect on Function
Enter Code	**A.** Ask resident: *"Over the past 5 days, has pain made it hard for you to sleep at night?"* 0. **No** 1. **Yes** 9. **Unable to answer**
Enter Code	**B.** Ask resident: *"Over the past 5 days, have you limited your day-to-day activities because of pain?"* 0. **No** 1. **Yes** 9. **Unable to answer**

Steps for Assessment

1. Ask the resident each of the two questions exactly as they are written.
2. If the resident's response does not lead to a clear "yes" or "no" answer, repeat the resident's response and then try to narrow the focus of the response. For example, if the resident responded to the question, "Has pain made it hard for you to sleep at night?" by saying, "I always have trouble sleeping," then the assessor might reply, "You always have trouble sleeping. Is it your pain that makes it hard for you to sleep?

Coding Instructions for J0500A, Over the Past 5 Days, Has Pain Made It Hard for You to Sleep at Night?

- **Code 0, no:** if the resident responds "no," indicating that pain did not interfere with sleep.
- **Code 1, yes:** if the resident responds "yes," indicating that pain interfered with sleep.
- **Code 9, unable to answer:** if the resident is unable to answer the question, does not respond or gives a nonsensical response. Proceed to items J0500B, J0600 AND J0700.

Coding Instructions for J0500B, Over the Past 5 Days, Have You Limited Your Day-to-day Activities because of Pain?

- **Code 0, no:** if the resident indicates that pain did not interfere with daily activities.
- **Code 1, yes:** if the resident indicates that pain interfered with daily activities.
- **Code 9, unable to answer:** if the resident is unable to answer the question, does not respond or gives a nonsensical response. Proceed to items J0600 AND J0700.

Examples for J0500A, Over the Past 5 Days, Has Pain Made It Hard for You to Sleep at Night?

1. Mrs. D. responds, "I had a little back pain from being in the wheelchair all day, but it felt so much better when I went to bed. I slept like a baby."

    Coding: J0500A would be **coded 0, no.**

    Rationale: Mrs. D. reports no sleep problems related to pain.

2. Mr. E. responds, "I can't sleep at all in this place."
    The interviewer clarifies by saying, "You can't sleep here. Would you say that was because pain made it hard for you to sleep at night?"
    Mr. E. responds, "No. It has nothing to do with me. I have no pain. It is because everyone is making so much noise."

    Coding: J0500A would be **coded 0, no.**

    Rationale: Mr. E. reports that his sleep problems are not related to pain.

3. Miss G. responds, "Yes, the back pain makes it hard to sleep. I have to ask for extra pain medicine, and I still wake up several times during the night because my back hurts so much."

    Coding: J0500A would be **coded 1, yes.**

    Rationale: The resident reports pain-related sleep problems.

Examples for J0500B, Over the Past 5 Days, Have You Limited Your Day-to-day Activities because of Pain?

1. Ms. L. responds, "No, I had some pain on Wednesday, but I didn't want to miss the shopping trip, so I went."

    Coding: J0500B would be **coded 0, no.**

    Rationale: Although Ms. L. reports pain, she did not limit her activity because of it.

2. Mrs. N. responds, "Yes, I haven't been able to play the piano, because my shoulder hurts."

    Coding: J0500B would be **coded 1, yes.**

    Rationale: Mrs. N. reports limiting her activities because of pain.

3. Mrs. S. responds, "I don't know. I have not tried to knit since my finger swelled up yesterday, because I am afraid it might hurt even more than it does now."

    Coding: J0500B would be **coded 1, yes.**

    Rationale: Resident avoided a usual activity because of fear that her pain would increase.

4. Mr. Q. responds, "I don't like painful activities."
    Interviewer repeats question and Mr. Q. responds, "I designed a plane one time."

    Coding: J0500B would be **coded 9, unable to answer**.

    Rationale: Resident has provided a nonsensical answer to the question. Proceed to items J0600 AND J0700.

J0600: Pain Intensity (5-Day Look Back)

J0600. Pain Intensity - Administer **ONLY ONE** of the following pain intensity questions (A or B)	
Enter Rating ☐☐	**A. Numeric Rating Scale (00-10)** Ask resident: *"Please rate your worst pain over the last 5 days on a zero to ten scale, with zero being no pain and ten as the worst pain you can imagine."* (Show resident 00-10 pain scale) **Enter two-digit response. Enter 99 if unable to answer.**
Enter Code ☐	**B. Verbal Descriptor Scale** Ask resident: *"Please rate the intensity of your worst pain over the last 5 days."* (Show resident verbal scale) 1. **Mild** 2. **Moderate** 3. **Severe** 4. **Very severe, horrible** 9. **Unable to answer**

Steps for Assessment

1. You may use either **Numeric Rating Scale** item (J0600A) or **Verbal Descriptor Scale** item (J0600B) to interview the resident about pain intensity.

    • For each resident, try to use the same scale used on prior assessments.

2. If the resident is unable to answer using one scale, the other scale should be attempted.
3. Record **either** the **Numeric Rating Scale** item (J0600A) **or** the **Verbal Descriptor Scale** item (J0600B). Leave the response for the unused scale blank.
4. Read the question and item choices slowly. While reading, you may show the resident the response options (the 0-10 or verbal descriptor scale) clearly printed on a piece of paper, such as a cue card. Use large, clear print.

    • For 0-10 scale, say, "Please rate your worst pain over the last 5 days with zero being no pain, and ten as the worst pain you can imagine."

    • For **Verbal Descriptor Scale**, say, "Please rate the intensity of your worst pain over the last 5 days."

5. The resident may provide a verbal response, point to the written response, or both.

Coding Instructions for J0600A. Numeric Rating Scale (00-10)

Enter the two digit number (00-10) indicated by the resident as corresponding to the intensity of his or her worst pain during the 5-day look-back period, where zero is no pain, and 10 is the worst pain imaginable.

• Enter 99 if unable to answer.
• If the Numeric Rating Scale is not used, leave the response box blank.

Coding Instructions for J0600B. Verbal Descriptor Scale

• **Code 1, mild:** if resident indicates that his or her pain is "mild."

• **Code 2, moderate:** if resident indicates that his or her pain is "moderate."

• **Code 3, severe:** if resident indicates that his or her pain is "severe."

• **Code 4, very severe, horrible:** if resident indicates that his or her pain is "very severe or horrible."

J0600: Pain Intensity (cont.)

- **Code 9, unable to answer:** if resident is unable to answer, chooses not to respond, does not respond or gives a nonsensical response. Proceed to item J0700.
- If the **Verbal Descriptor Scale** is not used, leave the response box blank.

Examples for J0600A. Numeric Rating Scale (00-10)

1. The nurse asks Ms. T. to rate her pain on a scale of 0 to 10. Ms. T. states that she is not sure, because she has shoulder pain and knee pain, and sometimes it is really bad, and sometimes it is OK. The nurse reminds Ms. T. to think about all the pain she had during the last 5 days and select the number that describes her worst pain. She reports that her pain is a "6."

   Coding: J0600A would be **coded 06**.

   Rationale: The resident said her pain was 6 on the 0 to 10 scale. Because a 2-digit number is required, it is entered as 06.

2. The nurse asks Mr. S. to rate his pain, reviews use of the scale, and provides the 0 to 10 visual aid. Mr. S. says, "My pain doesn't have any numbers." The nurse explains that the numbers help the staff understand how severe his pain is, and repeats that the "0" end is no pain and the "10" end is the worst pain imaginable. Mr. S. replies, "I don't know where it would fall."

   Coding: Item J0600A would be **coded 99, unable to answer.** The interviewer would go on to ask about pain intensity using the **Verbal Descriptor Scale** item (J0600B).

   Rationale: The resident was unable to select a number or point to a location on the 0-10 scale that represented his level of pain intensity.

Examples for J0600B. Verbal Descriptor Scale

1. The nurse asks Mr. R. to rate his pain using the verbal descriptor scale. He looks at the response options presented using a cue card and says his pain is "severe" sometimes, but most of the time it is "mild."

   Coding: J0600B would be **coded 3, severe.**

   Rationale: The resident said his worst pain was "Severe."

2. The nurse asks Ms. U. to rate her pain, reviews use of the verbal descriptor scale, and provides a cue card as a visual aid. Ms. U. says, "I'm not sure whether it's mild or moderate." The nurse reminds Ms. U. to think about her worst pain during the last 5 days. Ms. U. says "At its worst, it was moderate."

   Coding: Item J0600B would be **coded 2, moderate.**

   Rationale: The resident indicated that her worst pain was "Moderate."

J0700: Should the Staff Assessment for Pain be Conducted? (5-Day Look Back)

J0700. Should the Staff Assessment for Pain be Conducted?	
Enter Code ☐	0. No (J0400 = 1 thru 4) → Skip to J1100, Shortness of Breath (dyspnea) 1. Yes (J0400 = 9) → Continue to J0800, Indicators of Pain or Possible Pain

Item Rationale

Item J0700 closes the pain interview and determines if the resident interview was complete or incomplete and based on this determination, whether a staff assessment needs to be completed.

Health-related Quality of Life

- Resident interview for pain is preferred because it improves the detection of pain. However, a small percentage of residents are unable or unwilling to complete the pain interview.
- Persons unable to complete the pain interview may still have pain.

Planning for Care

- Resident self-report is the most reliable means of assessing pain. However, when a resident is unable to provide the information, staff assessment is necessary.

> **DEFINITIONS**
>
> **COMPLETED INTERVIEW**
> The pain interview is successfully completed if the resident reported no pain (answered No to J0300), or if the resident reported pain (J0300=yes) and the follow-up question J0400 is answered.

- Even though the resident was unable to complete the interview, important insights may be gained from the responses that were obtained, observing behaviors and observing the resident's affect during the interview.

Steps for Assessment

1. Review the resident's responses to items J0200-J0400.
2. The **Staff Assessment for Pain** should only be completed if the **Pain Assessment Interview** (J0200-J0600) was not completed.

Coding Instructions for J0700. Should the Staff Assessment for Pain be Conducted? This item is to be coded at the completion of items J0400-J0600.

- **Code 0, no:** if the resident completed the **Pain Assessment Interview** item (J0400 = 1, 2, 3, or 4. Skip to **Shortness of Breath (dyspnea)** item (J1100).
- **Code 1, yes:** if the resident was unable to complete the **Pain Assessment Interview** (J0400 = 9). Continue to **Indicators of Pain or Possible Pain** item (J0800).

J0800: Indicators of Pain (5-Day Look Back)

*Complete this item only if the **Pain Assessment Interview** (J0200-J0600) was not completed.*

Staff Assessment for Pain		
J0800. Indicators of Pain or Possible Pain in the last 5 days		
↓ Check all that apply		
☐	**A.**	**Non-verbal sounds** (e.g., crying, whining, gasping, moaning, or groaning)
☐	**B.**	**Vocal complaints of pain** (e.g., that hurts, ouch, stop)
☐	**C.**	**Facial expressions** (e.g., grimaces, winces, wrinkled forehead, furrowed brow, clenched teeth or jaw)
☐	**D.**	**Protective body movements or postures** (e.g., bracing, guarding, rubbing or massaging a body part/area, clutching or holding a body part during movement)
☐	**Z.**	**None of these signs observed or documented** → If checked, skip to J1100, Shortness of Breath (dyspnea)

Item Rationale

Health-related Quality of Life

- Residents who cannot verbally communicate about their pain are at particularly high risk for underdetection and undertreatment of pain.
- Severe cognitive impairment may affect the ability of residents to verbally communicate, thus limiting the availability of self-reported information about pain. In this population, fewer complaints may not mean less pain.
- Individuals who are unable to verbally communicate may be more likely to use alternative methods of expression to communicate their pain.
- Even in this population some verbal complaints of pain may be made and should be taken seriously.

Planning for Care

- Consistent approach to observation improves the accuracy of pain assessment for residents who are unable to verbally communicate their pain.
- Particular attention should be paid to using the indicators of pain during activities when pain is most likely to be demonstrated (e.g., bathing, transferring, dressing, walking and potentially during eating).
- Staff must carefully monitor, track, and document any possible signs and symptoms of pain.
- Identification of these pain indicators can:
  — provide a basis for more comprehensive pain assessment,
  — provide a basis for determining appropriate treatment, and
  — provide a basis for ongoing monitoring of pain presence and treatment response.
- If pain indicators are present, assessment should identify aggravating/alleviating factors related to pain.

J0800: Indicators of Pain (cont.)

Steps for Assessment

DEFINITIONS

NON VERBAL SOUNDS
e.g., crying, whining, gasping, moaning, groaning or other audible indications associated with pain.

VOCAL COMPLAINTS OF PAIN
e.g., "That hurts," "ouch," "stop," etc.

FACIAL EXPRESSIONS THAT MAY BE INDICATORS OF PAIN
e.g., grimaces, winces, wrinkled forehead, furrowed brow, clenched teeth or jaw, etc.

PROTECTIVE BODY MOVEMENTS OR POSTURES
e.g., bracing, guarding, rubbing or massaging a body part/area, clutching or holding a body part during movement, etc.

1. **Review the medical record** for documentation of each indicator of pain listed in J0800 that occurred during the 5-day look-back period. If the record documents the presence of any of the signs and symptoms listed, confirm your record review with the direct care staff on all shifts who work most closely with the resident during activities of daily living (ADL).

2. **Interview staff** because the medical record may fail to note all observable pain behaviors. For any indicators that were not noted as present in medical record review, interview direct care staff on all shifts who work with the resident during ADL. Ask directly about the presence of each indicator that was not noted as being present in the record.

3. **Observe resident** during care activities. If you observe additional indicators of pain during the 5-day look-back period, code the corresponding items.

   • Observations for pain indicators may be more sensitive if the resident is observed during ADL, or wound care.

Coding Instructions

Check all that apply in the past 5 days based on staff observation of pain indicators.

• If the medical record review and the interview with direct care providers and observation on all shifts provide no evidence of pain indicators, Check J0800Z, None of these **signs observed or documented**, and proceed to **Shortness of Breath** item (J1100).

• **Check J0800A, non-verbal sounds:** included but not limited to if crying, whining, gasping, moaning, or groaning were observed or reported during the look-back period.

• **Check J0800B, vocal complaints of pain:** included but not limited to if the resident was observed to make vocal complaints of pain (e.g. "that hurts," "ouch," or "stop").

• **Check J0800C, facial expressions:** included but not limited to if grimaces, winces, wrinkled forehead, furrowed brow, clenched teeth or jaw were observed or reported during the look-back period.

• **Check J0800D, protective body movements or postures:** included but not limited to if bracing, guarding, rubbing or massaging a body part/area, or clutching or holding a body part during movement were observed or reported during the look-back period.

J0800: Indicators of Pain (cont.)

- **Check J0800Z, none of these signs observed or documented:** if none of these signs were observed or reported during the look-back period.

Coding Tips

- Behavior change, depressed mood, rejection of care and decreased activity participation may be related to pain. These behaviors and symptoms are identified in other sections and not reported here as pain screening items. However, the contribution of pain should be considered when following up on those symptoms and behaviors.

Examples

1. Mr. P. has advanced dementia and is unable to verbally communicate. A note in his medical record documents that he has been awake during the last night crying and rubbing his elbow. When you go to his room to interview the certified nurse aide (CNA) caring for him, you observe Mr. P. grimacing and clenching his teeth. The CNA reports that he has been moaning and said "ouch" when she tried to move his arm.

   Coding: **Non-verbal Sounds** item (J0800A); **Vocal Complaints of Pain** item (J0800B); **Facial Expressions** item (J0800C); and **Protective Body Movements or Postures** item (J0800D), would be **checked**.

   Rationale: Mr. P. has demonstrated vocal complaints of pain (ouch), non-verbal sounds (crying and moaning), facial expression of pain (grimacing and clenched teeth), and protective body movements (rubbing his elbow).

2. Mrs. M. has end-stage Parkinson's disease and is unable to verbally communicate. There is no documentation of pain in her medical record during the 5-day look-back period. The CNAs caring for her report that on some mornings she moans and winces when her arms and legs are moved during morning care. During direct observation, you note that Mrs. M. cries and attempts to pull her hand away when the CNA tries to open the contracted hand to wash it.

   Coding: **Non-verbal Sounds** items (J0800A); **Facial Expressions** item (J0800C); and **Protective Body Movements or Postures** item (J0800D), would be **checked**.

   Rationale: Mrs. M. has demonstrated non-verbal sounds (crying, moaning); facial expression of pain (wince), and protective body movements (attempt to withdraw).

3. Mrs. E. has been unable to verbally communicate following a massive cerebrovascular accident (CVA) several months ago and has a Stage 3 pressure ulcer. There is no documentation of pain in her medical record. The CNA who cares for her reports that she does not seem to have any pain. You observe the resident during her pressure ulcer dressing change. During the treatment, you observe groaning, facial grimaces, and a wrinkled forehead.

   Coding: **Non-verbal Sounds** item (J0800A), and **Facial Expressions** item (J0800C), would be **checked**.

   Rationale: The resident has demonstrated non-verbal sounds (groaning) and facial expression of pain (wrinkled forehead and grimacing).

J0800: Indicators of Pain (cont.)

Examples (cont.)

4. Mr. S. is in a persistent vegetative state following a traumatic brain injury. He is unable to verbally communicate. There is no documentation of pain in his medical record during the 5-day look-back period. The CNA reports that he appears comfortable whenever she cares for him. You observe the CNA providing morning care and transferring him from bed to chair. No pain indicators are observed at any time.

   Coding: None of These Signs Observed or Documented item (J0800Z), would be **checked**.

   Rationale: All steps for the assessment have been followed and no pain indicators have been documented, reported or directly observed.

J0850: Frequency of Indicator of Pain or Possible Pain (5-Day Look Back)

J0850. Frequency of Indicator of Pain or Possible Pain in the last 5 days	
Enter Code	Frequency with which resident complains or shows evidence of pain or possible pain 1. **Indicators of pain** or possible pain observed **1 to 2 days** 2. **Indicators of pain** or possible pain observed **3 to 4 days** 3. **Indicators of pain** or possible pain observed **daily**

Item Rationale

Health-related Quality of Life

- Unrelieved pain adversely affects function and mobility contributing to dependence, skin breakdown, contractures, and weight loss.
- Pain significantly adversely affects a person's quality of life and is tightly linked to depression, diminished self-confidence and self-esteem, as well as to an increase in behavior problems, particularly for cognitively impaired residents.

Planning for Care

- Assessment of pain frequency provides:
  — A basis for evaluating treatment need and response to treatment.
  — Information to aide in identifying optimum timing of treatment.

Steps for Assessment

1. Review medical record and interview staff and direct caregivers to determine the number of days the resident either complained of pain or showed evidence of pain as described in J0800 over the past 5 days.

J0850: Frequency of Indicator of Pain or Possible Pain (cont.)

Coding Instructions

Code for pain frequency over the last 5 days.

- **Code 1:** if based on staff observation, the resident complained or showed evidence of pain 1 to 2 days.
- **Code 2:** if based on staff observation, the resident complained or showed evidence of pain on 3 to 4 of the last 5 days.
- **Code 3:** if based on staff observation, the resident complained or showed evidence of pain on a daily basis.

Examples

1. Mr. M. is an 80-year old male with advanced dementia. During the 5-day look-back period, Mr. M. was noted to be grimacing and verbalizing "ouch" over the past 2 days when his right shoulder was moved.

   Coding: Item J0850 would be **coded 1, indicators of pain observed 1 to 2 days.**
   Rationale: He has demonstrated vocal complaints of pain ("ouch"), facial expression of pain (grimacing) on 2 of the last 5 days.

2. Mrs. C. is a 78-year old female with a history of CVA with expressive aphasia and dementia. During the 5-day look-back period, the resident was noted on a daily basis to be rubbing her right knee and grimacing.

   Coding: Item J0850 would be **coded 3, indicators of pain observed daily.**
   Rationale: The resident was observed with a facial expression of pain (grimacing) and protective body movements (rubbing her knee) every day during the look-back period.

J1100: Shortness of Breath (dyspnea)

	J1100. Shortness of Breath (dyspnea)	
	↓ Check all that apply	
☐	A.	**Shortness of breath** or trouble breathing **with exertion** (e.g., walking, bathing, transferring)
☐	B.	**Shortness of breath** or trouble breathing **when sitting at rest**
☐	C.	**Shortness of breath** or trouble breathing **when lying flat**
☐	Z.	**None of the above**

Item Rationale

Health-related Quality of Life

- Shortness of breath can be an extremely distressing symptom to residents and lead to decreased interaction and quality of life.
- Some residents compensate for shortness of breath by limiting activity. They sometimes compensate for shortness of breath when lying flat by elevating the head of the bed and do not alert caregivers to the problem.

J1100: Shortness of Breath (dyspnea) (cont.)

Planning for Care

- Shortness of breath can be an indication of a change in condition requiring further assessment and should be explored.
- The care plan should address underlying illnesses that may exacerbate symptoms of shortness of breath as well as symptomatic treatment for shortness of breath when it is not quickly reversible.

Steps for Assessment

Interview the resident about shortness of breath. Many residents, including those with mild to moderate dementia, may be able to provide feedback about their own symptoms.

1. If the resident is not experiencing shortness of breath or trouble breathing during the interview, ask the resident if shortness of breath occurs when he or she engages in certain activities.
2. Review the medical record for staff documentation of the presence of shortness of breath or trouble breathing. Interview staff on all shifts, and family/significant other regarding resident history of shortness of breath, allergies or other environmental triggers of shortness of breath.
3. Observe the resident for shortness of breath or trouble breathing. Signs of shortness of breath include: increased respiratory rate, pursed lip breathing, a prolonged expiratory phase, audible respirations and gasping for air at rest, interrupted speech pattern (only able to say a few words before taking a breath) and use of shoulder and other accessory muscles to breathe.
4. If shortness of breath or trouble breathing is observed, note whether it occurs with certain positions or activities.

Coding Instructions

Check all that apply during the 7-day look-back period.

Any evidence of the presence of a symptom of shortness of breath should be captured in this item. A resident may have any combination of these symptoms.

- **Check J1100A:** if shortness of breath or trouble breathing is present when the resident is engaging in activity. Shortness of breath could be present during activity as limited as turning or moving in bed during daily care or with more strenuous activity such as transferring, walking, or bathing. If the resident avoids activity or is unable to engage in activity because of shortness of breath, then code this as present.
- **Check J1100B:** if shortness of breath or trouble breathing is present when the resident is sitting at rest.
- **Check J1100C:** if shortness of breath or trouble breathing is present when the resident attempts to lie flat. Also code this as present if the resident avoids lying flat because of shortness of breath.
- **Check J1100Z:** if the resident reports no shortness of breath or trouble breathing and the medical record and staff interviews indicate that shortness of breath appears to be absent or well controlled with current medication.

J1100: Shortness of Breath (dyspnea) (cont.)

Examples

1. Mrs. W. has diagnoses of chronic obstructive pulmonary disease (COPD) and heart failure. She is on 2 liters of oxygen and daily respiratory treatments. With oxygen she is able to ambulate and participate in most group activities. She reports feeling "winded" when going on outings that require walking one or more blocks and has been observed having to stop to rest several times under such circumstances. Recently, she describes feeling "out of breath" when she tries to lie down.

   Coding: J1100A and J1100C would be **checked.**
   Rationale: Mrs. W. reported being short of breath when lying down as well as during outings that required ambulating longer distances.

2. Mr. T. has used an inhaler for years. He is not typically noted to be short of breath. Three days ago, during a respiratory illness, he had mild trouble with his breathing, even when sitting in bed. His shortness of breath also caused him to limit group activities.

   Coding: J1100A and J1100B would be **checked.**
   Rationale: Mr. T. was short of breath at rest and was noted to avoid activities because of shortness of breath.

J1300: Current Tobacco Use

J1300. Current Tobacco Use	
Enter Code	Tobacco use
	0. No
	1. Yes

Item Rationale

Health-related Quality of Life

- The negative effects of smoking can shorten life expectancy and create health problems that interfere with daily activities and adversely affect quality of life.

Planning for Care

- This item opens the door to negotiation of a plan of care with the resident that includes support for smoking cessation.
- If cessation is declined, a care plan that allows safe and environmental accommodation of resident preferences is needed.

Steps for Assessment

1. Ask the resident if he or she used tobacco in any form during the 7-day look-back period.
2. If the resident states that he or she used tobacco in some form during the 7-day look-back period, **code 1, yes**.

DEFINITIONS

TOBACCO USE
Includes tobacco used in any form.

J1300: Current Tobacco Use (cont.)

3. If the resident is unable to answer or indicates that he or she did not use tobacco of any kind during the look-back period, review the medical record and interview staff for any indication of tobacco use by the resident during the look-back period.

Coding Instructions

- **Code 0, no:** if there are no indications that the resident used any form of tobacco.
- **Code 1, yes:** if the resident or any other source indicates that the resident used tobacco in some form during the look-back period.

J1400: Prognosis

J1400. Prognosis	
Enter Code ☐	Does the resident have a condition or chronic disease that may result in a **life expectancy of less than 6 months?** (Requires physician documentation) 0. No 1. Yes

Item Rationale

Health-related Quality of Life

- Residents with conditions or diseases that may result in a life expectancy of less than 6 months have special needs and may benefit from palliative or hospice services in the nursing home.

Planning for Care

- If life expectancy is less than 6 months, interdisciplinary team care planning should be based on the resident's preferences for goals and interventions of care whenever possible.

Steps for Assessment

1. Review the medical record for documentation by the physician that the resident's condition or chronic disease may result in a life expectancy of less than 6 months, or that they have a terminal illness.
2. If the physician states that the resident's life expectancy may be less than 6 months, request that he or she document this in the medical record. Do not code until there is documentation in the medical record.
3. Review the medical record to determine whether the resident is receiving hospice services.

> **DEFINITIONS**
>
> **CONDITION OR CHRONIC DISEASE THAT MAY RESULT IN A LIFE EXPECTANCY OF LESS THAN 6 MONTHS** In the physician's judgment, the resident has a diagnosis or combination of clinical conditions that have advanced (or will continue to deteriorate) to a point that the average resident with that level of illness would not be expected to survive more than 6 months.
>
> This judgment should be substantiated by a physician note. It can be difficult to pinpoint the exact life expectancy for a single resident. Physician judgment should be based on typical or average life expectancy of residents with similar level of disease burden as this resident.

J1400: Prognosis (cont.)

Coding Instructions

- **Code 0, no:** if the medical record does not contain physician documentation that the resident has a terminal disease or a condition or chronic disease that may result in a life expectancy of less than 6 months and the resident is not receiving hospice services.
- **Code 1, yes:** if the medical record includes physician documentation that the resident has a terminal disease or that the resident's condition or chronic disease may result in a life expectancy of less than 6 months or whether the resident is receiving hospice services.

Examples

1. Mrs. T. has a diagnosis of heart failure. During the past few months, she has had three hospital admissions for acute heart failure. Her heart has become significantly weaker despite maximum treatment with medications and oxygen. Her physician has discussed her deteriorating condition with her and her family and has documented that her prognosis for survival beyond the next couple of months is poor.

   Coding: J1400 would be **coded 1, yes**.
   Rationale: The physician documented that her life expectancy is likely to be less than 6 months.

> **DEFINITIONS**
>
> **HOSPICE SERVICES**
> A program for terminally ill persons where an array of services is provided for the palliation and management of terminal illness and related conditions. The hospice must be licensed by the state as a hospice provider and/or certified under the Medicare program as a hospice provider.

2. Mr. J. was diagnosed with non-small cell lung cancer that is metastatic to his bone. He is not a candidate for surgical or curative treatment. With his consent, Mr. J. has been referred to hospice by his physician, who documented that his life expectancy was less than 6 months.

   Coding: J1400 would be **coded 1, yes**.
   Rationale: The physician referred the resident to hospice and documented that his life expectancy is likely to be less than 6 months.

J1550: Problem Conditions

J1550. Problem Conditions	
↓ Check all that apply	
☐	A. Fever
☐	B. Vomiting
☐	C. Dehydrated
☐	D. Internal bleeding
☐	Z. None of the above

J1550: Problem Conditions (cont.)

Intent: This item provides an opportunity for screening in the areas of fever, vomiting, fluid deficits, and internal bleeding. Clinical screenings provide indications for further evaluation, diagnosis and clinical care planning.

Item Rationale

Health-related Quality of Life

- Timely assessment is needed to identify underlying causes and risk for complications.

Planning for Care

- Implementation of care plans to treat underlying causes and avoid complications is critical.

Steps for Assessment

1. Review the medical record, interview staff on all shifts and observe the resident for any indication that the resident had vomiting, fever, potential signs of dehydration, or internal bleeding during the 7-day look-back period.

Coding Instructions

Check all that apply (blue box)

- **J1550A,** fever
- **J1550B,** vomiting
- **J1550D,** dehydrated
- **J1550H,** internal bleeding
- **J1550Z,** none of the above

Coding Tips

- **Fever:** Fever is defined as a temperature 2.4 degrees F higher than baseline. The resident's baseline temperature should be established prior to the Assessment Reference Date.
- **Fever assessment prior to establishing base line temperature:** A temperature of 100.4 degrees F (38 degrees C) on admission (i.e., prior to the establishment of the baseline temperature) would be considered a fever.
- **Vomiting:** Regurgitation of stomach contents; may be caused by many factors (e.g., drug toxicity, infection, psychogenic).

J1550: Problem Conditions (cont.)

- **Dehydrated:** Check this item if the resident presents with two or more of the following potential indicators for dehydration:

  1. Resident takes in less than the recommended 1,500 ml of fluids daily (water or liquids in beverages and water in foods with high fluid content, such as gelatin and soups). Note: The recommended intake level has been changed from 2,500 ml to 1,500 ml to reflect current practice standards.
  2. Resident has one or more clinical signs of dehydration, **including but not limited to** dry mucous membranes, poor skin turgor, cracked lips, thirst, sunken eyes, dark urine, new onset or increased confusion, fever, or abnormal laboratory values (e.g., elevated hemoglobin and hematocrit, potassium chloride, sodium, albumin, blood urea nitrogen, or urine specific gravity).
  3. Resident's fluid loss exceeds the amount of fluids he or she takes in (e.g., loss from vomiting, fever, diarrhea that exceeds fluid replacement).

- **Internal Bleeding:** Bleeding may be frank (such as bright red blood) or occult (such as guaiac positive stools). Clinical indicators include black, tarry stools, vomiting "coffee grounds," hematuria (blood in urine), hemoptysis (coughing up blood), and severe epistaxis (nosebleed) that requires packing. However, nose bleeds that are easily controlled, menses, or a urinalysis that shows a small amount of red blood cells should not be coded as internal bleeding.

J1700: Fall History on Admission

J1700. Fall History on Admission	
Complete only if A0310A = 01 or A0310E = 1	
Enter Code	**A.** Did the resident have a fall any time in the **last month** prior to admission? 0. **No** 1. **Yes** 9. **Unable to determine**
Enter Code	**B.** Did the resident have a fall any time in the **last 2-6 months** prior to admission? 0. **No** 1. **Yes** 9. **Unable to determine**
Enter Code	**C.** Did the resident have any **fracture related to a fall in the 6 months** prior to admission? 0. **No** 1. **Yes** 9. **Unable to determine**

Item Rationale

Health-related Quality of Life

- Falls are a leading cause of injury, morbidity, and mortality in older adults.
- A previous fall, especially a recent fall, recurrent falls, and falls with significant injury are the most important predictors of risk for future falls and injurious falls.
- Persons with a history of falling may limit activities because of a fear of falling and should be evaluated for reversible causes of falling.

J1700: Fall History on Admission (cont.)

Planning for Care

- Determine the potential need for further assessment and intervention, including evaluation of the resident's need for rehabilitation or assistive devices.
- Evaluate the physical environment as well as staffing needs for residents who are at risk for falls.

Steps for Assessment

The period of review is 180 days (6 months) prior to admission, looking back from the resident's entry date (A1600).

1. Ask the resident and family or significant other about a history of falls in the month prior to admission and in the 6 months prior to admission. This would include any fall, no matter where it occurred.
2. Review inter-facility transfer information (if the resident is being admitted from another facility) for evidence of falls.
3. Review all relevant medical records received from facilities where the resident resided during the previous 6 months; also review any other medical records received for evidence of one or more falls.

Coding Instructions for J1700A, Did the Resident Have a Fall Any Time in the Last Month Prior to Admission?

> **DEFINITIONS**
>
> **FALL**
> Unintentional change in position coming to rest on the ground, floor or onto the next lower surface (e.g., onto a bed, chair, or bedside mat). The fall may be witnessed, reported by the resident or an observer or identified when a resident is found on the floor or ground. Falls include any fall, no matter whether it occurred at home, while out in the community, in an acute hospital or a nursing home. Falls are not a result of an overwhelming external force (e.g., a resident pushes another resident).
>
> An intercepted fall occurs when the resident would have fallen if he or she had not caught him/herself or had not been intercepted by another person – this is still considered a fall.

- **Code 0, no:** if resident and family report no falls and transfer records and medical records do not document a fall in the month preceding the resident's entry date item (A1600).

- **Code 1, yes:** if resident or family report or transfer records or medical records document a fall in the month preceding the resident's entry date item (A1600).

- **Code 9, unable to determine:** if the resident is unable to provide the information or if the resident and family are not available or do not have the information and medical record information is inadequate to determine whether a fall occurred.

J1700: Fall History on Admission (cont.)

Coding Instructions for J1700B, Did the Resident Have a Fall Any Time in the Last 2-6 Months prior to Admission?

- **Code 0, no:** if resident and family report no falls and transfer records and medical records do not document a fall in the 2-6 months prior to the resident's entry date item (A1600).

- **Code 1, yes:** if resident or family report or transfer records or medical records document a fall in the 2-6 months prior to the resident's entry date item (A1600).

- **Code 9, unable to determine:** if the resident is unable to provide the information, **or** if the resident and family are not available or do not have the information, and medical record information is inadequate to determine whether a fall occurred.

Coding Instructions for J1700C. Did the Resident Have Any Fracture Related to a Fall in the 6 Months prior to Admission?

- **Code 0, no:** if resident and family report no fractures related to falls and transfer records and medical records do not document a fracture related to fall in the 6 months (0-180 days) preceding the resident's entry date item (A1600).

- **Code 1, yes:** if resident or family report or transfer records or medical records document a fracture related to fall in the 6 months (0-180 days) preceding the resident's entry date item (A1600).

- **Code 9, unable to determine:** if the resident is unable to provide the information, **or** if the resident and family are not available or do not have the information, and medical record information is inadequate to determine whether a fall occurred.

> **DEFINITIONS**
>
> **FRACTURE RELATED TO A FALL**
> Any documented bone fracture (in a problem list from a medical record, an x-ray report, or by history of the resident or caregiver) that occurred as a direct result of a fall or was recognized and later attributed to the fall. Do not include fractures caused by trauma related to car crashes or pedestrian versus car accidents or impact of another person or object against the resident.

Examples

1. On admission interview, Mrs. J. is asked about falls and says she has "not really fallen." However, she goes on to say that when she went shopping with her daughter about 2 weeks ago, her walker got tangled with the shopping cart and she slipped down to the floor.

   Coding: J1700A would be **coded 1, yes**.
   Rationale: Falls caused by slipping meet the definition of falls.

J1700: Fall History on Admission (cont.)

2. On admission interview a resident denies a history of falling. However, her daughter says that she found her mother on the floor near her toilet twice about 3-4 months ago.

   Coding: J1700B would be **coded 1, yes**.
   Rationale: If the individual is found on the floor, a fall is assumed to have occurred.

3. On admission interview, Mr. M. and his family deny any history of falling. However, nursing notes in the transferring hospital record document that Mr. M. repeatedly tried to get out of bed unassisted at night to go to the bathroom and was found on a mat placed at his bedside to prevent injury the week prior to nursing home transfer.

   Coding: J1700A would be **coded 1, yes**.
   Rationale: Medical records from an outside facility document that Mr. M. was found on a mat on the floor. This is defined as a fall.

4. Medical records note that Miss K. had hip surgery 5 months prior to admission to the nursing home. Miss K.'s daughter says the surgery was needed to fix a broken hip due to a fall.

   Coding: Both J1700B and J1700C would be **coded 1, yes**.
   Rationale: Miss K. had a fall related fracture 1-6 months prior to nursing home entry.

5. Mr. O.'s hospital transfer record includes a history of osteoporosis and vertebral compression fractures. The record does not mention falls, and Mr. O. denies any history of falling.

   Coding: J1700C would be **coded 0, no**.
   Rationale: The fractures were not related to a fall.

6. Ms. P. has a history of a "Colle's fracture" of her left wrist about 3 weeks before nursing home admission. Her son recalls that the fracture occurred when Ms. P. tripped on a rug and fell forward on her outstretched hands.

   Coding: Both J1700A and J1700C would be **coded 1, yes**.
   Rationale: Ms. P. had a fall-related fracture less than 1 month prior to entry.

J1800: Any Falls Since Admission or Prior Assessment (OBRA or PPS), whichever is more recent

J1800. Any Falls Since Admission or Prior Assessment (OBRA, PPS, or Discharge), whichever is more recent	
Enter Code ☐	Has the resident had any falls since admission or the prior assessment (OBRA, PPS, or Discharge), whichever is more recent? 0. No → Skip to K0100, Swallowing Disorder 1. Yes → Continue to J1900, Number of Falls Since Admission or Prior Assessment (OBRA, PPS, or Discharge)

Item Rationale

Health-related Quality of Life

- Falls are a leading cause of morbidity and mortality among nursing home residents.

- Falls result in serious injury, especially hip fractures.

- Fear of falling can limit an individual's activity and negatively impact quality of life.

> **DEFINITIONS**
>
> **PRIOR ASSESSMENT**
> Most recent MDS assessment that reported on falls.

J1800: Any Falls Since Admission or Prior Assessment (cont.)

Planning for Care

- Identification of residents who are at high risk of falling is a top priority for care planning. A previous fall is the most important predictor of risk for future falls.
- Falls may be an indicator of functional decline and development of other serious conditions such as delirium, adverse drug reactions, dehydration, and infections.
- External risk factors include medication side effects, use of appliances and restraints, and environmental conditions.
- A fall should stimulate evaluation of the resident's need for rehabilitation, ambulation aids, modification of the physical environment, or additional monitoring (e.g., toileting, to avoid incontinence).

Steps for Assessment

1. If this is the first assessment (A0310E = 1), review the medical record for the time period from the admission date to the ARD.
2. If this is not the first assessment (A0310E = 0), the review period is from the day after the ARD of the last MDS assessment to the ARD of the current assessment.
3. Review all available sources for any fall since the last assessment, no matter whether it occurred while out in the community, in an acute hospital, or in the nursing home. Include medical records generated in any health care setting since last assessment.
4. Review nursing home incident reports, fall logs and the medical record (physician, nursing, therapy, and nursing assistant notes).
5. Ask the resident and family about falls during the look-back period. Resident and family reports of falls should be captured here whether or not these incidents are documented in the medical record.

Coding Instructions

- **Code 0, no:** if the resident has not had any fall since the last assessment. Skip to **Swallowing Disorder** item (K0100).
- **Code 1, yes:** if the resident has fallen since the last assessment. Continue to **Number of Falls Since Admission or Prior Assessment (OBRA or PPS)** item (J1900), whichever is more recent.

Examples

1. An incident report describes an event in which Mr. S. was walking down the hall and appeared to slip on a wet spot on the floor. He lost his balance and bumped into the wall, but was able to grab onto the hand rail and steady himself.

   Coding: J1800 would be **coded 1, yes**.
   Rationale: An intercepted fall is considered a fall.

J1900: Number of Falls Since Admission or Prior Assessment (OBRA or PPS), whichever is more recent

J1900. Number of Falls Since Admission or Prior Assessment (OBRA, PPS, or Discharge), whichever is more recent		
	↓ Enter Codes in Boxes	
Coding: 0. None 1. One 2. Two or more	☐	**A. No injury** - no evidence of any injury is noted on physical assessment by the nurse or primary care clinician; no complaints of pain or injury by the resident; no change in the resident's behavior is noted after the fall
	☐	**B. Injury (except major)** - skin tears, abrasions, lacerations, superficial bruises, hematomas and sprains; or any fall-related injury that causes the resident to complain of pain
	☐	**C. Major injury** - bone fractures, joint dislocations, closed head injuries with altered consciousness, subdural hematoma

Item Rationale

Health-related Quality of Life

- Falls are a leading cause of morbidity and mortality among nursing home residents.
- Falls result in serious injury, especially hip fractures.
- Previous falls, especially recurrent falls and falls with injury, are the most important predictor of future falls and injurious falls.

> **DEFINITIONS**
>
> **INJURY RELATED TO A FALL**
> Any documented injury that occurred as a result of, or was recognized within a short period of time (e.g., hours to a few days) after the fall and attributed to the fall.

Planning for Care

- Identification of residents who are at high risk of falling is a top priority for care planning.
- Falls indicate functional decline and other serious conditions such as delirium, adverse drug reactions, dehydration, and infections.
- External risk factors include medication side effects, use of appliances and restraints, and environmental conditions.
- A fall should stimulate evaluation of the resident's need for rehabilitation or ambulation aids and of the need for monitoring or modification of the physical environment.

Steps for Assessment

1. If this is the first assessment (A0310E = 1), review the medical record for the time period from the admission date to the ARD.
2. If this is not the first assessment (A0310E = 0), the review period is from the day after the ARD of the last MDS assessment to the ARD of the current assessment.

> **DEFINITIONS**
>
> **INJURY (EXCEPT MAJOR)**
> Includes skin tears, abrasions, lacerations, superficial bruises, hematomas, and sprains; or any fall-related injury that causes the resident to complain of pain.
>
> **MAJOR INJURY**
> Includes bone fractures, joint dislocations, closed head injuries with altered consciousness, subdural hematoma.

J1900: Number of Falls Since Admission or Prior Assessment (cont.)

3. Review all available sources for any fall since the last assessment, no matter whether it occurred while out in the community, in an acute hospital, or in the nursing home. Include medical records generated in any health care setting since last assessment. All relevant records received from acute and post-acute facilities where the resident was admitted during the look-back period should be reviewed for evidence of one or more falls.

4. Review nursing home incident reports and medical record (physician, nursing, therapy, and nursing assistant notes) for falls and level of injury.

5. Ask the resident, staff, and family about falls during the look-back period. Resident and family reports of falls should be captured here, whether or not these incidents are documented in the medical record.

Coding Instructions for J1900

Determine the number of falls that occurred since admission or prior assessment and code the level of fall-related injury for each. Code each fall only once.

- If the resident has multiple injuries in a single fall, code the fall for the highest level of injury.

Coding Instructions for J1900A, No Injury

- **Code 0, none:** if the resident had no injurious fall since the admission or prior assessment.

- **Code 1, one:** if the resident had one injurious fall since admission or prior assessment.

- **Code 2, two or more:** if the resident had two or more injurious falls since admission or prior assessment.

Coding Instructions for J1900B, Injury (Except Major)

- **Code 0, none:** if the resident had no injurious fall (except major) since admission or prior assessment.

- **Code 1, one:** if the resident had one injurious fall (except major) since admission or prior assessment.

- **Code 2, two or more:** if the resident had two or more injurious falls (except major) since admission or prior assessment.

Coding Instructions for J1900C, Major Injury

- **Code 0, none:** if the resident had no major injurious fall since admission or prior assessment.

- **Code 1, one:** if the resident had one major injurious fall since admission or prior assessment.

J1900: Number of Falls Since Admission or Prior Assessment (cont.)

- **Code 2, two or more:** if the resident had two or more major injurious falls since admission or prior assessment.

Examples

1. A nursing note states that Mrs. K. slipped out of her wheelchair onto the floor while at the dining room table. Before being assisted back into her chair, an assessment was completed that indicated no injury.

   Coding: J1900A would be **coded 1, one**

   Rationale: Slipping to the floor is a fall. No injury was noted.

2. Nurse's notes describe a situation in which Ms. Z. went out with her family for dinner. When they returned, her son stated that while at the restaurant, she went to the bathroom and the door closed against her walker, causing her to lose balance and fall. No injury was noted when she returned from dinner.

   Coding: J1900A would be **coded 1, one**

   Rationale: Falls during the nursing home stay, even if on outings, are captured here.

3. A nurse's note describes a resident who, while being treated for pneumonia, climbed over his bedrails and fell to the floor. He had a cut over his left eye and some swelling on his arm. He was sent to the emergency room, where X-rays revealed no injury and neurological checks revealed no changes in mental status.

   Coding: J1900B would be **coded 1, one**

   Rationale: Lacerations and swelling without fracture are classified as injury (except major).

4. A resident fell, lacerated his head, and head CT scan indicated a subdural hematoma.

   Coding: J1900C would be **coded 1, one**

   Rationale: Subdural hematoma is a major injury. The injury occurred as a result of a fall.

SECTION K: SWALLOWING/NUTRITIONAL STATUS

Intent: The items in this section are intended to assess the many conditions that could affect the resident's ability to maintain adequate nutrition and hydration. This section covers swallowing disorders, height and weight, weight loss, and nutritional approaches. Nurse assessors should collaborate with the dietitian and dietary staff to ensure that items in this section have been assessed and calculated accurately.

K0100: Swallowing Disorder

K0100. Swallowing Disorder	
Signs and symptoms of possible swallowing disorder	
↓ Check all that apply	
☐	A. Loss of liquids/solids from mouth when eating or drinking
☐	B. Holding food in mouth/cheeks or residual food in mouth after meals
☐	C. Coughing or choking during meals or when swallowing medications
☐	D. Complaints of difficulty or pain with swallowing
☐	Z. None of the above

Item Rationale

Health-related Quality of Life

- The ability to swallow safely can be affected by many disease processes and functional decline.

- Alterations in the ability to swallow can result in choking and aspiration, which can increase the resident's risk for malnutrition, dehydration, and aspiration pneumonia.

Planning for Care

- Care planning should include provisions for monitoring the resident during mealtimes and during functions/activities that include the consumption of food and liquids.

- When necessary, the resident should be evaluated by the physician, speech language pathologist and/or occupational therapist to assess for any need for swallowing therapy and/or to provide recommendations regarding the consistency of food and liquids.

- Assess for signs and symptoms that suggest a swallowing disorder that has not been successfully treated or managed with diet modifications or other interventions (e.g., tube feeding, double swallow, turning head to swallow, etc.) and therefore represents a functional problem for the resident.

- Care plan should be developed to assist resident to maintain safe and effective swallow using compensatory techniques, alteration in diet consistency, and positioning during and following meals.

K0100: Swallowing/Nutritional Status (cont.)

Steps for Assessment

1. Ask the resident if he or she has had any difficulty swallowing during the 7-day look-back period. Ask about each of the symptoms in K0100A through K0100D.

   Observe the resident during meals or at other times when he or she is eating, drinking, or swallowing to determine whether any of the listed symptoms of possible swallowing disorder are exhibited.

2. Interview staff members on all shifts who work with the resident and ask if any of the four listed symptoms were evident during the 7-day look-back period.

3. Review the medical record, including nursing, physician, dietician, and speech language pathologist notes, and any available information on dental history or problems. Dental problems may include poor fitting dentures, dental caries, edentulous, mouth sores, tumors and/or pain with food consumption.

Coding Instructions

Check all that apply.

- **K0100A, loss of liquids/solids from mouth when eating or drinking.** When the resident has food or liquid in his or her mouth, the food or liquid dribbles down chin or falls out of the mouth.

- **K0100B, holding food in mouth/cheeks or residual food in mouth after meals.** Holding food in mouth or cheeks for prolonged periods of time (sometimes labeled pocketing) or food left in mouth because resident failed to empty mouth completely.

- **K0100C, coughing or choking during meals or when swallowing medications.** The resident may cough or gag, turn red, have more labored breathing, or have difficulty speaking when eating, drinking, or taking medications. The resident may frequently complain of food or medications "going down the wrong way."

- **K0100D, complaints of difficulty or pain with swallowing.** Resident may refuse food because it is painful or difficult to swallow.

- **K0100Z, none of the above:** if none of the K0100A through K0100D signs or symptoms were present during the look-back.

Coding Tips

- Do not code a swallowing problem when interventions have been successful in treating the problem and therefore the signs/symptoms of the problem (K0100A through K0100D) did not occur during the 7-day look-back period.

- Code even if the symptom occurred only once in the 7-day look-back period.

K0200: Height and Weight

K0200. Height and Weight - While measuring, if the number is X.1 - X.4 round down; X.5 or greater round up

☐☐ inches	**A. Height** (in inches). Record most recent height measure since admission
☐☐☐ pounds	**B. Weight** (in pounds). Base weight on most recent measure in last 30 days; measure weight consistently, according to standard facility practice (e.g., in a.m. after voiding, before meal, with shoes off, etc.)

Item Rationale

Health-related Quality of Life

- Diminished nutritional and hydration status can lead to debility that can adversely affect health and safety as well as quality of life.

Planning for Care

- Height and weight measurements assist staff with assessing the resident's nutrition and hydration status by providing a mechanism for monitoring stability of weight over a period of time. The measurement of weight is one guide for determining nutritional status.

Steps for Assessment for K0200A, **Height**

1. On admission, measure and record height in inches.
2. Measure height consistently over time in accordance with the facility policy and procedure, which should reflect current standards of practice (shoes off, etc.).
3. For subsequent assessments, check the medical record. If the last height recorded was more than one year ago, measure and record the resident's height again.

Coding Instructions for K0200A, **Height**

- Record height to the nearest whole inch.
- Use mathematical rounding (i.e., if height measurement is X.5 inches or greater, round height upward to the nearest whole inch. If height measurement number is X.1 to X.4 inches, round down to the nearest whole inch). For example, a height of 62.5 inches would be rounded to 63 inches and a height of 62.4 inches would be rounded to 62 inches.

Steps for Assessment for K0200B, **Weight**

1. On admission, weigh the resident and record results.
2. For subsequent assessments, check the medical record and enter the weight taken within 30 days of the ARD of this assessment.
3. If the last recorded weight was taken more than 30 days prior to the ARD of this assessment or previous weight is not available, weigh the resident again.
4. If the resident's weight was taken more than once during the preceding month, record the most recent weight.

K0200: Height and Weight (cont.)

5. Measure weight consistently over time in accordance with standard nursing home practice including time of day or scale (e.g., after voiding, before meal).

Coding Instructions for K0200B, **Weight**

- Use mathematical rounding (i.e., If weight is X.5 pounds [lbs] or more, round weight upward to the nearest whole pound. If weight is X.1 to X.4 lbs, round down to the nearest whole pound). For example, a weight of 152.5 lbs would be rounded to 153 lbs and a weight of 152.4 lbs would be rounded to 152 lbs.
- If a resident cannot be weighed, for example because of extreme pain, immobility, or risk of pathological fractures, use the standard no-information code (-) and document rationale on the resident's medical record.

K0300: Weight Loss

K0300. Weight Loss	
Enter Code	**Loss of 5% or more in the last month or loss of 10% or more in last 6 months**
	0. **No** or unknown
	1. **Yes, on** physician-prescribed weight-loss regimen
	2. **Yes, not on** physician-prescribed weight-loss regimen

Item Rationale

Health-related Quality of Life

- Weight loss can result in debility and adversely affect health, safety, and quality of life.
- For persons with morbid obesity, controlled and careful weight loss can improve mobility and health status.
- For persons with a large volume (fluid) overload, controlled and careful diuresis can improve health status.

Planning for Care

- Weight loss may be an important indicator of a change in the resident's health status or environment.
- If significant weight loss is noted, the interdisciplinary team should review for possible causes of changed intake, changed caloric need, change in medication (e.g., diuretics), or changed fluid volume status.
- Weight loss should be monitored on a continuing basis; weight loss should be assessed and care planned at the time of detection and not delayed until the next MDS assessment.

> **DEFINITIONS**
>
> **5% WEIGHT LOSS IN 30 DAYS**
> Start with the resident's weight closest to 30 days ago and multiply it by .95 (or 95%). The resulting figure represents a 5% loss from the weight 30 days ago. If the resident's current weight is equal to or less than the resulting figure, the resident has lost more than 5% body weight.

K0300: Weight Loss (cont.)

Steps for Assessment

This item compares the resident's weight in the current observation period with his or her weight at two snapshots in time:

- At a point closest to 30-days preceding the current weight.
- At a point closest to 180-days preceding the current weight.

This item does not consider weight fluctuation outside of these two time points, although the resident's weight should be monitored on a continual basis and weight gain or loss assessed and addressed on the care plan as necessary.

For a New Admission

1. Ask the resident, family, or significant other about weight loss over the past 30 and 180 days.
2. Consult the resident's physician, review transfer documentation, and compare with admission weight.
3. If the admission weight is less than the previous weight, calculate the percentage of weight loss.
4. Complete the same process to determine and calculate weight loss comparing the admission weight to the weight 30 and 180 days ago.

For Subsequent Assessments

1. From the medical record, compare the resident's weight in the current observation period to his or her weight in the observation period 30 days ago.
2. If the current weight is less than the weight in the observation period 30 days ago, calculate the percentage of weight loss.
3. From the medical record, compare the resident's weight in the current observation period to his or her weight in the observation period 180 days ago.
4. If the current weight is less than the weight in the observation period 180 days ago, calculate the percentage of weight loss.

DEFINITIONS

10% WEIGHT LOSS IN 180 DAYS
Start with the resident's weight closest to 180 days ago and multiply it by .90 (or 90%). The resulting figure represents a 10% loss from the weight 180 days ago. If the resident's current weight is equal to or less than the resulting figure, the resident has lost 10% or more body weight.

DEFINITIONS

PHYSICIAN-PRESCRIBED WEIGHT-LOSS REGIMEN
A weight reduction plan ordered by the resident's physician with the care plan goal of weight reduction. May employ a calorie-restricted diet or other weight loss diets and exercise. Also includes planned diuresis.
It is important that weight loss is intentional.

BODY MASS INDEX (BMI) Number calculated from a person's weight and height. BMI is used as a screening tool to identify possible weight problems for adults. Visit http://www.cdc.gov/healthyweight/assessing/bmi/adult_bmi/index.html

K0300: Weight Loss (cont.)

Coding Instructions

Mathematically round weights as described in Section K0200B before completing the weight loss calculation.

- **Code 0, no or unknown:** if the resident has not experienced weight loss of 5% or more in the past 30 days or 10% or more in the last 180 days or if information about prior weight is not available.
- **Code 1, yes on physician-prescribed weight loss regimen:** if the resident has experienced a weight loss of 5% or more in the past 30 days or 10% or more in the last 180 days, and the weight loss was planned and pursuant to a physician's order.
- **Code 2, yes, not on physician-prescribed weight-loss regimen:** if the resident has experienced a weight loss of 5% or more in the past 30 days or 10% or more in the last 180 days, and the weight loss was not planned and prescribed by a physician.

Coding Tips

- A resident may experience weight variances in between the snapshot time periods. Although these require follow up at the time, they are not captured on the MDS.
- If the resident is losing/gaining a significant amount of weight, the facility should not wait for the 30- or 180-day timeframe to address the problem. Weight changes of 5% in 1 month, 7.5% in 3 months, or 10% in 6 months should prompt a thorough assessment of the resident's nutritional status.
- To code K0300 as **1, yes**, the expressed goal of the diet must be inducing weight loss.
- On occasion, a resident with normal BMI or even low BMI is placed on a diabetic or otherwise calorie-restricted diet. In this instance, the intent of the diet is not to induce weight loss, and it would not be considered a physician-ordered weight-loss regimen.

Examples

1. Mrs. J has been on a physician ordered calorie-restricted diet for the past year. She and her physician agreed to a plan of weight reduction. Her current weight is 169 lbs. Her weight 30 days ago was 172 lbs. Her weight 180 days ago was 192 lbs.

   Coding: K0300 would be **coded 1, yes, on physician-prescribed weight-loss regimen.**
   Rationale:
   - 30-day calculation: $172 \times 0.95 = 163.4$. Since the resident's current weight of 169 lbs is more than 163.4 lbs, which is the 5% point, she **has not** lost 5% body weight in the last 30 days.
   - 180-day calculation: $192 \times .90 = 172.8$. Since the resident's current weight of 169 lbs **is** less than 172.8 lbs, which is the 10% point, she **has** lost 10% or more of body weight in the last 180 days.

K0300: Weight Loss (cont.)

2. Mr. S has had increasing need for assistance with eating over the past 6 months. His current weight is 195 lbs. His weight 30 days ago was 197 lbs. His weight 180 days ago was 185 lbs.

> **Coding:** K0300 would be **coded 0, No.**
> **Rationale:**
> - 30-day calculation: 197 x 0.95 = 187.15. Because the resident's current weight of 195 lbs is more than 187.15 lbs, which is the 5% point, he **has not** lost 5% body weight in the last 30 days.
> - 180-day calculation: Mr. S's current weight of 195 lbs is greater than his weight 180 days ago, so there is no need to calculate his weight loss. He has gained weight over this time period.

3. Ms. K underwent a BKA (below the knee amputation). Her preoperative weight 30 days ago was 130 lbs. Her most recent postoperative weight is 102 lbs. The amputated leg weighed 8 lbs. Her weight 180 days ago was 125 lbs.

Was the change in weight significant? Calculation of change in weight must take into account the weight of the amputated limb (which in this case is 6% of 130 lbs = 7.8 lbs).

- 30-day calculation:
  Step 1: Add the weight of the amputated limb to the current weight to obtain the weight if no amputation occurred:
  102 lbs (current weight) + 8 lbs (weight of leg) = 110 lbs (current body weight taking the amputated leg into account)
  Step 2: Calculate the difference between the most recent weight (including weight of the limb) and the previous weight (at 30 days)
  130 lbs (preoperative weight) - 110 lbs (present weight if had two legs) = 20 lbs (weight lost)
  Step 3: Calculate the percent weight change relative to the initial weight:
  20 lbs (weight change) /130 lbs (preoperative weight) = 6% weight loss
  Step 4: The percent weight change is significant if >5% at 30 days
  Therefore, the most recent postoperative weight of 102 lbs (110 lbs, taking the amputated limb into account) is >5% weight loss (significant at 30 days).

- 180-day calculation:
  Step 1: Add the weight of the amputated limb to the current weight to obtain the weight if no amputation occurred:
  102 lbs (current weight) + 8 lbs (weight of leg) = 110 lbs (current body weight taking the amputated leg into account)
  Step 2: Calculate the difference between the most recent weight (including weight of the limb) and the previous weight (at 180 days):
  125 lbs (preoperative weight 180 days ago) - 110 lbs (present weight if had two legs) = 15 lbs (weight lost)
  Step 3: Calculate the percent weight change relative to the initial weight:

K0300: Weight Loss (cont.)

15 lbs (weight change) / 130 lbs (preoperative weight) = 8.6% weight loss

Step 4: The percent weight change is significant if >10% at 180 days

Therefore, the most recent postoperative weight of 110 lbs (110 lbs, taking the amputated limb into account) is <10% weight loss (**not** significant at 180 days). **Present weight of 110 lbs <10% weight loss (not significant at 180 days).**

Coding: K0300 would be **coded 2, yes, weight change is significant; not on physician-prescribed weight-loss regimen.**

Rationale: The resident had a significant weight loss of 5% in 30 days and did not have a weight loss of 10% in 180 days, the item would be coded as 2, yes weight change is significant; not on physician-prescribed weight –loss regime, with one of the items being triggered.

K0500: Nutritional Approaches

K0500. Nutritional Approaches	
↓ Check all that apply	
☐	A. Parenteral/IV feeding
☐	B. Feeding tube - nasogastric or abdominal (PEG)
☐	C. Mechanically altered diet - require change in texture of food or liquids (e.g., pureed food, thickened liquids)
☐	D. Therapeutic diet (e.g., low salt, diabetic, low cholesterol)
☐	Z. None of the above

Item Rationale

Health-related Quality of Life

- Nutritional approaches that vary from the normal (e.g., mechanically altered food) or that rely on alternative methods (e.g., parenteral/IV or feeding tubes) can diminish an individual's sense of dignity and self-worth as well as diminish pleasure from eating.

- The resident's clinical condition may potentially benefit from the various nutritional approaches included here. It is important to work with the resident and family members to establish nutritional support goals that balance the resident's preferences and overall clinical goals.

Planning for Care

- Alternative nutritional approaches should be monitored to validate effectiveness.

- Care planning should include periodic reevaluation of the appropriateness of the approach.

DEFINITIONS

PARENTERAL/IV FEEDING Introduction of a nutritive substance into the body by means other than the intestinal tract (e.g., subcutaneous, intravenous).

FEEDING TUBE Presence of any type of tube that can deliver food/ nutritional substances/ fluids/ medications directly into the gastrointestinal system. Examples include, but are not limited to, nasogastric tubes, gastrostomy tubes, jejunostomy tubes, percutaneous endoscopic gastrotomy (PEG) tubes.

K0500: Nutritional Approaches (cont.)

Steps for Assessment

- Review the medical record to determine if any of the listed nutritional approaches were received by the resident during the 7-day look-back period.

Coding Instructions

Check all that apply. If none apply, check K0500Z. None of the above.

- **K0500A,** parenteral/IV feeding
- **K0500B,** feeding tube
- **K0500C,** mechanically altered diet
- **K0500D,** therapeutic diet
- **K0500Z,** none of the above

Coding Tips

*K0500 includes any and all nutrition and hydration received by the nursing home resident in the last 7 days either at the nursing home, at the hospital as an outpatient or an inpatient, **provided they were administered for nutrition or hydration**.*

- Parenteral/IV feeding—The following fluids may be included **when there is supporting documentation that reflects the need for additional fluid intake specifically addressing a nutrition or hydration need. This supporting documentation should be noted in the resident's medical record according to State and/or internal facility policy:**
  — IV fluids or hyperalimentation, including total parenteral nutrition (TPN), administered continuously or intermittently
  — IV fluids running at KVO (Keep Vein Open)
  — IV fluids contained in IV Piggybacks
  — Hypodermoclysis and subcutaneous ports in hydration therapy
- **The following items are NOT to be coded in K0500A:**
  — IV Medications—**Code these when appropriate in O0100H, IV Medications.**
  — IV fluids administered solely for the purpose of "prevention" of dehydration. Active diagnosis of dehydration must be present in order to code this fluid in K0500A.
  — IV fluids administered as a routine part of an operative or diagnostic procedure or recovery room stay.
  — IV fluids administered solely as flushes.
  — Parenteral/IV fluids administered in conjunction with chemotherapy or dialysis.

> **DEFINITIONS**
>
> **MECHANICALLY ALTERED DIET** A diet specifically prepared to alter the texture or consistency of food to facilitate oral intake. Examples include soft solids, puréed foods, ground meat, and thickened liquids. A mechanically altered diet should not automatically be considered a therapeutic diet.
>
> **THERAPEUTIC DIET** A diet ordered to manage problematic health conditions. Therapeutic refers to the nutritional content of the food. Examples include calorie-specific, low-salt, low-fat, lactose free, no added sugar, and supplements during meals.

K0500: Nutritional Approaches (cont.)

- Guidelines on basic fluid and electrolyte replacement can be found online at http://www.merck.com/mmpe/sec19/ch276/ch276b.html.
- Enteral feeding formulas:
  - Should not be coded as a mechanically altered diet.
  - Should only be coded as **K0400D, Therapeutic Diet** when the enteral formula is to manage problematic health conditions, e.g. enteral formulas specific to diabetics.

Examples

1. Mrs. H is receiving an antibiotic in 100 cc of normal saline via IV. She has a urinary tract infection (UTI), fever, abnormal lab results (e.g., new pyuria, microscopic hematuria, urine culture with growth >100,000 colony forming units of a urinary pathogen), and documented inadequate fluid intake (i.e., output of fluids far exceeds fluid intake) with signs and symptoms of dehydration. She is placed on the nursing home's hydration plan to ensure adequate hydration. Documentation shows IV fluids are being administered as part of the already identified need for additional hydration.

   Coding: K0500A would **be checked.** The IV medication would be coded at **IV Medications** item (O0100H).
   Rationale: The resident received 100 cc of IV fluid **and** there is supporting documentation that reflected an identified need for additional fluid intake for hydration.

2. Mr. J is receiving an antibiotic in 100 cc of normal saline via IV. He has a UTI, no fever, and documented adequate fluid intake. He is placed on the nursing home's hydration plan to ensure adequate hydration.

   Coding: K0500A would **NOT be checked.** The IV medication would be coded at **IV Medications** item (O0100H).
   Rationale: Although the resident received the additional fluid, there is no documentation to support a need for additional fluid intake.

K0700: Percent Intake by Artificial Route

Complete only if K0500A or K0500B is checked. Skip to Section L, Oral/Dental Status, if neither is checked.

K0700. Percent Intake by Artificial Route - Complete K0700 only if K0500A or K0500B is checked	
Enter Code ☐	A. Proportion of total calories the resident received through parenteral or tube feeding 1. 25% or less 2. 26-50% 3. 51% or more
Enter Code ☐	B. Average fluid intake per day by IV or tube feeding 1. 500 cc/day or less 2. 501 cc/day or more

K0700: Percent Intake by Artificial Route (cont.)

Item Rationale

Health-related Quality of Life

* Nutritional approaches that vary from the normal, such as parenteral/IV or feeding tubes, can diminish an individual's sense of dignity and self-worth as well as diminish pleasure from eating.

Planning for Care

* The proportion of calories received through artificial routes should be monitored with periodic reassessment to ensure adequate nutrition and hydration.
* Periodic reassessment is necessary to facilitate transition to increased oral intake as indicated by the resident's condition.

K0700A, Proportion of Total Calories the Resident Received through Parental or Tube Feedings in the Last 7 Days

Steps for Assessment

1. Review intake records to determine actual intake through parenteral or tube feeding routes.
2. Calculate proportion of total calories received through these routes.
   * If the resident took no food or fluids by mouth or took just sips of fluid, stop here and **code 3, 51% or more.**
   * If the resident had more substantial oral intake than this, consult with the dietician.

Coding Instructions

* Select the best response:
  1. 25% or less
  2. 26% to 50%
  3. 51% or more

Example

1. Calculation for Proportion of Total Calories from IV or Tube Feeding
   Mr. H has had a feeding tube since his surgery. He is currently more alert and feeling much better. He is very motivated to have the tube removed. He has been taking soft solids by mouth, but only in small to medium amounts. For the past 7 days, he has been receiving tube feedings for nutritional supplementation. The dietitian has totaled his calories per day as follows:

Oral and Tube Feeding Intake		
	Oral	Tube
Sun.	500	2,000
Mon.	250	2,250
Tues.	250	2,250
Wed.	350	2,250
Thurs.	500	2,000
Fri.	250	2,250
Sat.	350	2,000
Total	2,450	15,000

K0700: Percent Intake by Artificial Route (cont.)

Coding: K0700A would be coded **3, 51% or more.**

Rationale: Total Oral intake is 2,450 calories

Total Tube intake is 15,000 calories

Total calories is 2,450 + 15,000 = 17,450

Calculation of the percentage of total calories by tube feeding:

15,000/17,450 = .859 X 100 = 85.9%

Mr. H received 85.9% of his calories by tube feeding, therefore K0700A **code 3, 51% or more** is correct.

K0700B, Average Fluid Intake per Day by IV or Tube Feeding in the Last 7 Days.

Steps for Assessment

1. Review intake records from the last 7 days.
2. Add up the total amount of fluid received each day by IV and/or tube feedings only.
3. Divide the week's total fluid intake by 7 to calculate the average of fluid intake per day.
4. Divide by 7 even if the resident did not receive IV fluids and/or tube feeding on each of the 7 days.

Coding Instructions

Code for the average number of cc's of fluid the resident received per day by IV or tube feeding. Record what was actually received by the resident, not what was ordered.

- **Code 1:** 500 cc/day or less
- **Code 2:** 501 cc/day or more

Examples

1. **Calculation for Average Daily Fluid Intake**

   Ms. A has swallowing difficulties secondary to Huntington's disease. She is able to take oral fluids by mouth with supervision, but not enough to maintain hydration. She received the following daily fluid totals by supplemental tube feedings (including water, prepared nutritional supplements, juices) during the last 7 days.

IV Fluid Intake	
Sun.	1250 cc
Mon.	775 cc
Tues.	925 cc
Wed.	1200 cc
Thurs.	1200 cc
Fri.	500 cc
Sat.	450 cc
Total	6,300 cc

K0700: Percent Intake by Artificial Route (cont.)

Coding: K0700B would be coded **2, 501cc/day or more**.

Rationale: The total fluid intake by supplemental tube feedings = 6,300 cc
6,300 cc divided by 7 days = 900 cc/day
900 cc is greater than 500 cc, therefore **code 2, 501 cc/day or more** is correct.

2. **Calculation for Average Daily Fluid Intake**

Mrs. G. received 1 liter of IV fluids during the 7-day assessment period. She received no other intake via IV or tube feeding during the assessment period.

IV Fluid Intake	
Sun.	0 cc
Mon.	0 cc
Tues.	1,000 cc
Wed.	0 cc
Thurs.	0 cc
Fri.	0 cc
Sat.	0 cc
Total	1,000 cc

Coding: K0500b would be coded **1, 500 cc/day or less**.

Rationale: The total fluid intake by supplemental tube feedings = 1000 cc
1000 cc divided by 7 days = 142.9 cc/day
142.9 cc is less than 500 cc, therefore **code 1, 500 cc/day or less** is correct.

SECTION L: ORAL/DENTAL STATUS

Intent: This item is intended to record any dental **problems** present in the 7-day look-back period.

L0200: Dental

L0200. Dental	
↓ Check all that apply	
☐	A. **Broken or loosely fitting full or partial denture** (chipped, cracked, uncleanable, or loose)
☐	B. **No natural teeth or tooth fragment(s)** (edentulous)
☐	C. **Abnormal mouth tissue** (ulcers, masses, oral lesions, including under denture or partial if one is worn)
☐	D. **Obvious or likely cavity or broken natural teeth**
☐	E. **Inflamed or bleeding gums or loose natural teeth**
☐	F. **Mouth or facial pain, discomfort or difficulty with chewing**
☐	G. **Unable to examine**
☐	Z. **None of the above were present**

Item Rationale

Health-related Quality of Life

- Poor oral health has a negative impact on:
  — quality of life
  — overall health
  — nutritional status
- Assessment can identify periodontal disease that can contribute to or cause systemic diseases and conditions, such as aspiration, malnutrition, pneumonia, endocarditis, and poor control of diabetes.

Planning for Care

- Assessing dental status can help identify residents who may be at risk for aspiration, malnutrition, pneumonia, endocarditis, and poor control of diabetes.

DEFINITIONS

CAVITY
A tooth with a discolored hole or area of decay that may have debris in it.

BROKEN NATURAL TEETH OR TOOTH FRAGMENT
Very large cavity, tooth broken off or decayed to gum line, or broken teeth (from a fall or trauma)

ORAL LESIONS
A discolored area of tissue (red, white, yellow, or darkened) on the lips, gums, tongue, palate, cheek lining, or throat.

L0200: Dental (cont.)

Steps for Assessment

1. Ask the resident about the presence of chewing problems or mouth or facial pain/discomfort.
2. Ask the resident, family, or significant other whether the resident has or recently had dentures or partials. (If resident or family/significant other reports that the resident recently had dentures or partials, but they do not have them at the facility, ask for a reason.)
3. If the resident has dentures or partials, examine for loose fit. Ask him or her to remove, and examine for chips, cracks, and cleanliness. Removal of dentures and/or partials is necessary for adequate assessment.

> **DEFINITIONS**
>
> **ORAL MASS**
> A swollen or raised lump, bump, or nodule on any oral surface. May be hard or soft, and with or without pain.
>
> **ULCER**
> Mouth sore, blister or eroded area of tissue on any oral surface.

4. Conduct exam of the resident's lips and oral cavity with dentures or partials removed, if applicable. Use a light source that is adequate to visualize the back of the mouth. Visually observe and feel all oral surfaces including lips, gums, tongue, palate, mouth floor, and cheek lining. Check for abnormal mouth tissue, abnormal teeth, or inflamed or bleeding gums. The assessor should use his or her gloved fingers to adequately feel for masses or loose teeth.
5. If the resident is unable to self-report, then observe him or her while eating with dentures or partials, if indicated, to determine if chewing problems or mouth pain are present.
6. Oral examination of residents who are uncooperative and do not allow for a thorough oral exam may result in medical conditions being missed. Referral for dental evaluation should be considered for these residents and any resident who exhibits dental or oral issues.

Coding Instructions

- **Check L0200 A, broken or loosely fitting full or partial denture:** if the denture or partial is chipped, cracked, uncleanable, or loose. A denture is coded as loose if the resident complains that it is loose, the denture visibly moves when the resident opens his or her mouth, or the denture moves when the resident tries to talk.

- **Check L0200 B, no natural teeth or tooth fragment(s) (edentulous):** if the resident is edentulous or lacks all natural teeth or parts of teeth.

- **Check L0200 C, abnormal mouth tissue (ulcers, masses, oral lesions):** Select if any ulcer, mass, or oral lesion is noted on any oral surface.

- **Check L0200 D, obvious or likely cavity or broken natural teeth:** if any cavity or broken tooth is seen.

- **Check L0200 E, inflamed or bleeding gums or loose natural teeth:** if gums appear irritated, red, swollen, or bleeding. Teeth are coded as loose if they readily move when light pressure is applied with a fingertip.

- **Check L0200 F, mouth or facial pain or discomfort with chewing:** if the resident reports any pain in the mouth or face, or discomfort with chewing.

- **Check L0200 G, unable to examine:** if the resident's mouth cannot be examined.

- **Check L0200 Z, none of the above:** if none of conditions A through F is present.

L0200: Dental (cont.)

Coding Tips

- Mouth or facial pain coded for this item should also be coded in Section J, items J0100 through J0850.

SECTION M: SKIN CONDITIONS

Intent: The items in this section document the risk, presence, appearance, and change of pressure ulcers. This section also notes other skin ulcers, wounds, or lesions, and documents some treatment categories related to skin injury or avoiding injury. It is important to recognize and evaluate each resident's risk factors and to identify and evaluate all areas at risk of constant pressure. A complete assessment of skin is essential to an effective pressure ulcer prevention and skin treatment program. Be certain to include in the assessment process, a holistic approach. It is imperative to determine the etiology of all wounds and lesions, as this will determine and direct the proper treatment and management of the wound.

M0100: Determination of Pressure Ulcer Risk

M0100. Determination of Pressure Ulcer Risk	
↓ Check all that apply	
☐	A. Resident has a stage 1 or greater, a scar over bony prominence, or a non-removable dressing/device
☐	B. Formal assessment instrument/tool (e.g., Braden, Norton, or other)
☐	C. Clinical assessment
☐	Z. None of the above

Item Rationale

Health-related Quality of Life

- Pressure ulcers occur when tissue is compressed between a bony prominence and an external surface. In addition to pressure, shear force, and friction are important contributors to pressure ulcer development.
- The underlying health of a resident's soft tissue affects how much pressure, shear force, or friction is needed to damage tissue. Skin and soft tissue changes associated with aging, illness, small blood vessel disease, and malnutrition increase vulnerability to pressure ulcers.
- Additional external factors, such as excess moisture, and tissue exposure to urine or feces, can increase risk.

Planning for Care

- The care planning process should include efforts to stabilize, reduce, or remove underlying risk factors; to monitor the impact of the interventions; and to modify the interventions as appropriate based on the individualized needs of the resident.
- Throughout this section, terminology referring to "healed" vs. "unhealed" ulcers refers to whether or not the ulcer is "closed" vs. "open." When considering this, recognize that Stage 1, DTI, and unstageable pressure ulcers although "closed," (i.e. may be covered with tissue, eschar, slough, etc.) would not be considered "healed."
- Facilities should be aware that the resident is at higher risk of having the area of a closed pressure ulcer open up due to damage, injury, or pressure, because of the loss of tensile strength of the overlying tissue. Tensile strength of the skin overlying a closed pressure ulcer is 80% of normal skin tensile strength. Facilities should put preventative measures in place that will mitigate the opening of a closed ulcer due to the fragility of the overlying tissue.

M0100: Determination of Pressure Ulcer Risk (cont.)

Steps for Assessment

1. Review the medical record, including skin care flow sheets or other skin tracking forms, nurses' notes, and pressure ulcer risk assessments.
2. Speak with the treatment nurse and direct care staff on all shifts to confirm conclusions from the medical record review and observations of the resident.
3. Examine the resident and determine whether any ulcers, scars, or non-removable dressings/devices are present. Assess key areas for pressure ulcer development (e.g., sacrum, coccyx, trochanters, ischial tuberosities, and heels). Also assess bony prominences (e.g. elbows and ankles) and skin that is under braces or subjected to pressure (e.g., ears from oxygen tubing).

Coding Instructions

*For this item, **check all that apply**:*

- **Check A if resident has a Stage 1 or greater pressure ulcer, a scar over bony prominence, or a non-removable dressing/ device.** Review descriptions of pressure ulcer stages and information obtained during physical examination and medical record review. Examples of non-removable dressings/devices include a primary surgical dressing, a cast, or a brace.

- **Check B if a formal assessment has been completed.** An example of an established pressure ulcer risk tool is the *Braden Scale for Predicting Pressure Sore Risk*©. Other tools may be used.

- **Check C if the resident's risk for pressure ulcer development is based on clinical assessment.** A clinical assessment could include a head-to-toe physical examination of the skin and observation or medical record review of pressure ulcer risk factors. Examples of risk factors include the following:
  — impaired/decreased mobility and decreased functional ability
  — co-morbid conditions, such as end stage renal disease, thyroid disease, or diabetes mellitus;
  — drugs, such as steroids, that may affect wound healing;
  — impaired diffuse or localized blood flow (e.g., generalized atherosclerosis or lower extremity arterial insufficiency);

DEFINITIONS

PRESSURE ULCER RISK FACTOR
Examples of risk factors include immobility and decreased functional ability; co-morbid conditions such as end-stage renal disease, thyroid disease, or diabetes; drugs such as steroids; impaired diffuse or localized blood flow; resident refusal of care and treatment; cognitive impairment; exposure of skin to urinary and fecal incontinence; under nutrition, malnutrition, and hydration deficits; and a healed ulcer.

PRESSURE ULCER RISK TOOLS
Screening tools that are designed to help identify residents who might develop a pressure ulcer. A common risk assessment tool is the Braden Scale for Predicting Pressure Sore Risk©.

M0100: Determination of Pressure Ulcer Risk (cont.)

- — resident refusal of some aspects of care and treatment;
- — cognitive impairment;
- — urinary and fecal incontinence;
- — under nutrition, malnutrition, and hydration deficits; and
- — healed pressure ulcers, especially Stage 3 or 4 which are more likely to have recurrent breakdown.

- **Check Z if none of the above apply.**

M0150: Risk of Pressure Ulcers

M0150. Risk of Pressure Ulcers	
Enter Code	Is this resident at risk of developing pressure ulcers? 0. No 1. Yes

Item Rationale

Health-related Quality of Life

- It is important to recognize and evaluate each resident's risk factors and to identify and evaluate all areas at risk of constant pressure.

Planning for Care

- The care process should include efforts to stabilize, reduce, or remove underlying risk factors; to monitor the impact of the interventions; and to modify the interventions as appropriate.

Steps for Assessment

1. Based on the item(s) reviewed for M0100, determine if the resident is at risk for developing a pressure ulcer.
2. If the medical record reveals that the resident currently has a Stage 1 or greater pressure ulcer, a scar over a bony prominence, or a non-removable dressing or device, the resident is at risk for worsening or new pressure ulcers.
3. Review formal risk assessment tools to determine the resident's "risk score."
4. Review the components of the clinical assessment conducted for evidence of pressure ulcer risk.

Coding Instructions

- **Code 0, no:** if the resident is not at risk for developing pressure ulcers based on a review of information gathered for M0100.

- **Code 1, yes:** if the resident is at risk for developing pressure ulcers based on a review of information gathered for M0100.

M0210: Unhealed Pressure Ulcer(s)

M0210. Unhealed Pressure Ulcer(s)	
Enter Code ☐	**Does this resident have one or more unhealed pressure ulcer(s) at Stage 1 or higher?** 0. **No →** Skip to M0900, Healed Pressure Ulcers 1. **Yes →** Continue to M0300, Current Number of Unhealed (non-epithelialized) Pressure Ulcers at Each Stage

Item Rationale

Health-related Quality of Life

- Pressure ulcers and other wounds or lesions affect quality of life for residents because they may limit activity, may be painful, and may require time-consuming treatments and dressing changes.

Planning for Care

> **DEFINITIONS**
>
> **PRESSURE ULCER**
> A pressure ulcer is localized injury to the skin and/or underlying tissue usually over a bony prominence, as a result of pressure, or pressure in combination with shear and/or friction.

- The pressure ulcer definitions used in the RAI Manual have been adapted from those recommended by the National Pressure Ulcer Advisory Panel (NPUAP) 2007 Pressure Ulcer Stages.

- An existing pressure ulcer identifies residents at risk for further complications or skin injury. Risk factors described in M0100 should be addressed.

- For MDS assessment, staging of ulcers should be coded in terms of what is assessed (seen and palpated, i.e. visible tissue, palpable bone) during the look-back period. Nursing homes may adopt the NPUAP guidelines in their clinical practice and nursing documentation. However, since CMS has adapted the NPUAP guidelines for MDS purposes, the definitions do not perfectly correlate with each stage as described by NPUAP. Therefore, you cannot use the NPUAP definitions to code the MDS. You must code the MDS according to the instructions in this manual.

- Pressure ulcer staging provides a description of the extent of visible tissue damage or palpable bone and informs expectations for healing times.

Steps for Assessment

1. Review the medical record, including skin care flow sheets or other skin tracking forms.
2. Speak with direct care staff and the treatment nurse to confirm conclusions from the medical record review.
3. Examine the resident and determine whether any ulcers are present.
   - Key areas for pressure ulcer development include sacrum, coccyx, trochanters, ischial tuberosities, and heels. Other areas, such as bony deformities, skin under braces, and skin subjected to excess pressure, shear or friction, are also at risk for pressure ulcers.
   - Without a full body skin assessment, a pressure ulcer can be missed.
   - Examine the resident in a well-lit room. Adequate lighting is important for detecting skin changes.
   - For any pressure ulcers identified, measure and record the deepest anatomical stage (see instructions on page M-5).

4. Identify any known or likely unstageable pressure ulcers (see instructions beginning on page M-6).

M0210: Unhealed Pressure Ulcer(s) (cont.)

Coding Instructions

Code based on the presence of any pressure ulcer (regardless of stage) in the past 7 days.

- **Code 0, no:** if the resident did not have a pressure ulcer in the 7-day look-back period. Then skip Items M0300–M0800.
- **Code 1, yes:** if the resident had any pressure ulcer (Stage 1, 2, 3, 4, or unstageable) in the 7-day look-back period. Proceed to **Current Number of Unhealed Pressure Ulcers at Each Stage** item (M0300).

Coding Tips

- If an ulcer arises from a combination of factors which are primarily caused by pressure, then the ulcer should be included in this section as a pressure ulcer. Each ulcer should be coded only once, either as a pressure ulcer or an ulcer due to another cause.
- If a pressure ulcer is surgically repaired with a flap or graft, it should be coded as a surgical wound and not as a pressure ulcer. If the flap or graft fails, continue to code it as a surgical wound until healed.
- If a resident had a pressure ulcer that healed before the look-back period, **code 0** and then complete **Healed Pressure Ulcers** item (M0900).
- Residents with diabetes mellitus (DM) can have a pressure, venous, arterial, or diabetic neuropathic ulcer. The primary etiology should be considered when coding whether the diabetic has an ulcer that is caused by pressure or other factors.
- If a resident with DM has a heel ulcer from pressure and the ulcer is present in the 7-day look-back period, **code 1** and proceed to code items M0300–M0900 as appropriate for the pressure ulcer.
- If a resident with DM has an ulcer on the plantar (bottom) surface of the foot closer to the metatarsal and the ulcer is present in the 7-day look-back period, **code 0** and proceed to M1040 to code the ulcer as a diabetic foot ulcer.

M0300: Current Number of Unhealed Pressure Ulcers at Each Stage

Steps for completing M0300A–G

Step 1: Determine Deepest Anatomical Stage

For each pressure ulcer, determine the deepest anatomical stage. Do not reverse or back stage. Consider current and historical levels of tissue involvement.

1. Observe the base of any pressure ulcers present to determine the depth of tissue layers involved.

M0300: Current Number of Unhealed Pressure Ulcers at Each Stage (cont.)

2. Ulcer staging should be based on the ulcer's deepest visible anatomical level. Review the history of each pressure ulcer in the medical record. If the pressure ulcer has ever been classified at a deeper stage than what is observed now, it should continue to be classified at the deeper stage. Nursing homes that carefully document and track ulcers will be able to more accurately code this item.
3. Pressure ulcers that are healed before the look-back period are not coded in this section. Code under **Healed Pressure Ulcers** item (M0900).
4. Guidance on staging pressure ulcers may be obtained in Appendix C - CAA Resources.

Step 2: Identify Unstageable Pressure Ulcers

1. Visualization of the wound bed is necessary for accurate staging. However, if the wound bed is partially covered by eschar or slough, but the depth of tissue loss can be measured, do not code as unstageable.
2. Pressure ulcers that have necrotic or eschar (tan, black, or brown) tissue present such that the tissue layers involved with the pressure ulcer cannot be determined, should be classified as unstageable, as illustrated at http://www.npuap.org/images/NPUAP-Unstage2.jpg
3. Pressure ulcers in which the base of the ulcer is covered by slough (yellow, tan, gray, green or brown) are unstageable.
4. A pressure ulcer with intact skin that is a suspected deep tissue injury should not be coded as a Stage 1 pressure ulcer. It should be coded as unstageable, as illustrated at http://www.npuap.org/images/NPUAP-SuspectDTI.jpg
5. Known pressure ulcers covered by a non-removable dressing/device (e.g., primary surgical dressing, cast) should be coded as unstageable.

Step 3: Determine "Present on Admission"

*For **each** pressure ulcer, determine if the pressure ulcer was present at the time of admission and **not** acquired while the resident was in the care of the nursing home. Consider current and historical levels of tissue involvement.*

1. Review the medical record for the history of the ulcer.
2. Review for location and stage at the time of admission or reentry. If the pressure ulcer was present on admission and subsequently worsened to a higher stage during the resident's stay, the pressure ulcer is coded at that higher stage, and that higher stage **should not be considered as "present on admission."**
3. If the pressure ulcer was unstageable on admission, but becomes stageable later, it should be considered as "present on admission" at the stage at which it first becomes stageable. If it subsequently worsens to a higher stage, that higher stage **should not be considered "present on admission."**
4. If a resident who has a pressure ulcer is hospitalized and returns with that pressure ulcer at the same stage, the pressure ulcer **should not be coded as "present on admission"** because it was present at the facility prior to the hospitalization.
5. If a current pressure ulcer worsens to a higher stage during a hospitalization, it is coded at the higher stage upon reentry and **should be coded as "present on admission."**

M0300A: Number of Stage 1 Pressure Ulcers

M0300. Current Number of Unhealed (non-epithelialized) Pressure Ulcers at Each Stage	
Enter Number ☐	**A. Number of Stage 1 pressure ulcers** **Stage 1:** Intact skin with non-blanchable redness of a localized area usually over a bony prominence. Darkly pigmented skin may not have a visible blanching; in dark skin tones only it may appear with persistent blue or purple hues

Item Rationale

Health-related Quality of Care

- Stage 1 pressure ulcers may deteriorate to more severe pressure ulcers without adequate intervention; as such, they are an important risk factor for further tissue damage.

Planning for Care

- Development of a Stage 1 pressure ulcer should be one of multiple factors that initiate pressure ulcer prevention interventions.

Steps for Assessment

1. Perform head-to-toe assessment. Conduct a full body skin assessment focusing on bony prominences and pressure-bearing areas (sacrum, buttocks, heels, ankles, etc).
2. For the purposes of coding, determine that the lesion being assessed is **primarily** related to pressure and that other conditions have been ruled out. If pressure is NOT the **primary** cause, do NOT code here.
3. Reliance on only one descriptor is inadequate to determine the staging of the pressure ulcer between Stage 1 and suspected deep tissue ulcers. The descriptors are similar for these two types of ulcers (e.g., temperature (warmth or coolness); tissue consistency (firm or boggy).
4. Check any reddened areas for ability to blanch by firmly pressing a finger into the reddened tissues and then removing it. In non-blanchable reddened areas, there is no loss of skin color or pressure-induced pallor at the compressed site.
5. Search for other areas of skin that differ from surrounding tissue that may be painful, firm, soft, warmer, or cooler compared to adjacent tissue. Stage 1 may be difficult to detect in individuals with dark skin tones. Look for temperature or color changes.

> **DEFINITIONS**
>
> **STAGE 1 PRESSURE ULCER**
> An observable, pressure-related alteration of intact skin, whose indicators as compared to an adjacent or opposite area on the body may include changes in one or more of the following parameters: skin temperature (warmth or coolness); tissue consistency (firm or boggy); sensation (pain, itching); and/or a define area of persistent redness in lightly pigmented skin, whereas in darker skin tones, the ulcer may appear with persistent red, blue, or purple hues.
>
> **NON-BLANCHABLE**
> Reddened areas of tissue that do not turn white or pale when pressed firmly with a finger or device.

Coding Instructions for M0300A

- **Enter the number** of Stage 1 pressure ulcers that are currently present.
- **Enter 0** if no Stage 1 pressure ulcers are present.

M0300A: Number of Stage 1 Pressure Ulcers (cont.)

Coding Tips

- Pressure ulcers with intact skin that are suspected deep tissue injury should **not** be coded as Stage 1 pressure ulcers. They should be coded as **Unstageable – Deep tissue** item (M0300G).

M0300B: Stage 2 Pressure Ulcers

M0300. Current Number of Unhealed (non-epithelialized) **Pressure Ulcers at Each Stage**

B. Stage 2: Partial thickness loss of dermis presenting as a shallow open ulcer with a red or pink wound bed, without slough. May also present as an intact or open/ruptured blister

Enter Number [ ]

1. **Number of Stage 2 pressure ulcers** - If 0 → Skip to M0300C, Stage 3

Enter Number [ ]

2. **Number of these Stage 2 pressure ulcers that were present upon admission/reentry** - enter how many were noted at the time of admission

3. **Date of oldest Stage 2 pressure ulcer** - Enter dashes if date is unknown:

[ ][ ] – [ ][ ] – [ ][ ][ ][ ]
Month   Day   Year

Item Rationale

Health-related Quality of Life

- Stage 2 pressure ulcers may worsen without proper interventions.
- These residents are at risk for further complications or skin injury.

Planning for Care

- **Most Stage 2** pressure ulcers should heal in a reasonable time frame (e.g., 60 days).
- Stage 2 pressure ulcers are often related to friction and/or shearing force, and the care plan should incorporate efforts to limit these forces on the skin and tissues.
- Stage 2 pressure ulcers may be more likely to heal with treatment than higher stage pressure ulcers.
- The care plan should include individualized interventions and evidence that the interventions have been monitored and modified as appropriate.

> **DEFINITIONS**
>
> **STAGE 2 PRESSURE ULCER**
> Partial thickness loss of dermis presenting as a shallow open ulcer with a red-pink wound bed, **without slough.**
>
> May also present as an intact or open/ruptured blister.

Steps for Assessment

1. Perform head-to-toe assessment. Conduct a full body skin assessment focusing on bony prominences and pressure-bearing areas (sacrum, buttocks, heels, ankles, etc).
2. For the purposes of coding, determine that the lesion being assessed is primarily related to pressure and that other conditions have been ruled out. If pressure is NOT the primary cause, do NOT code here.

M0300B: Stage 2 Pressure Ulcers (cont.)

3. Examine the area adjacent to or surrounding an intact blister for evidence of tissue damage. **If other conditions are ruled out and the tissue adjacent to, or surrounding the blister demonstrates signs of tissue damage, (e.g., color change, tenderness, bogginess or firmness, warmth or coolness) these characteristics suggest a suspected deep tissue injury rather than a Stage 2 Pressure Ulcer.**
4. Stage 2 pressure ulcers will **generally** lack the surrounding characteristics found with a deep tissue injury.
5. Identify the number of these pressure ulcers that were present on admission (see instructions on page M-6).
6. Identify the oldest Stage 2 pressure ulcer and the date it was first noted at that stage.

Coding Instructions for M0300B

- **Enter the number** of pressure ulcers that are currently present and whose deepest anatomical stage is Stage 2.

- **Enter 0** if no Stage 2 pressure ulcers are present and skip to **Current Number of Unhealed Pressure Ulcers at Each Stage** item (M0300C).

- **Enter the number** of Stage 2 pressure ulcers that were first noted at the time of admission AND—for residents who are reentering the facility after a hospital stay, enter the number of Stage 2 pressure ulcers that were acquired during the hospitalization (i.e., the Stage 2 pressure ulcer was not acquired in the nursing facility prior to admission to the hospital).

- **Enter 0** if no Stage 2 pressure ulcers were first noted at the time of admission.

- **Enter the date of the oldest Stage 2 pressure ulcer.** Do not leave any boxes blank. If the month or day contains only a single digit, fill the first box in with a "0." For example, January 2, 2011, should be entered as 01-02-2011. If the date is unknown, enter a dash in every block.

Coding Tips

- A Stage 2 pressure ulcer presents as a shiny or dry shallow ulcer without slough or bruising.

- If the oldest Stage 2 pressure ulcer was present on admission and the date it was first noted is unknown, enter a dash in every block.

- Do NOT code skin tears, tape burns, perineal dermatitis, maceration, excoriation, or suspected deep tissue injury here.

- When a lesion that is related to pressure presents with an intact blister, examine the adjacent and surrounding area for signs of deep tissue injury. When a deep tissue injury **is** determined, do NOT code as a Stage 2.

M0300C: Stage 3 Pressure Ulcers

M0300. Current Number of Unhealed (non-epithelialized) Pressure Ulcers at Each Stage	
Enter Number ☐ Enter Number ☐	**C. Stage 3:** Full thickness tissue loss. Subcutaneous fat may be visible but bone, tendon or muscle is not exposed. Slough may be present but does not obscure the depth of tissue loss. May include undermining and tunneling **1. Number of Stage 3 pressure ulcers** - If 0 → Skip to M0300D, Stage 4 **2. Number of these Stage 3 pressure ulcers that were present upon admission/reentry** - enter how many were noted at the time of admission

Item Rationale

Health-related Quality of Life

- Pressure ulcers affect quality of life for residents because they may limit activity, may be painful, and may require time-consuming treatments and dressing changes.

Planning for Care

- Pressure ulcers at more advanced stages typically require more aggressive interventions, including more frequent repositioning, attention to nutritional status, and care that may be more time or staff intensive.

> **DEFINITIONS**
>
> **STAGE 3 PRESSURE ULCER**
> Full thickness tissue loss. Subcutaneous fat may be visible but bone, tendon or muscle is not exposed. Slough may be present but does not obscure the depth of tissue loss. May include undermining or tunneling.

- An existing pressure ulcer may put residents at risk for further complications or skin injury.
- If a pressure ulcer fails to show some evidence toward healing within 14 days, the pressure ulcer (including potential complications) and the resident's overall clinical condition should be reassessed.

Steps for Assessment

1. Perform head-to-toe assessment. Conduct a full body skin assessment focusing on bony prominences and pressure-bearing areas (sacrum, buttocks, heels, ankles, etc).
2. For the purposes of coding, determine that the lesion being assessed is primarily related to pressure and that other conditions have been ruled out. If pressure is NOT the primary cause, do NOT code here.
3. Identify all Stage 3 pressure ulcers currently present.
4. Identify the number of these pressure ulcers that were present on admission.

Coding Instructions for M0300C

- **Enter the number** of pressure ulcers that are currently present and whose deepest anatomical stage is Stage 3.

- **Enter 0** if no Stage 3 pressure ulcers are present and skip to **Current Number of Unhealed Pressures Ulcers at Each Stage** item (M0300D).

M0300C: Stage 3 Pressure Ulcers (cont.)

- **Enter the number** of Stage 3 pressure ulcers that were first noted at Stage 3 at the time of admission AND—for residents who are reentering the facility after a hospital stay, enter the number of Stage 3 pressure ulcers that were acquired during the hospitalization (i.e., the Stage 3 pressure ulcer was not acquired in the nursing facility prior to admission to the hospital).

- **Enter 0** if no Stage 3 pressure ulcers were first noted at the time of admission.

Coding Tips

- The depth of a Stage 3 pressure ulcer varies by anatomical location. Stage 3 pressure ulcers can be shallow, particularly on areas that do not have subcutaneous tissue, such as the bridge of the nose, ear, occiput, and malleolus.

- In contrast, areas of significant adiposity can develop extremely deep Stage 3 pressure ulcers. Therefore, observation and assessment of skin folds should be part of overall skin assessment.

- Bone/tendon/muscle is not visible or directly palpable in a Stage 3 pressure ulcer.

Examples

1. A pressure ulcer described as a Stage 2 was noted and documented in the resident's medical record at the time of admission. On a later assessment, the wound is noted to be a full thickness ulcer, thus it is now a Stage 3 pressure ulcer.

   Coding: The current Stage 3 pressure ulcer would be coded at **M0300C1 as Code1, and at M0300C2 as 0 not present on admission.**

   Rationale: The designation of "present on admission" requires that the pressure ulcer be at the same location **and** not have worsened to a deeper anatomical stage. This pressure ulcer worsened after admission.

2. A resident develops a Stage 2 pressure ulcer while at the nursing facility. The resident is hospitalized due to pneumonia for 8 days and returns with a Stage 3 pressure ulcer in the same location.

   Coding: The pressure ulcer would be coded at **M0300C1 as Code 1, and at M0300C2 as 1, present on admission.**

   Rationale: Even though the resident had a pressure ulcer in the same anatomical location prior to transfer, because it worsened to a Stage 3 during hospitalization it should be coded as a Stage 3, present on admission.

3. On admission, the resident has three small Stage 2 pressure ulcers on her coccyx. Two weeks later, the coccyx is assessed. Two of the Stage 2 pressure ulcers have merged and the third has worsened to a Stage 3 pressure ulcer.

   Coding: The two merged pressure ulcers would be coded at **M0300B1 as 1, and at M0300B2 as 1, present on admission**. The **Stage 3 pressure ulcer** would be **coded at M0300C1 as 1, and at M0300C2 as 0, not present on admission.**

   Rationale: Two of the pressure ulcers on the coccyx have merged, but have remained at the same stage as they were at the time of admission; the one that increased to a Stage 3 has increased in stage since admission and hence cannot be coded as present on admission.

4. A resident developed two Stage 2 pressure ulcers during her stay; one on the coccyx and the other on the left lateral malleolus. At some point she is hospitalized and returns with two pressure ulcers. One is the previous Stage 2 on the coccyx, which has not changed; the other is a new Stage 3 on the left trochanter. The Stage 2 previously on the left lateral malleolus has healed.

   Coding: The **Stage 2** pressure ulcer would be coded at **M0300B1 as 1, and at M0300B2 as 0, not present on admission; the Stage 3** would be coded at **M0300C1 as 1, and at M0300C2 as 1, present on admission.**

   Rationale: The Stage 2 pressure ulcer on the coccyx was present prior to hospitalization; the Stage 3 developed during hospitalization and is coded as present on admission. The Stage 2 on the left lateral malleolus has healed and is therefore no longer coded here but in Item M0900, Healed Pressure Ulcers.

M0300D: Stage 4 Pressure Ulcers

M0300. Current Number of Unhealed (non-epithelialized) Pressure Ulcers at Each Stage	
Enter Number ☐ Enter Number ☐	**D. Stage 4:** Full thickness tissue loss with exposed bone, tendon or muscle. Slough or eschar may be present on some parts of the wound bed. Often includes undermining and tunneling 1. **Number of Stage 4 pressure ulcers** - If 0 → Skip to M0300E, Unstageable: Non-removable dressing 2. **Number of these Stage 4 pressure ulcers that were present upon admission/reentry** - enter how many were noted at the time of admission

Item Rationale

Health-related Quality of Life

- Pressure ulcers affect quality of life for residents because they may limit activity, may be painful, and may require time-consuming treatments and dressing changes.

M0300D: Stage 4 Pressure Ulcers (cont.)

Planning for Care

- Pressure ulcers at more advanced stages typically require more aggressive interventions, including more frequent repositioning, attention to nutritional status, more frequent dressing changes, and treatment that is more time-consuming than with routine preventive care.

- An existing pressure ulcer may put residents at risk for further complications or skin injury.

- If a pressure ulcer fails to show some evidence toward healing within 14 days, the pressure ulcer (including potential complications) and the resident's overall clinical condition should be reassessed.

> **DEFINITIONS**
>
> **STAGE 4 PRESSURE ULCER**
> Full thickness tissue loss with exposed bone, tendon or muscle. Slough or eschar may be present on some parts of the wound bed. Often includes undermining and tunneling.

Steps for Assessment

1. Perform head-to-toe assessment. Conduct a full body skin assessment focusing on bony prominences and pressure-bearing areas (sacrum, buttocks, heels, ankles, etc).
2. For the purposes of coding, determine that the lesion being assessed is primarily related to pressure and that other conditions have been ruled out. If pressure is NOT the primary cause, do NOT code here.
3. Identify all Stage 4 pressure ulcers currently present.
4. Identify the number of these pressure ulcers that were present on admission.

Coding Instructions for M0300D

- **Enter the number** of pressure ulcers that are currently present and whose deepest anatomical stage is Stage 4.

- **Enter 0** if no Stage 4 pressure ulcers are present and skip to **Current Number of Unhealed Pressure Ulcers at Each Stage** item (M0300E).

- **Enter the number** of Stage 4 pressure ulcers that were first noted at Stage 4 at the time of admission AND—for residents who are reentering the facility after a hospital stay, enter the number of Stage 4 pressure ulcers that were acquired during the hospitalization (e.g., the Stage 4 pressure ulcer was not acquired in the nursing facility prior to admission to the hospital).

- **Enter 0** if no Stage 4 pressure ulcers were first noted at the time of admission.

> **DEFINITIONS**
>
> **TUNNELING**
> A passage way of tissue destruction under the skin surface that has an opening at the skin level from the edge of the wound.
>
> **UNDERMINING**
> The destruction of tissue or ulceration extending under the skin edges (margins) so that the pressure ulcer is larger at its base than at the skin surface.

M0300D: Stage 4 Pressure Ulcers (cont.)

Coding Tips

- The depth of a Stage 4 pressure ulcer varies by anatomical location. The bridge of the nose, ear, occiput, and malleolus do not have subcutaneous tissue, and these ulcers can be shallow.
- Stage 4 pressure ulcers can extend into muscle and/or supporting structures (e.g., fascia, tendon, or joint capsule) making osteomyelitis possible.
- Exposed bone/tendon/muscle is visible or directly palpable.

M0300E: Unstageable Pressure Ulcers Related to Non-removable Dressing/Device

	M0300. Current Number of Unhealed (non-epithelialized) Pressure Ulcers at Each Stage - Continued
	E. Unstageable - Non-removable dressing: Known but not stageable due to non-removable dressing/device
Enter Number ☐	**1. Number of unstageable pressure ulcers due to non-removable dressing/device** - If 0 → Skip to M0300F, Unstageable: Slough and/or eschar
Enter Number ☐	**2. Number of these unstageable pressure ulcers that were present upon admission/reentry** - enter how many were noted at the time of admission

Item Rationale

Health-related Quality of Life

- Although the wound bed cannot be visualized, and hence the pressure ulcer cannot be staged, the pressure ulcer may affect quality of life for residents because it may limit activity and may be painful.

Planning for Care

- Although the pressure ulcer itself cannot be observed, the surrounding area is monitored for signs of redness, swelling, increased drainage, or tenderness to touch, and the resident is monitored for adequate pain control.

> **DEFINITIONS**
>
> **NON-REMOVABLE DRESSING/ DEVICE**
> Includes, for example, a primary surgical dressing that cannot be removed, an orthopedic device, or cast.

Steps for Assessment

1. Review the medical record for documentation of a pressure ulcer covered by a non-removable dressing.
2. Determine the number of pressure ulcers unstageable related to a non-removable dressing/device. Examples of non-removable dressings/devices include a dressing that is not to be removed per physician's order, an orthopedic device, or a cast.
3. Identify the number of these pressure ulcers that were present on admission (see page M-6 for assessment process).

M0300E: Unstageable Pressure Ulcers Related to Non-removable Dressing/Device (cont.)

Coding Instructions for M0300E

- **Enter the number** of pressure ulcers that are unstageable related to non-removable dressing/device.

- **Enter 0** if no unstageable pressure ulcers are present and skip to **Current Number of Unhealed Pressure Ulcers at Each Stage** item (M0300F).

- **Enter the number** of unstageable pressure ulcers related to a non-removable dressing/device that were first noted at the time of admission AND—for residents who are reentering the facility after a hospital stay, that were acquired during the hospitalization.

- **Enter 0** if no unstageable pressure ulcers were first noted at the time of admission.

M0300F: Unstageable Pressure Ulcers Related to Slough and/or Eschar

M0300. Current Number of Unhealed (non-epithelialized) Pressure Ulcers at Each Stage - Continued	
	F. Unstageable - Slough and/or eschar: Known but not stageable due to coverage of wound bed by slough and/or eschar
Enter Number ☐	1. **Number of unstageable pressure ulcers due to coverage of wound bed by slough and/or eschar** - If 0 ➔ Skip to M0300G, Unstageable: Deep tissue
Enter Number ☐	2. **Number of these unstageable pressure ulcers that were present upon admission/reentry** - enter how many were noted at the time of admission

Item Rationale

Health-related Quality of Life

- Although the wound bed cannot be visualized, and hence the pressure ulcer cannot be staged, the pressure ulcer may affect quality of life for residents because it may limit activity, may be painful, and may require time-consuming treatments and dressing changes.

Planning for Care

- Visualization of the wound bed is necessary for accurate staging.
- The presence of pressure ulcers and other skin changes should be accounted for in the interdisciplinary care plan.
- Pressure ulcers that present as unstageable require care planning that includes, in the absence of ischemia, debridement of necrotic and dead tissue and restaging once the necrotic tissue is removed.

DEFINITIONS

SLOUGH TISSUE
Non-viable yellow, tan, gray, green or brown tissue; usually moist, can be soft, stringy and mucinous in texture. Slough may be adherent to the base of the wound or present in clumps throughout the wound bed.

ESCHAR TISSUE
Dead or devitalized tissue that is hard or soft in texture; usually black, brown, or tan in color, and may appear scab-like. Necrotic tissue and eschar are usually firmly adherent to the base of the wound and often the sides/ edges of the wound.

M0300F: Unstageable Pressure Ulcers Related to Slough and/or Eschar (cont.)

Steps for Assessment

1. Determine the number of pressure ulcers that are unstageable due to slough/eschar.
2. Identify the number of these pressure ulcers that were present on admission (see page M-6 for assessment process).

DEFINITIONS

FLUCTUANCE
Used to describe the texture of wound tissue indicative of underlying unexposed fluid.

Coding Instructions for M0300F

- **Enter the number** of pressure ulcers that are unstageable related to slough and/or eschar.
- **Enter 0** if no unstageable pressure ulcers are present and skip to **Current Number of Unhealed Pressure Ulcers at Each Stage** item (M0300G).
- **Enter the number** of unstageable pressure ulcers related to slough and/or eschar that were first noted at the time of admission AND—for residents who are reentering the facility after a hospital stay that were acquired during the hospitalization.
- **Enter 0** if no unstageable pressure ulcers were first noted at the time of admission.

Coding Tips

- Pressure ulcers that are covered with slough and/or eschar should be coded as unstageable because the true depth (and therefore stage) cannot be determined. Only until enough slough and/or eschar is removed to expose the depth of the tissue layers involved, can the stage of the wound be determined.

- Stable eschar (i.e., dry, adherent, intact without erythema or fluctuance) on the heels serves as "the body's natural (biological) cover" and should only be removed after careful clinical consideration, including ruling out ischemia, and consultation with the resident's physician, or nurse practitioner, physician assistant, or clinical nurse specialist if allowable under state licensure laws.

- Once the pressure ulcer is debrided of slough and/or eschar such that the tissues involved can be determined, then code the ulcer for the reclassified stage. The pressure ulcer does not have to be completely debrided or free of all slough and/or eschar tissue in order for reclassification of stage to occur.

Examples

1. A resident is admitted with a sacral pressure ulcer that is 100% covered with black eschar.

   Coding: The pressure ulcer would be coded at **M0300F1 as 1, and at M0300F2 as 1, present on admission.**

   Rationale: The pressure ulcer depth is not observable because it is covered with eschar so it is unstageable. It was present on admission.

M0300F: Unstageable Pressure Ulcers Related to Slough and/or Eschar (cont.)

2. A pressure ulcer on the sacrum was present on admission, and was 100% covered with black eschar. On the admission assessment, it was coded as unstageable and present on admission. The pressure ulcer is later debrided using conservative methods and after 4 weeks the ulcer has 50% to 75% eschar present. The assessor can now see that the damage extends down to the bone.

    Coding: The ulcer is reclassified as a Stage 4 pressure ulcer. On the subsequent MDS, it is coded at **M0300D1 as 1, and at M0300D2 as 1, present on admission.**

    Rationale: After debridement, the pressure ulcer is no longer unstageable because it can be observed to be a Stage 4 pressure ulcer and should be coded at M0300D. This pressure ulcer's dimensions would also be entered at M0610 if this pressure ulcer has the largest surface area of all Stage 3 or 4 pressure ulcers for this resident.

3. Miss J. was admitted with one small Stage 2 pressure ulcer. Despite treatment, it is not improving. In fact, it now appears deeper than originally observed, and the wound bed is covered with slough.

    Coding: Code at **M0300F1 as 1, and at M0300F2 as 0**, **not present on admission.**

    Rationale: The pressure ulcer is coded as unstageable due to coverage of the wound bed by slough but not coded as present on admission because it can no longer be coded as a Stage 2.

M0300G: Unstageable Pressure Ulcers Related to Suspected Deep Tissue Injury

M0300. Current Number of Unhealed (non-epithelialized) Pressure Ulcers at Each Stage - Continued	
	G. **Unstageable - Deep tissue:** Suspected deep tissue injury in evolution
Enter Number ☐	1. **Number of unstageable pressure ulcers with suspected deep tissue injury in evolution** - If 0 → Skip to M0610, Dimension of Unhealed Stage 3 or 4 Pressure Ulcers or Eschar
Enter Number ☐	2. **Number of these unstageable pressure ulcers that were present upon admission/reentry** - enter how many were noted at the time of admission

Item Rationale

Health-related Quality of Life

- Deep tissue injury may precede the development of a Stage 3 or 4 pressure ulcer even with optimal treatment.

M0300G: Unstageable Pressure Ulcers Related to Suspected Deep Tissue Injury (cont.)

- Quality health care begins with prevention and risk assessment, and care planning begins with prevention. Appropriate care planning is essential in optimizing a resident's ability to avoid, as well as recover from, pressure (as well as all) wounds. Deep tissue injuries may sometimes indicate severe damage. Identification and management of Deep Tissue Injury (DTI) is imperative.

> **DEFINITIONS**
>
> **SUSPECTED DEEP TISSUE INJURY**
> Purple or maroon area of discolored intact skin due to damage of underlying soft tissue damage. The area may be preceded by tissue that is painful, firm, mushy, boggy, warmer or cooler as compared to adjacent tissue.

Planning for Care

- Suspected deep tissue injury requires vigilant monitoring because of the potential for rapid deterioration. Such monitoring should be reflected in the care plan.

Steps for Assessment

1. Perform head-to-toe assessment. Conduct a full body skin assessment focusing on bony prominences and pressure-bearing areas (sacrum, buttocks, heels, ankles, etc.).
2. For the purposes of coding, determine that the lesion being assessed is primarily a result of pressure and that other conditions have been ruled out. If pressure is NOT the primary cause, do NOT code here.
3. Examine the area adjacent to, or surrounding, an intact blister for evidence of tissue damage. If the tissue adjacent to, or surrounding, the blister **does not show** signs of tissue damage (e.g., color change, tenderness, bogginess or firmness, warmth or coolness), do NOT code as a suspected Deep Tissue Injury.
4. In dark-skinned individuals, the area of injury is probably not purple/maroon, but rather darker than the surrounding tissue.
5. Determine the number of pressure ulcers that are unstageable related to suspected Deep Tissue Injury.
6. Identify the number of these pressure ulcers that were present on admission (see page M-6 for instructions).
7. Clearly document assessment findings in the resident's medical record, and track and document appropriate wound care planning and management.

Coding Instructions for M0300G

- **Enter the number** of unstageable pressure ulcer related to suspected deep tissue injury. Based on skin tone, the injured tissue area may present as a darker tone than the surrounding intact skin. These areas of discoloration are potentially areas of suspected deep tissue injury.

- **Enter 0** if no unstageable pressure ulcers are present and skip to **Dimensions of Unhealed Stage 3 or Stage 4 Pressure Ulcers or Eschar** item (M0610).

M0300G: Unstageable Pressure Ulcers Related to Suspected Deep Tissue Injury (cont.)

- **Enter the number** of unstageable pressure ulcers related to suspected deep tissue injury that were first noted at the time of admission AND—for residents who are reentering the facility after a hospital stay, that were acquired during the hospitalization.
- **Enter 0** if no unstageable pressure ulcers were first noted at the time of admission.

Coding Tips

- Once suspected deep tissue injury has opened to an ulcer, reclassify the ulcer into the appropriate stage. Then code the ulcer for the reclassified stage.
- Deep tissue injury may be difficult to detect in individuals with dark skin tones.
- Evolution may be rapid, exposing additional layers of tissue even with optimal treatment.
- When a lesion due to pressure presents with an intact blister AND the surrounding or adjacent soft tissue does NOT have the characteristics of Deep Tissue Injury, do NOT code here.

M0610: Dimensions of Unhealed Stage 3 or 4 Pressure Ulcers or Unstageable Pressure Ulcer Due to Slough or Eschar

M0610. Dimensions of Unhealed Stage 3 or 4 Pressure Ulcers or Eschar
Complete only if M0300C1, M0300D1 or M0300F1 is greater than 0
If the resident has one or more unhealed (non-epithelialized) Stage 3 or 4 pressure ulcers or an unstageable pressure ulcer due to slough or eschar, identify the pressure ulcer with the largest surface area (length x width) and record in centimeters:
☐☐.☐ cm   **A. Pressure ulcer length:** Longest length from head to toe
☐☐.☐ cm   **B. Pressure ulcer width:** Widest width of the same pressure ulcer, side-to-side perpendicular (90-degree angle) to length
☐☐.☐ cm   **C. Pressure ulcer depth:** Depth of the same pressure ulcer from the visible surface to the deepest area (if depth is unknown, enter a dash in each box)

Item Rationale

Health-related Quality of Life

- Pressure ulcer dimensions are an important characteristic used to assess and monitor healing.

Planning for Care

- Evaluating the dimensions of the pressure ulcer is one aspect of the process of monitoring response to treatment.
- Pressure ulcer measurement findings are used to plan interventions that will best prepare the wound bed for healing.

M0610: Dimensions of Unhealed Stage 3 or 4 Pressure Ulcers or Unstageable Pressure Ulcer Due to Slough or Eschar (cont.)

Steps for Assessment

*If the resident has **one or more** unhealed (non-epithelialized) Stage 3 or 4 pressure ulcers or an unstageable pressure ulcer due to slough or eschar, **identify the pressure ulcer with the largest surface area** (length × width) and record in centimeters. **Complete only if a pressure ulcer is coded in M0300C1, M0300D1, or M0300F1.** The Figure (right) illustrates the measurement process.*

1. Measurement is based on observation of the Stage 3, Stage 4, or unstageable pressure ulcer due to slough or eschar **after** the dressing and any exudate are removed.
2. Use a disposable measuring device or a cotton-tipped applicator.
3. Determine longest length (white arrow line) head to toe and greatest width (black arrow line) of each Stage 3, Stage 4, or unstageable pressure ulcer due to slough or eschar.
4. Measure the longest length of the pressure ulcer. If using a cotton-tipped applicator, mark on the applicator the distance between healthy skin tissue at each margin and lay the applicator next to a centimeter ruler to determine length.
5. Using a similar approach, measure the longest width (perpendicular to the length forming a "+," side to side).
6. Measure every Stage 3, Stage 4, and unstageable pressure ulcer due to slough or eschar that is present. **The clinician must be aware of all pressure ulcers present in order to determine which pressure ulcer is the largest.** Use a skin tracking sheet or other worksheet to record the dimensions for each pressure ulcer. Select the largest one by comparing the surface areas (length x width) of each.
7. Considering **only** the largest Stage 3 or 4 pressure ulcer due to slough or eschar, determine the deepest area and record the depth in centimeters. To measure wound depth, moisten a sterile, cotton-tipped applicator with 0.9% sodium chloride (NaCl) solution or sterile water. Place the applicator tip in the deepest aspect of the ulcer and measure the distance to the skin level. If the depth is uneven, measure several areas and document the depth of the ulcer that is the deepest. If depth cannot be assessed due to slough or eschar, enter dashes in M0610C.
8. If two pressure ulcers occur on the same bony prominence and are separated, at least superficially, by skin, then count them as two separate pressure ulcers. Classify the stage and measure each pressure ulcer separately.

M0610: Dimensions of Unhealed Stage 3 or 4 Pressure Ulcers or Unstageable Pressure Ulcer Due to Slough or Eschar (cont.)

Coding Instructions for M0610 Dimensions of Unhealed Stage 3 or 4 Pressure Ulcers or Unstageable Due to Slough or Eschar

- **Enter the current longest length** of the largest Stage 3, Stage 4, or unstageable pressure ulcer due to slough or eschar in centimeters to one decimal point (e.g., 2.3 cm).
- **Enter the widest width** in centimeters of the largest Stage 3, Stage 4, or unstageable pressure ulcer due to slough or eschar. Record the width in centimeters to one decimal point.
- **Enter the depth** measured in centimeters of the largest Stage 3 or 4. Record the depth in centimeters to one decimal point. Note that depth cannot be assessed if wound bed is unstageable due to being covered with slough or eschar. If a pressure ulcer covered with slough or eschar is the largest unhealed pressure ulcer identified for measurement, enter dashes in item M0610C.

Coding Tips

- Place the resident in the most appropriate position which will allow for accurate wound measurement.
- Select a uniform, consistent method for measuring wound length, width, and depth to facilitate meaningful comparisons of wound measurements across time.
- Assessment of the pressure ulcer for tunneling and undermining is an important part of the complete pressure ulcer assessment. Measurement of tunneling and undermining is not recorded on the MDS but should be assessed, monitored, and treated as part of the comprehensive care plan.

M0700: Most Severe Tissue Type for Any Pressure Ulcer

M0700. Most Severe Tissue Type for Any Pressure Ulcer	
Enter Code [ ]	Select the best description of the most severe type of tissue present in any pressure ulcer bed 1. **Epithelial tissue** - new skin growing in superficial ulcer. It can be light pink and shiny, even in persons with darkly pigmented skin 2. **Granulation tissue** - pink or red tissue with shiny, moist, granular appearance 3. **Slough** - yellow or white tissue that adheres to the ulcer bed in strings or thick clumps, or is mucinous 4. **Necrotic tissue (Eschar)** - black, brown, or tan tissue that adheres firmly to the wound bed or ulcer edges, may be softer or harder than surrounding skin

Item Rationale

Health-related Quality of Life

- The presence of a pressure ulcer may affect quality of life for residents because it may limit activity, may be painful, and may require time-consuming treatments and dressing changes.

M0700: Most Severe Tissue Type for Any Pressure Ulcer (cont.)

Planning for Care

- Identify tissue type.
- Tissue characteristics of pressure ulcers should be considered when determining treatment options and choices.
- Changes in tissue characteristics over time are indicative of wound healing or degeneration.

Steps for Assessment

1. Examine the wound bed or base of each pressure ulcer. Adequate lighting is important to detect skin changes.
2. Determine the type(s) of tissue in the wound bed (e.g., epithelial, granulation, slough, eschar).

Coding Instructions for M0700

- **Code 1, epithelial tissue:** if the wound is superficial and is re-epithelializing.
- **Code 2, granulation tissue:** if the wound is clean (e.g., free of slough and necrotic tissue) and contains granulation tissue.
- **Code 3, slough:** if there is any amount of slough present and necrotic tissue is absent.
- **Code 4, necrotic tissue (eschar):** if there is any necrotic tissue (eschar) present.

Coding Tips and Special Populations

- All Stage 2 pressure ulcers should be **coded as 1** for this item.
- Stage 2 pressure ulcers should **not** be coded with granulation, slough, or necrotic tissue.
- Code for the most severe type of tissue present in the pressure ulcer wound bed.
- If the wound bed is covered with a mix of different types of tissue, code for the most severe type. For example, if a mixture of necrotic tissue (eschar) and slough is present, code for necrotic tissue (eschar).

DEFINITIONS

EPITHELIAL TISSUE
New skin that is light pink and shiny (even in person's with darkly pigmented skin). In Stage 2 pressure ulcers, epithelial tissue is seen in the center and edges of the ulcer. In full thickness Stage 3 and 4 pressure ulcers, epithelial tissue advances from the edges of the wound.

GRANULATION TISSUE
Red tissue with "cobblestone" or bumpy appearance, bleeds easily when injured.

SLOUGH TISSUE
Non-viable yellow, tan, gray, green or brown tissue; usually moist, can be soft, stringy and mucinous in texture. Slough may be adherent to the base of the wound or present in clumps throughout the wound bed.

NECROTIC TISSUE (ESCHAR)
Dead or devitalized tissue that is hard or soft in texture; usually black, brown, or tan in color, and may appear scab-like. Necrotic tissue and eschar are usually firmly adherent to the base of the wound and often the sides/edges of the wound.

M0700: Most Severe Tissue Type for Any Pressure Ulcer (cont.)

Examples

1. A resident has a Stage 2 pressure ulcer on the right ischial tuberosity that is healing and a Stage 3 pressure ulcer on the sacrum that is also healing with red granulation tissue that has filled 75% of the ulcer and epithelial tissue that has resurfaced 25% of the ulcer.

   Coding: Code **M0700 as 2, granulation tissue.**

   Rationale: Coding for M0700 is based on the sacral ulcer, because it is the pressure ulcer with the most severe tissue type. Code 2, (Granulation tissue), is selected because this is the most severe tissue present in the wound.

2. A resident has a Stage 2 pressure ulcer on the right heel and no other pressure ulcers.

   Coding: Code **M0700 as 1, epithelial tissue**.

   Rationale: Coding for M0700 is Code 1, (Epithelial tissue) because epithelial tissue is consistent with identification of this pressure ulcer as a Stage 2 pressure ulcer.

3. A resident has a pressure ulcer on the left trochanter that has 25% black necrotic tissue present, 75% granulation tissue present, and some epithelialization at the edges of the wound.

   Coding: Code **M0700 as 4, necrotic tissue.**

   Rationale: Coding is for the most severe tissue type present, which is not always the majority of type of tissue. Therefore, Coding for M0700 is Code 4, (Necrotic tissue).

M0800: Worsening in Pressure Ulcer Status Since Prior Assessment (OBRA, PPS, or Discharge)

M0800. Worsening in Pressure Ulcer Status Since Prior Assessment (OBRA, PPS, or Discharge) Complete only if A0310E = 0
Indicate the number of current pressure ulcers that were **not present or were at a lesser stage** on prior assessment (OBRA, PPS, or Discharge). If no current pressure ulcer at a given stage, enter 0
Enter Number ☐ A. Stage 2
Enter Number ☐ B. Stage 3
Enter Number ☐ C. Stage 4

Item Rationale

Health-related Quality of Life

- This item documents whether skin status, overall, has worsened since the last assessment. To track increasing skin damage, this item documents the number of new pressure ulcers and whether any pressure ulcers have worsened to a higher (deeper) stage since the last assessment. Such tracking of pressure ulcers is consistent with good clinical care.

M0800: Worsening in Pressure Ulcer Status Since Prior Assessment (OBRA, PPS, or Discharge) (cont.)

Planning for Care

- Pressure ulcers that degenerate or worsen to a higher (deeper) stage require a reevaluation of the interdisciplinary care plan.

Steps for Assessment

*Look-back period for this item is back to the ARD of the prior assessment. **If there was no prior assessment (i.e., if this is the first OBRA or PPS assessment), do not complete this item.** Skip to M1030, **Number of Venous and Arterial Ulcers.***

1. Review the history of each current pressure ulcer. Specifically, compare the current stage to past stages to determine whether any pressure ulcer on the current assessment is new or at a higher (deeper) stage when compared to the last MDS assessment. This allows a more accurate assessment than simply comparing total counts on the current and prior MDS assessment.
2. For each current stage, count the number of current pressure ulcers that are new or have worsened since the last MDS assessment was completed.

Coding Instructions for M0800

- **Enter the number** of pressure ulcers that were not present OR were at a lesser stage on prior assessment.
- **Code 0:** if no pressure ulcers have worsened OR there are no new pressure ulcers.

Coding Tips

- Coding this item will be easier for nursing homes that document and follow pressure ulcer status on a routine basis.
- Coding unstageable pressure ulcers:
  — If an ulcer was unstageable on admission, do not consider it to be worse on the first assessment. However, if it worsens after that assessment, it should be included.
  — If a previously staged pressure ulcer becomes unstageable and then is debrided sufficiently to be staged, compare its stage before and after it was unstageable. If the pressure ulcer's stage has worsened, code it as such in this item.
  — If a pressure ulcer is acquired during a hospital admission, it is coded as "present on admission" and not included in a count of worsening pressure ulcers.
  — **If a pressure ulcer worsens to a more severe stage during a hospital admission, it should also be coded as "present on admission" and not included in counts of worsening pressure ulcers.** While not included in counts of worsening pressure ulcers, it is important to recognize clinically on reentry that the resident's overall skin status deteriorated while in the hospital. In either case, if the pressure ulcer deteriorates (worsens) to a higher (deeper) stage on subsequent MDS assessments, it would then be included in counts of worsening pressure ulcers.

M0800: Worsening in Pressure Ulcer Status Since Prior Assessment (OBRA, PPS, or Discharge) (cont.)

Examples

1. A resident has a pressure ulcer on the right ischial tuberosity that was Stage 2 on the previous MDS assessment and has now deteriorated (worsened) to a Stage 3 pressure ulcer.

   Coding: Code **M0800A as 0, M0800B as 1**, and **M0800C as 0.**

   Rationale: The pressure ulcer was at a lesser stage on the prior assessment.

2. A resident is admitted with an unstageable pressure ulcer on the sacrum, which is debrided and reclassified as a Stage 4 pressure ulcer 3 weeks later. The initial MDS assessment listed the pressure ulcer as unstageable.

   Coding: Code **M0800A as 0**, **M0800B as 0**, and **M0800C as 0.**

   Rationale: The unstageable pressure ulcer was present on the initial MDS assessment. After debridement it was a Stage 4. This is the first staging since debridement and should not be counted as worsening on the MDS assessment.

3. A resident has previous medical record and MDS documentation of a Stage 2 pressure ulcer on the sacrum and a Stage 3 pressure ulcer on the right heel. Current skin care flow sheets indicate a Stage 3 pressure ulcer on the sacrum, a Stage 4 pressure ulcer on the right hccl, and a Stage 2 pressure ulcer on the left trochanter.

   Coding: Code **M0800A as 1, M0800B as 1**, and **M0800C as 1.**

   Rationale: M0800A would be coded 1 because the new Stage 2 pressure ulcer on the left trochanter was not present on the prior assessment. M0800B would be coded 1 and M0800C would be coded 1 for the worsening in pressure ulcer status (i.e. increased severity) of the sacrum and right heel pressure ulcers.

4. A resident develops a Stage 3 pressure ulcer while at the nursing home. The wound bed is subsequently covered with slough and is coded on the next assessment as unstageable. After debridement, the wound bed is clean and the pressure ulcer is coded as a Stage 3.

   Coding: Code **M0800A as 0**, **M0800B as 0**, and **M0800C as 0.**

   Rationale: M0800B would be coded 0 because the current Stage 3 pressure ulcer is the same stage as it was prior to the period it became unstageable.

M0900: Healed Pressure Ulcers

	M0900. Healed Pressure Ulcers Complete only if A0310E = 0

Enter Code
[ ]
	A. Were pressure ulcers present on the prior assessment (OBRA, PPS, or Discharge)?
	  0. **No** → Skip to M1030, Number of Venous and Arterial Ulcers
	  1. **Yes** → Continue to M0900B, Stage 2

	Indicate the number of pressure ulcers that were noted on the prior assessment (OBRA, PPS, or Discharge) that have completely closed (resurfaced with epithelium). If no healed pressure ulcer at a given stage since the prior assessment (OBRA, PPS, or Discharge), enter 0
Enter Number [ ]	**B. Stage 2**
Enter Number [ ]	**C. Stage 3**
Enter Number [ ]	**D. Stage 4**

Item Rationale

Health-related Quality of Life

- Pressure ulcers do not heal in a reverse sequence, that is, the body does not replace the types and layers of tissue (e.g., muscle, fat, and dermis) that were lost during the pressure ulcer development. Replacement tissue is never as strong as the tissue that was lost and hence is more prone to future breakdown.

Planning for Care

- Pressure ulcers that heal require continued prevention interventions as the site is always at risk for future damage.

- **Most Stage 2** pressure ulcers should heal in a reasonable timeframe (e.g. 60 days). Full thickness Stage 3 and 4 pressure ulcers may require longer healing times.

- Current clinical standards do not support reverse staging or backstaging. For example, over time, a Stage 4 pressure ulcer has been healing such that it is less deep, wide, and long. Previous standards using reverse or backstaging would have permitted identification of the pressure ulcer as a Stage 2 pressure ulcer when it reached a depth consistent with Stage 2 pressure ulcers. Current standards require that it continue to be documented as a Stage 4 pressure ulcer until it has completely healed. For care planning purposes, a healed Stage 4 pressure ulcer will remain at increased risk for future breakdown or injury and will require continued monitoring.

> **DEFINITIONS**
>
> **HEALED PRESSURE ULCER**
> Completely closed, fully epithelialized, covered completely with epithelial tissue, or resurfaced with new skin, *even if* the area continues to have some surface discoloration.

M0900: Healed Pressure Ulcers (cont.)

Steps for Assessment

Complete on all residents, including those without a current pressure ulcer.

*Look-back period for this item is the ARD of the prior assessment. **If no prior assessment (i.e., if this is the first OBRA or PPS assessment), do not complete this item.** Skip to M1030.*

1. Review medical records to identify whether any pressure ulcers that were noted on the prior MDS assessment have completely closed by the ARD (A2300) of the current assessment.
2. Identify the deepest anatomical stage (see definition on page M-5) of each resurfaced (or healed) pressure ulcer.
3. Count the number of healed pressure ulcers for each stage.

Coding Instructions for M0900A

Complete on all residents (even if M0210 = 0)

- **Enter 0:** if there were no pressure ulcers on the prior assessment and skip to **Number of Venous and Arterial Ulcers** item (M1030).

- **Enter 1:** if there were pressure ulcers noted on the prior assessment.

Coding Instructions for M0900B, C, and D.

- **Enter the number** of pressure ulcers that have healed since the last assessment for each Stage 2 through 4.

- **Enter 0:** if there were no pressure ulcers at the given stage or no pressure ulcers that have healed.

Coding Tips

- Coding this item will be easier for nursing homes that systematically document and follow pressure ulcer status.

- If the prior assessment documents that a pressure ulcer healed between MDS assessments, but another pressure ulcer occurred at the same location, do not consider the first pressure ulcer to have healed, and do NOT record the pressure ulcer as healed.

M1030: Number of Venous and Arterial Ulcers

M1030. Number of Venous and Arterial Ulcers	
Enter Number ☐	Enter the total number of venous and arterial ulcers present

Item Rationale

Health-related Quality of Life

- Skin wounds and lesions affect quality of life for residents because they may limit activity, may be painful, and may require time-consuming treatments and dressing changes.

Planning for Care

- The presence of venous and arterial ulcers should be accounted for in the interdisciplinary care plan.
- This information identifies residents at risk for further complications or skin injury.

Steps for Assessment

1. Review the medical record, including skin care flow sheet or other skin tracking form.
2. Speak with direct care staff and the treatment nurse to confirm conclusions from the medical record review.
3. Examine the resident and determine whether any venous or arterial ulcers are present.

   - Key areas for venous ulcer development include the area proximal to the lateral and medial malleolus (e.g., above the inner and outer ankle area).
   - Key areas for arterial ulcer development include the distal part of the foot, dorsum or tops of the foot, or tips and tops of the toes.
   - Venous ulcers may or may not be painful and are typically shallow with irregular wound edges, a red granular (e.g., bumpy) wound bed, minimal to moderate amounts of yellow fibrinous material, and moderate to large amounts of exudate. The surrounding tissues may be erythematous or reddened, or appear brown-tinged due to hemosiderin staining. Leg edema may also be present.
   - Arterial ulcers are often painful and have a pale pink wound bed, necrotic tissue, minimal exudate, and minimal bleeding.

> **DEFINITIONS**
>
> **VENOUS ULCERS**
> Ulcers caused by peripheral venous disease, which most commonly occur proximal to the medial or lateral malleolus, above the inner or outer ankle, or on the lower calf area of the leg.
>
> **ARTERIAL ULCERS**
> Ulcers caused by peripheral arterial disease, which commonly occur on the tips and tops of the toes, tops of the foot, or distal to the medial malleolus.

> **DEFINITIONS**
>
> **HEMOSIDERIN**
> An intracellular storage form of iron; the granules consist of an ill-defined complex of ferric hydroxides, polysaccharides, and proteins having an iron content of approximately 33% by weight. It appears as a dark yellow-brown pigment.

M1030: Number of Venous and Arterial Ulcers (cont.)

Coding Instructions

Check all that apply in the last 7 days.

Pressure ulcers coded in M0210 through M0900 should NOT be coded here.

- **Enter the number** of venous and arterial ulcers present.
- **Enter 0:** if there were no venous or arterial ulcers present.

Coding Tips

Arterial Ulcers

- Trophic skin changes (e.g., dry skin, loss of hair growth, muscle atrophy, brittle nails) may also be present. The wound may start with some kind of minor trauma, such as hitting the leg on a wheelchair. The wound does not typically occur over a bony prominence, however, can occur on the tops of the toes. Pressure forces play virtually no role in the development of the ulcer, however, for some residents, pressure may play a part. Ischemia is the major etiology of these ulcers. Lower extremity and foot pulses may be diminished or absent.

Venous Ulcers

- The wound may start with some kind of minor trauma, such as hitting the leg on a wheelchair. The wound does not typically occur over a bony prominence, and pressure forces play virtually **no** role in the development of the ulcer.

Example

1. A resident has three toes on her right foot that have black tips. She does not have diabetes, but has been diagnosed with peripheral vascular disease.

   Coding: Code **M1030 as 3.**

   Rationale: Ischemic changes point to the ulcer being vascular.

M1040: Other Ulcers, Wounds and Skin Problems

M1040. Other Ulcers, Wounds and Skin Problems	
↓ Check all that apply	
Foot Problems	
☐	A. **Infection of the foot** (e.g., cellulitis, purulent drainage)
☐	B. **Diabetic foot ulcer(s)**
☐	C. **Other open lesion(s) on the foot**
Other Problems	
☐	D. **Open lesion(s) other than ulcers, rashes, cuts** (e.g., cancer lesion)
☐	E. **Surgical wound(s)**
☐	F. **Burn(s)** (second or third degree)
None of the Above	
☐	Z. **None of the above** were present

Item Rationale

Health-related Quality of Life

- Skin wounds and lesions affect quality of life for residents because they may limit activity, may be painful, and may require time-consuming treatments and dressing changes.
- Many of these ulcers, wounds and skin problems can worsen or increase risk for local and systemic infections.

Planning for Care

- This list represents only a subset of skin conditions or changes that nursing homes will assess and evaluate in residents.
- The presence of wounds and skin changes should be accounted for in the interdisciplinary care plan.
- This information identifies residents at risk for further complications or skin injury.

Steps for Assessment

1. Review the medical record, including skin care flow sheets or other skin tracking forms.
2. Speak with direct care staff and the treatment nurse to confirm conclusions from the medical record review.
3. Examine the resident and determine whether any ulcers, wounds, or skin problems are present.

- Key areas for diabetic foot ulcers include the plantar (bottom) surface of the foot, especially the metatarsal heads (the ball of the foot).

Coding Instructions

Check all that apply in the last 7 days. If there is no evidence of such problems in the last 7 days, check none of the above. Pressure ulcers coded in M0200 through M0900 should NOT be coded here.

- **M1040A,** infection of the foot (e.g., cellulitis, purulent drainage)
- **M1040B,** diabetic foot ulcer(s)
- **M1040C,** other open lesion(s) on the foot

DEFINITIONS

DIABETIC FOOT ULCERS
Ulcers caused by the neuropathic and small blood vessel complications of diabetes. Diabetic foot ulcers typically occur over the plantar (bottom) surface of the foot on load bearing areas such as the ball of the foot. Ulcers are usually deep, with necrotic tissue, moderate amounts of exudate, and callused wound edges. The wounds are very regular in shape and the wound edges are even with a punched-out appearance. These wounds are typically not painful.

SURGICAL WOUNDS
Any healing and non-healing, open or closed surgical incisions, skin grafts or drainage sites.

OPEN LESION OTHER THAN ULCERS, RASHES, CUTS
Most typically skin ulcers that develop as a result of diseases and conditions such as syphilis and cancer.

BURNS (SECOND OR THIRD DEGREE)
Skin and tissue injury caused by heat or chemicals and may be in any stage of healing.

M1040: Other Ulcers, Wounds and Skin Problems (cont.)

- **M1040D,** open lesion(s) other than ulcers, rashes, cuts (e.g., cancer lesion)
- **M1040E,** surgical wound(s)
- **M1040F,** burn(s)(second or third degree)
- **M1040Z,** none of the above were present

Coding Tips

M1040B Diabetic Foot Ulcers

- Diabetic neuropathy affects the lower extremities of individuals with diabetes. Individuals with diabetic neuropathy can have decreased awareness of pain in their feet. This means they are at high risk for foot injury, such as burns from hot water or heating pads, cuts or scrapes from stepping on foreign objects, and blisters from inappropriate or tight-fitting shoes. Because of decreased circulation and sensation, the resident may not be aware of the wound.

- Neuropathy can also cause changes in the structure of the bones and tissue in the foot. This means the individual with diabetes experiences pressure on the foot in areas not meant to bear pressure. Neuropathy can also cause changes in normal sweating, which means the individual with diabetes can have dry, cracked skin on his other foot.

- Do NOT include pressure ulcers that occur on residents with diabetes mellitus here. For example, an ulcer caused by pressure on the heel of a diabetic resident is a pressure ulcer and not a diabetic foot ulcer.

M1040D Open Lesion Other than Ulcers, Rashes, Cuts

- Do NOT code rashes, skin tears, cuts/lacerations here. Although not recorded on the MDS assessment, these skin conditions should be considered in the plan of care.

M1040E Surgical Wounds

- This category does not include healed surgical sites and stomas or lacerations that require suturing or butterfly closure as surgical wounds. PICC sites, central line sites, and peripheral IV sites are not coded as surgical wounds.

- Do not code pressure ulcers that have been surgically debrided as surgical wounds. They continue to be coded as pressure ulcers.

- This coding is appropriate for pressure ulcers that are surgically repaired with grafts and flap procedures.

M1040F Burns (Second or Third Degree)

- Do NOT include first degree burns (changes in skin color only).

M1040: Other Ulcers, Wounds and Skin Problems (cont.)

Examples

1. A resident with diabetes mellitus presents with an ulcer on the heel that is due to pressure.

    Coding: This ulcer is **not checked at M1040B. This ulcer should be coded where appropriate under the Pressure Ulcers items (M0210-M0900).**
    Rationale: Persons with diabetes can still develop pressure ulcers.

2. A resident is readmitted from the hospital after flap surgery to repair a sacral pressure ulcer.

    Coding: Check **M1040E**, (Surgical Wound(s)).

    Rationale: A surgical flap procedure to repair pressure ulcers changes the coding to a surgical wound.

M1200: Skin and Ulcer Treatments

	M1200. Skin and Ulcer Treatments
	↓ Check all that apply
☐	A. Pressure reducing device for chair
☐	B. Pressure reducing device for bed
☐	C. Turning/repositioning program
☐	D. Nutrition or hydration intervention to manage skin problems
☐	E. Ulcer care
☐	F. Surgical wound care
☐	G. Application of nonsurgical dressings (with or without topical medications) other than to feet
☐	H. Applications of ointments/medications other than to feet
☐	I. Application of dressings to feet (with or without topical medications)
☐	Z. None of the above were provided

Item Rationale

Health-related Quality of Life

- Appropriate prevention and treatment of skin changes and ulcers reduce complications and promote healing.

Planning for Care

- These general skin treatments include basic pressure ulcer prevention and skin health interventions that are a part of providing quality care and consistent with good clinical practice for those with skin health problems.
- These general treatments should guide more individualized and specific interventions in the care plan.

> **DEFINITIONS**
>
> **PRESSURE REDUCING DEVICE(S)**
> Equipment that aims to relieve pressure away from areas of high risk. May include foam, air, water gel, or other cushioning placed on a chair, wheelchair, or bed. Include pressure relieving, pressure reducing, and pressure redistributing devices. Devices are available for use with beds and seating.

M1200: Skin and Ulcer Treatments (cont.)

- If skin changes are not improving or are worsening, this information may be helpful in determining more appropriate care.

Steps for Assessment

1. Review the medical record, including treatment records and health care provider orders for documented skin treatments during the past 7 days. Some skin treatments may be part of routine standard care for residents, so check the nursing facility's policies and procedures and indicate here if administered during the look-back period.
2. Speak with direct care staff and the treatment nurse to confirm conclusions from the medical record review.
3. Some skin treatments can be determined by observation. For example, observation of the resident's wheelchair and bed will reveal if the resident is using pressure-reducing devices for the bed or wheelchair.

Coding Instructions

*Check all that apply in the last 7 days. **Check Z, None of the above were provided,** if none applied in the past 7 days.*

- **M1200A,** pressure reducing device for chair
- **M1200B,** pressure reducing device for bed
- **M1200C,** turning/repositioning program
- **M1200D,** nutrition or hydration intervention to manage skin problems
- **M1200E,** ulcer care
- **M1200F,** surgical wound care
- **M1200G,** application of non-surgical dressings (with or without topical medications) other than to feet
- **M1200H,** application of ointments/medications other than to feet
- **M1200I,** application of dressings to feet (with or without topical medications)
- **M1200Z,** none of the above were provided

Coding Tips

M1200A/M1200B Pressure Reducing Devices

- Pressure reducing devices redistribute pressure so that there is some relief on or near the area of the ulcer. The appropriate reducing (redistribution) device should be selected based on the individualized needs of the resident.

> **DEFINITIONS**
>
> **TURNING/ REPOSITIONING PROGRAM**
> Includes a consistent program for changing the resident's position and realigning the body. "Program" is defined as a specific approach that is organized, planned, documented, monitored, and evaluated based on an assessment of the resident's needs.
>
> **NUTRITION OR HYDRATION INTERVENTION TO MANAGE SKIN PROBLEMS**
> Dietary measures received by the resident for the purpose of preventing or treating specific skin conditions, e.g., wheat-free diet to prevent allergic dermatitis, high calorie diet with added supplements to prevent skin breakdown, high-protein supplements for wound healing.

M1200: Skin and Ulcer Treatments (cont.)

- Do not include egg crate cushions of any type in this category.
- Do NOT include doughnut or ring devices in chairs.

M1200C Turning/Repositioning Program

- The turning/repositioning program is specific as to the approaches for changing the resident's position and realigning the body. The program should specify the intervention (e.g., reposition on side, pillows between knees) and frequency (e.g., every 2 hours).
- Progress notes, assessments, and other documentation (as dictated by facility policy) should support that the turning/repositioning program is monitored and reassessed to determine the effectiveness of the intervention.

M1200E Ulcer Care

- Ulcer care includes **any** intervention for treating pressure ulcers coded in **Current Number of Unhealed Pressure Ulcers at Each Stage** item (M0300). Examples may include the use of topical dressings, chemical or surgical debridement, wound irrigations, negative pressure wound therapy (NPWT), and/or hydrotherapy.

M1200F Surgical Wound Care

- Do not include post-operative care following eye or oral surgery.
- Surgical debridement of a pressure ulcer continues to be coded as a pressure ulcer.
- Surgical would care may include any intervention for treating or protecting any type of surgical wound. Examples may include topical cleansing, wound irrigation, application of antimicrobial ointments, application of dressings of any type, suture/staple removal, and warm soaks or heat application.

M1200G Application of Non-surgical Dressings (with or without Topical Medications) Other than to Feet

- Do NOT code application of non-surgical dressings for pressure ulcer(s) on the foot in this item; use **Ulcer Care** item (M1200E).
- Dressings do not have to be applied daily in order to be coded on the MDS assessment. If any dressing meeting the MDS definitions was applied even once during the 7-day look-back period, the assessor should check that MDS item.
- This category may include but is not limited to: dry gauze dressings, dressings moistened with saline or other solutions, transparent dressings, hydrogel dressings, and dressings with hydrocolloid or hydroactive particles used to treat a skin condition, compression bandages, etc.

M1200H Application of Ointments/Medications Other than to Feet

- Do NOT code application of ointments/medications (e.g. chemical or enzymatic debridement) for pressure ulcers here; use **Ulcer Care**, item (M1200E).

271

M1200: Skin and Ulcer Treatments (cont.)

- This category may include ointments or medications used to treat a skin condition (e.g., cortisone, antifungal preparations, chemotherapeutic agents).
- **Ointments/medications may include topical creams, powders, and liquid sealants used to treat or prevent skin conditions.**
- This definition does not include ointments used to treat non-skin conditions (e.g., nitropaste for chest pain).

M1200I Application of Dressings to the Feet (with or without Topical Medications)

- Includes interventions to treat any foot wound or ulcer **other than a pressure ulcer**.
- Do NOT code application of dressings to pressure ulcers on the foot, use **Ulcer Care** item (M1200E).
- Do not code application of dressings to the ankle. The ankle is not part of the foot.

Examples

1. A resident is admitted with a Stage 3 pressure ulcer on the sacrum. Care during the last 7 days has included one debridement by the wound care consultant, application of daily dressings with enzymatic ointment for continued debridement, use of oral liquid nutritional supplements, and use of a pressure reducing (redistribution) pad on the wheelchair. The medical record documents delivery of care and notes that the resident is on a 2-hour turning/repositioning program that is organized, planned, documented, monitored and evaluated based on an individualized assessment of her needs. The nursing home has a policy that all residents with a pressure ulcer receive a multivitamin with vitamin C and zinc in recommended daily allowances and all mattresses in the nursing home are pressure reducing (redistribution) mattresses.

   Coding: Check items **M1200A, M1200B, M1200C, M1200D, and M1200E.**

   Rationale: Interventions include pressure reducing (redistribution) pad in the wheelchair (M1200A) and pressure reducing (redistribution) mattress on the bed (M1200B), turning and repositioning program (M1200C), nutritional supplements (M1200D), enzymatic debridement and application of dressings (M1200E).

2. A resident has a venous ulcer on the right leg. During the past 7 days the resident has had a three layer compression bandaging system applied once (orders are to reapply the compression bandages every 5 days). The resident also has a pressure redistributing mattress and pad for the wheelchair.

   Coding: Check items **M1200A, M1200B, and M1200G**.

   Rationale: Treatments include pressure reducing (redistribution) mattress (M1200B) and pad (M1200A) in the wheelchair and application of the compression bandaging system (M1200G).

M1200: Skin and Ulcer Treatments (cont.)

3. Mrs. S. has a diagnosis of right-sided hemiplegia from a previous stroke. As part of her assessment, it was noted that while in bed Mrs. S. is able to tolerate pressure on each side for approximately 3 hours before showing signs of the effects of pressure on her skin. Staff assist her to turn every 3 hours while in bed. When she is in her wheelchair, it is difficult for her to offload the pressure to her buttocks. Her assessment indicates that her skin cannot tolerate pressure for more than 1 hour without showing signs of the effect of the pressure when she is sitting, and therefore, Mrs. S. is assisted hourly by staff to stand for at least 1 full minute to relieve pressure. Staff document all of these interventions in the medical record and note the resident's response to the interventions.

   Coding: Check **M1200C.**

   Rationale: Treatments meet the criteria for a turning/repositioning program (i.e., it is organized, planned, documented, monitored, and evaluated), that is based on an assessment of the resident's unique needs.

4. Mr. J. has a diagnosis of Advanced Alzheimer's and is totally dependent on staff for all of his care. His care plan states that he is to be turned and repositioned, per facility policy, every 2 hours.

   Coding: DO NOT check item **M1200C.**

   Rationale: Treatments provided do not meet the criteria for a turning/repositioning program. There is no notation in the medical record about an assessed need for turning/repositioning, nor is there a specific approach or plan related to positioning and realigning of the body. There is no reassessment of the resident's response to turning and repositioning. There are not any skin or ulcer treatments being provided.

Scenarios for Pressure Ulcer Coding

Examples M0300, M0610, M0700 and M0800

1. Mr. S was admitted to the nursing home on January 22, 2011 with a Stage 2 pressure ulcer. The pressure ulcer history was not available due to resident being admitted to the hospital from home prior to coming to the nursing home. On Mr. S' quarterly assessment, it was noted that the Stage 2 pressure ulcer had neither worsened nor improved. On the second quarterly assessment the Stage 2 pressure ulcer was noted to have worsened to a Stage 3. The current dimensions of the Stage 3 pressure ulcer are L 3.0cm, W 2.4cm, and D 0.2cm with 100% granulation tissue noted in the wound bed.

   Admission Assessment:
   Coding:
   — **M0300A** (Number of Stage 1 pressure ulcers), Code 0.
   — **M0300B1** (Number of Stage 2 pressure ulcers), Code 1.
   — **M0300B2** (Number of Stage 2 pressure ulcers present on admission/re-entry), Code 1.
   — **M0300B3** (Date of the oldest Stage 2 pressure ulcer), code with dashes.

Scenarios for Pressure Ulcer Coding (cont.)

Rationale: The resident had one Stage 2 pressure ulcer on admission and the date of the oldest pressure ulcer was unknown.

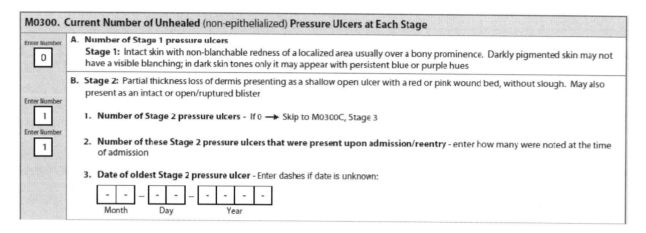

Quarterly Assessment #1:

Coding:

— **M0300A** (Number of Stage 1 pressure ulcers), Code 0.

— **M0300B1** (Number of Stage 2 pressure ulcers), Code 1.

— **M0300B2** (Number of Stage 2 pressure ulcers present upon admission/re-entry), Code 1.

— **M0300B3** (Date of the oldest Stage 2 pressure ulcer), Code 01/22/2011.

Rationale: On the quarterly assessment the Stage 2 pressure ulcer is still present so **M0300B3** is coded with the first date that the Stage 2 pressure ulcer was identified as the oldest, which was the date of admission.

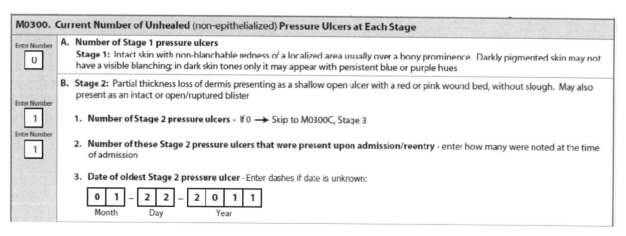

Quarterly Assessment #2:

Coding:

— **M0300A** (Number of Stage 1 pressure ulcers), Code 0.

Scenarios for Pressure Ulcer Coding (cont.)

— **M0300B1** (Number of Stage 2 pressure ulcers), Code 0 and skip to **M0300C**, Stage 3 pressure ulcers.
— **M0300C1** (Number of Stage 3 pressure ulcers). Code 1.
— **M0300C2** (Number of these Stage 3 pressure ulcers that were present upon admission/reentry). Code 0.
— **M0300D1, M0300E1, M0300F1, and M0300G1** Code 0's and proceed to code **M0610** (Dimensions of unhealed Stage 3 or 4 pressure ulcers or unstageable pressure ulcer related to slough or eschar) with the dimensions of the Stage 3 ulcer.
— **M0610A** (Pressure ulcer length), Code 03.0, **M0610B** (Pressure ulcer width), Code 02.4, **M0610C** (Pressure ulcer depth) Code 00.2.
— **M0700** (Most severe tissue type for any pressure ulcer), Code 2, Granulation tissue.
— **M0800** (Worsening in pressure ulcer status since prior assessment – OBRA, PPS, or Discharge) – **M0800A** (Stage 2) Code 0, **M0800B** (Stage 3) Code 1, **M0800C** (Stage 4) Code 0.

Rationale:

— **M0300B1** is coded 0 due to the fact that the resident now has a Stage 3 pressure ulcer and no longer has a Stage 2 pressure ulcer. Therefore, you are required to skip to **M0300C** (Stage 3 pressure ulcer).
— **M0300C1** is coded as 1 due to the fact the resident has one Stage 3 pressure ulcer.
— **M0300C2** is coded as 0 due to the fact that the Stage 3 pressure ulcer was not present on admission or reentry, but worsened from a Stage 2 to a Stage 3 in the facility.
— **M0300D1, M0300E1, M0300F1, and M0300G1** are coded as zeros (due to the fact the resident does not have any Stage 4 or unstageable ulcers). Proceed to code **M0610** with the dimensions of the Stage 3 ulcer.
— **M0610A** is coded, 03.0 for length, **M0610B** is coded 02.4 for width, and **M0610C** is coded 00.2 for depth. Since this resident only had one Stage 3 pressure ulcer at the time of second quarterly assessment, these are the dimensions that would be coded here as the largest ulcer.
— **M0700** is coded as 2 (Granulation tissue) because this is the most severe type of tissue present.
— **M0800A** is coded as 0, **M0800B** is coded as 1, and **M0800C** is coded as 0 because the Stage 2 pressure ulcer that was present on admission has now worsened to a Stage 3 pressure ulcer since the last assessment.

Scenarios for Pressure Ulcer Coding (cont.)

M0300. Current Number of Unhealed (non-epithelialized) **Pressure Ulcers at Each Stage**	
Enter Number `0`	**A. Number of Stage 1 pressure ulcers** **Stage 1:** Intact skin with non-blanchable redness of a localized area usually over a bony prominence. Darkly pigmented skin may not have a visible blanching; in dark skin tones only it may appear with persistent blue or purple hues

Enter Number
 	
`0`
 	
Enter Number
 	
`☐`
	B. Stage 2: Partial thickness loss of dermis presenting as a shallow open ulcer with a red or pink wound bed, without slough. May also present as an intact or open/ruptured blister
	
	1. Number of Stage 2 pressure ulcers - If 0 → Skip to M0300C, Stage 3
	
	2. Number of these Stage 2 pressure ulcers that were present upon admission/reentry - enter how many were noted at the time of admission
	
	3. Date of oldest Stage 2 pressure ulcer - Enter dashes if date is unknown:
	
	☐☐ ☐☐ ☐☐☐☐
	Month Day Year

Enter Number
 	
`1`
 	
Enter Number
 	
`0`
	C. Stage 3: Full thickness tissue loss. Subcutaneous fat may be visible but bone, tendon or muscle is not exposed. Slough may be present but does not obscure the depth of tissue loss. May include undermining and tunneling
	
	1. Number of Stage 3 pressure ulcers - If 0 → Skip to M0300D, Stage 4
	
	2. Number of these Stage 3 pressure ulcers that were present upon admission/reentry - enter how many were noted at the time of admission

Enter Number
 	
`0`
 	
Enter Number
 	
`☐`
	D. Stage 4: Full thickness tissue loss with exposed bone, tendon or muscle. Slough or eschar may be present on some parts of the wound bed. Often includes undermining and tunneling
	
	1. Number of Stage 4 pressure ulcers - If 0 → Skip to M0300E, Unstageable: Non-removable dressing
	
	2. Number of these Stage 4 pressure ulcers that were present upon admission/reentry - enter how many were noted at the time of admission

M0300 continued on next page	

Scenarios for Pressure Ulcer Coding (cont.)

	M0300. Current Number of Unhealed (non-epithelialized) Pressure Ulcers at Each Stage - Continued
	E. Unstageable - Non-removable dressing: Known but not stageable due to non-removable dressing/device
Enter Number **0** Enter Number	1. **Number of unstageable pressure ulcers due to non-removable dressing/device** - If 0 → Skip to M0300F, Unstageable: Slough and/or eschar
	2. **Number of these unstageable pressure ulcers that were present upon admission/reentry** - enter how many were noted at the time of admission
	F. Unstageable - Slough and/or eschar: Known but not stageable due to coverage of wound bed by slough and/or eschar
Enter Number **0** Enter Number	1. **Number of unstageable pressure ulcers due to coverage of wound bed by slough and/or eschar** - If 0 → Skip to M0300G, Unstageable: Deep tissue
	2. **Number of these unstageable pressure ulcers that were present upon admission/reentry** - enter how many were noted at the time of admission
	G. Unstageable - Deep tissue: Suspected deep tissue injury in evolution
Enter Number **0** Enter Number	1. **Number of unstageable pressure ulcers with suspected deep tissue injury in evolution** - If 0 → Skip to M0610, Dimension of Unhealed Stage 3 or 4 Pressure Ulcers or Eschar
	2. **Number of these unstageable pressure ulcers that were present upon admission/reentry** - enter how many were noted at the time of admission

	M0610. Dimensions of Unhealed Stage 3 or 4 Pressure Ulcers or Eschar Complete only if M0300C1, M0300D1 or M0300F1 is greater than 0
	If the resident has one or more unhealed (non-epithelialized) Stage 3 or 4 pressure ulcers or an unstageable pressure ulcer due to slough or eschar, identify the pressure ulcer with the largest surface area (length x width) and record in centimeters:
0 3 . 0 cm	**A. Pressure ulcer length:** Longest length from head to toe
0 2 . 4 cm	**B. Pressure ulcer width:** Widest width of the same pressure ulcer, side-to-side perpendicular (90-degree angle) to length
0 0 . 2 cm	**C. Pressure ulcer depth:** Depth of the same pressure ulcer from the visible surface to the deepest area (if depth is unknown, enter a dash in each box)

	M0700. Most Severe Tissue Type for Any Pressure Ulcer
Enter Code **2**	Select the best description of the most severe type of tissue present in any pressure ulcer bed 1. **Epithelial tissue** - new skin growing in superficial ulcer. It can be light pink and shiny, even in persons with darkly pigmented skin 2. **Granulation tissue** - pink or red tissue with shiny, moist, granular appearance 3. **Slough** - yellow or white tissue that adheres to the ulcer bed in strings or thick clumps, or is mucinous 4. **Necrotic tissue (Eschar)** - black, brown, or tan tissue that adheres firmly to the wound bed or ulcer edges, may be softer or harder than surrounding skin

	M0800. Worsening in Pressure Ulcer Status Since Prior Assessment (OBRA, PPS, or Discharge) Complete only if A0310E = 0
	Indicate the number of current pressure ulcers that were **not present or were at a lesser stage** on prior assessment (OBRA, PPS, or Discharge). If no current pressure ulcer at a given stage, enter 0
Enter Number **0**	**A. Stage 2**
Enter Number **1**	**B. Stage 3**
Enter Number **0**	**C. Stage 4**

Scenarios for Pressure Ulcer Coding (cont.)

Example M0100-M1200

1. Mrs. P is admitted to the nursing home on 10/23/2010 for a Medicare stay. In completing the PPS 5-day assessment, it was noted that the resident had a head-to-toe skin assessment and her skin was intact, but upon assessment using the Braden scale, was found to be at risk for skin break down. On the 14-day PPS (ARD of 11/5/2010), the resident was noted to have a Stage 2 pressure ulcer that was identified on her coccyx on 11/1/2010. This Stage 2 pressure ulcer was noted to have pink tissue with some epithelialization present in the wound bed. Dimensions of the ulcer were length 01.1 cm, width 00.5 cm, and no measurable depth. Mrs. P does not have any arterial or venous ulcers, wounds, or skin problems. She is receiving ulcer care with application of a dressing applied to the coccygeal ulcer. Mrs. P. also has pressure redistribution devices on both her bed and chair, and has been placed on a 1½ hour turning and repositioning schedule per tissue tolerance. On 11/13/2010 the resident was discharged return anticipated and reentered the facility on 11/15/10. Upon reentry the 5-day PPS ARD was set at 11/19/2010. In reviewing the record for this 5-day PPS assessment, it was noted that the resident had the same Stage 2 pressure ulcer on her coccyx, however, the measurements were now length 01.2 cm, width 00.6 cm, and still no measurable depth. It was also noted upon reentry that the resident had a suspected deep tissue injury of the right heel that was measured at length 01.9cm, width 02.5cm, and no visible depth.

5-Day PPS #1:

Coding:
  — **M0100B** (Formal assessment instrument), Check box.
  — **M0100C** (Clinical assessment), Check box.
  — **M0150** (Risk of Pressure Ulcers), Code 1.
  — **M0210** (One or more unhealed pressure ulcer(s) at Stage 1 or higher), Code 0 and skip to **M0900** (Healed pressure ulcers).
  — **M0900** (Healed pressure ulcers). Skip to M1030 since this item is only completed if **A0310E=0**. The 5-Day PPS Assessment is the first assessment since the most recent entry of any kind (admission or reentry), therefore, **A0310E=1**.
  — **M1030** (Number of Venous and Arterial ulcers), Code 0.
  — **M1040** (Other ulcers, wounds and skin problems), Check Z (None of the above).
  — **M1200** (Skin and Ulcer Treatments), Check Z (None of the above were provided).

Rationale: The resident had a formal assessment using the Braden scale and also had a head-to-toe skin assessment completed. Pressure ulcer risk was identified via formal assessment. Upon assessment the resident's skin was noted to be intact, therefore, M0210 was coded 0, M0900 was skipped because the 5-Day PPS is the first assessment. M1030 was coded 0 due to the resident not having any of these conditions. M1040Z was checked since none of these problems were noted. M1200Z was checked because none of these treatments were provided.

Scenarios for Pressure Ulcer Coding (cont.)

M1030. Number of Venous and Arterial Ulcers	
Enter Number `0`	**Enter the total number of venous and arterial ulcers present**

M1040. Other Ulcers, Wounds and Skin Problems

↓ **Check all that apply**

	Foot Problems
☐	**A. Infection of the foot** (e.g., cellulitis, purulent drainage)
☐	**B. Diabetic foot ulcer(s)**
☐	**C. Other open lesion(s) on the foot**
	Other Problems
☐	**D. Open lesion(s) other than ulcers, rashes, cuts** (e.g., cancer lesion)
☐	**E. Surgical wound(s)**
☐	**F. Burn(s)** (second or third degree)
	None of the Above
☒	**Z. None of the above** were present

M1200. Skin and Ulcer Treatments

↓ **Check all that apply**

☐	**A. Pressure reducing device for chair**
☐	**B. Pressure reducing device for bed**
☐	**C. Turning/repositioning program**
☐	**D. Nutrition or hydration intervention** to manage skin problems
☐	**E. Ulcer care**
☐	**F. Surgical wound care**
☐	**G. Application of nonsurgical dressings** (with or without topical medications) other than to feet
☐	**H. Applications of ointments/medications** other than to feet
☐	**I. Application of dressings to feet** (with or without topical medications)
☒	**Z. None of the above** were provided

Scenarios for Pressure Ulcer Coding (cont.)

14-Day PPS:

Coding:

- **M0100A** (Resident has a Stage 1 or greater, a scar over bony prominence, or a non-removable dressing/device), Check box.
- **M0100B** (Formal assessment instrument), Check box.
- **M0100C** (Clinical assessment), Check box.
- **M0150** (Risk of Pressure Ulcers), Code 1.
- **M0210** (One or more unhealed pressure ulcer(s) at Stage 1 or higher), Code 1.
- **M0300A** (Number of Stage 1 pressure ulcers), Code 0.
- **M0300B1** (Number of Stage 2 pressure ulcers), Code 1.
- **M0300B2** (Number of Stage 2 pressure ulcers present on admission/re-entry), Code 0.
- **M0300B3** (Date of the oldest Stage 2 pressure ulcer), Enter 11-01-2010.
- **M0300C1** (Number of Stage 3 pressure ulcers), Code 0 and skip to **M0300D** (Stage 4).
- **M0300D1** (Number of Stage 4 pressure ulcers), Code 0 and skip to **M0300E** (Unstageable: Non-removable dressing).
- **M0300E1** (Unstageable: Non-removable dressing), Code 0 and skip to **M0300F** (Unstageable: Slough and/or eschar).
- **M0300F1** (Unstageable: Slough and/or eschar), Code 0 and skip to **M0300G** (Unstageable: Deep tissue).
- **M0300G1** (Unstageable: Deep tissue), Code 0 and skip to **M0610** (Dimension of Unhealed Stage 3 or 4 Pressure Ulcers or Eschar).
- **M0610** (Dimension of Unhealed Stage 3 or 4 Pressure Ulcers or Eschar), is NOT completed, as the resident has a Stage 2 pressure ulcer.
- **M0700** (Most severe tissue type for any pressure ulcer), Code 1 (Epithelial tissue).
- **M0800** (Worsening in pressure ulcer status since prior assessment (OBRA, PPS, or Discharge)), **M0800A**, Code 1; **M0800B**, Code 0; **M0800C**, Code 0. This item is completed because the 14-Day PPS is NOT the first assessment since the most recent entry of any kind (admission or reentry). Therefore, **A0310E=0**. **M0800A** is coded 1 because the resident has a new Stage 2 pressure ulcer that was not present on the prior assessment.
- **M0900A** (Healed pressure ulcers), Code 0. This is completed because the 14- Day PPS is NOT the first assessment since the most recent entry of any kind (admission or reentry). Therefore **A0310E=0**. Since there were no pressure ulcers noted on the 5-Day PPS assessment, this is coded 0, and skip to **M1030**.
- **M1030** (Number of Venous and Arterial ulcers), Code 0.
- **M1040** (Other ulcers, wounds and skin problems), Check Z (None of the above).
- **M1200A** (Pressure reducing device for chair), **M1200B** (Pressure reducing device for bed), **M1200C** (Turning/repositioning program), and **M1200E** (Ulcer care) are all checked.

Rationale: The resident had a formal assessment using the Braden scale and also had a head-to-toe skin assessment completed. Pressure ulcer risk was identified via formal assessment. On the 5-Day PPS assessment the resident's skin was noted to be intact, however, on the 14-Day PPS assessment, it was noted that the resident had a new Stage 2 pressure ulcer. Since the resident has had both a 5-day and 14-Day PPS completed, the 14-Day PPS would be coded 0 at **A0310E**. This is because the 14-Day PPS is NOT the first assessment since the most recent admission. Since **A0310E=0**, items **M0800** (Worsening in pressure ulcer status) and **M0900** (Healed pressure ulcers) would be completed. Since the resident did not have a pressure ulcer on the 5-Day PPS and did have one on the 14-Day PPS, the new Stage 2 pressure ulcer is documented under **M0800** (Worsening in pressure ulcer status). **M0900** (Healed pressure ulcers) is coded as 0 because there were no pressure ulcers noted on the prior assessment (5-Day PPS). There were no other skin problems noted. However the resident, since she is at an even higher risk of breakdown since the development of a new ulcer, has preventative measures put in place with pressure redistribution devices for her chair and bed. She was also placed on a turning and repositioning program based on tissue tolerance. Therefore **M1200A, M1200B, and M1200C** were all checked. She also now requires ulcer care and application of a dressing to the coccygeal ulcer, so **M1200E** is also checked. **M1200G** (Application of nonsurgical dressings – with or without topical medications) would **NOT** be coded here because **any** intervention for treating pressure ulcers is coded in **M1200E** (Ulcer care).

Scenarios for Pressure Ulcer Coding (cont.)

M0100. Determination of Pressure Ulcer Risk	
↓ **Check all that apply**	
☒	A. Resident has a stage 1 or greater, a scar over bony prominence, or a non-removable dressing/device
☒	B. Formal assessment instrument/tool (e.g., Braden, Norton, or other)
☒	C. Clinical assessment
☐	Z. None of the above

M0150. Risk of Pressure Ulcers	
Enter Code **1**	**Is this resident at risk of developing pressure ulcers?** 0. No 1. Yes

M0210. Unhealed Pressure Ulcer(s)	
Enter Code **1**	**Does this resident have one or more unhealed pressure ulcer(s) at Stage 1 or higher?** 0. No → Skip to M0900, Healed Pressure Ulcers 1. Yes → Continue to M0300, Current Number of Unhealed (non-epithelialized) Pressure Ulcers at Each Stage

M0300. Current Number of Unhealed (non-epithelialized) Pressure Ulcers at Each Stage	
Enter Number **0**	A. **Number of Stage 1 pressure ulcers** **Stage 1:** Intact skin with non-blanchable redness of a localized area usually over a bony prominence. Darkly pigmented skin may not have a visible blanching; in dark skin tones only it may appear with persistent blue or purple hues
	B. **Stage 2:** Partial thickness loss of dermis presenting as a shallow open ulcer with a red or pink wound bed, without slough. May also present as an intact or open/ruptured blister
Enter Number **1**	1. **Number of Stage 2 pressure ulcers** - If 0 → Skip to M0300C, Stage 3
Enter Number **0**	2. **Number of these Stage 2 pressure ulcers that were present upon admission/reentry** - enter how many were noted at the time of admission
	3. **Date of oldest Stage 2 pressure ulcer** - Enter dashes if date is unknown: `1 1 - 0 1 - 2 0 1 0` Month Day Year
	C. **Stage 3:** Full thickness tissue loss. Subcutaneous fat may be visible but bone, tendon or muscle is not exposed. Slough may be present but does not obscure the depth of tissue loss. May include undermining and tunneling
Enter Number **0**	1. **Number of Stage 3 pressure ulcers** - If 0 → Skip to M0300D, Stage 4
Enter Number ☐	2. **Number of these Stage 3 pressure ulcers that were present upon admission/reentry** - enter how many were noted at the time of admission
	D. **Stage 4:** Full thickness tissue loss with exposed bone, tendon or muscle. Slough or eschar may be present on some parts of the wound bed. Often includes undermining and tunneling
Enter Number **0**	1. **Number of Stage 4 pressure ulcers** - If 0 → Skip to M0300E, Unstageable: Non-removable dressing
Enter Number ☐	2. **Number of these Stage 4 pressure ulcers that were present upon admission/reentry** - enter how many were noted at the time of admission
M0300 continued on next page	

Scenarios for Pressure Ulcer Coding (cont.)

M0300. Current Number of Unhealed (non-epithelialized) **Pressure Ulcers at Each Stage** - Continued

E. Unstageable - Non-removable dressing: Known but not stageable due to non-removable dressing/device

Enter Number
| 0 |

1. **Number of unstageable pressure ulcers due to non-removable dressing/device** - If 0 → Skip to M0300F, Unstageable: Slough and/or eschar

Enter Number
| |

2. **Number of these unstageable pressure ulcers that were present upon admission/reentry** - enter how many were noted at the time of admission

F. Unstageable - Slough and/or eschar: Known but not stageable due to coverage of wound bed by slough and/or eschar

Enter Number
| 0 |

1. **Number of unstageable pressure ulcers due to coverage of wound bed by slough and/or eschar** - If 0 → Skip to M0300G, Unstageable: Deep tissue

Enter Number
| |

2. **Number of these unstageable pressure ulcers that were present upon admission/reentry** - enter how many were noted at the time of admission

G. Unstageable - Deep tissue: Suspected deep tissue injury in evolution

Enter Number
| 0 |

1. **Number of unstageable pressure ulcers with suspected deep tissue injury in evolution** - If 0 → Skip to M0610, Dimension of Unhealed Stage 3 or 4 Pressure Ulcers or Eschar

Enter Number
| |

2. **Number of these unstageable pressure ulcers that were present upon admission/reentry** - enter how many were noted at the time of admission

---

M0700. Most Severe Tissue Type for Any Pressure Ulcer

Enter Code
| 1 |

Select the best description of the most severe type of tissue present in any pressure ulcer bed
1. **Epithelial tissue** - new skin growing in superficial ulcer. It can be light pink and shiny, even in persons with darkly pigmented skin
2. **Granulation tissue** - pink or red tissue with shiny, moist, granular appearance
3. **Slough** - yellow or white tissue that adheres to the ulcer bed in strings or thick clumps, or is mucinous
4. **Necrotic tissue (Eschar)** - black, brown, or tan tissue that adheres firmly to the wound bed or ulcer edges, may be softer or harder than surrounding skin

M0800. Worsening in Pressure Ulcer Status Since Prior Assessment (OBRA, PPS, or Discharge)
Complete only if A0310E = 0

Indicate the number of current pressure ulcers that were **not present or were at a lesser stage** on prior assessment (OBRA, PPS, or Discharge). If no current pressure ulcer at a given stage, enter 0

Enter Number
| 1 |

A. Stage 2

Enter Number
| 0 |

B. Stage 3

Enter Number
| 0 |

C. Stage 4

Scenarios for Pressure Ulcer Coding (cont.)

M0900. Healed Pressure Ulcers Complete only if A0310E = 0	

Enter Code
`0`
	A. Were pressure ulcers present on the prior assessment (OBRA, PPS, or Discharge)?
	    0. **No** → Skip to M1030, Number of Venous and Arterial Ulcers
	    1. **Yes** → Continue to M0900B, Stage 2

	Indicate the number of pressure ulcers that were noted on the prior assessment (OBRA, PPS, or Discharge) that have completely closed (resurfaced with epithelium). If no healed pressure ulcer at a given stage since the prior assessment (OBRA, PPS, or Discharge), enter 0
Enter Number	**B. Stage 2**
Enter Number	**C. Stage 3**
Enter Number	**D. Stage 4**

M1030. Number of Venous and Arterial Ulcers	
Enter Number `0`	**Enter the total number of venous and arterial ulcers present**

M1040. Other Ulcers, Wounds and Skin Problems	
↓ **Check all that apply**	
	Foot Problems
☐	**A. Infection of the foot** (e.g., cellulitis, purulent drainage)
☐	**B. Diabetic foot ulcer(s)**
☐	**C. Other open lesion(s) on the foot**
	Other Problems
☐	**D. Open lesion(s) other than ulcers, rashes, cuts** (e.g., cancer lesion)
☐	**E. Surgical wound(s)**
☐	**F. Burn(s)** (second or third degree)
	None of the Above
☒	**Z. None of the above** were present

M1200. Skin and Ulcer Treatments	
↓ **Check all that apply**	
☒	**A. Pressure reducing device for chair**
☒	**B. Pressure reducing device for bed**
☒	**C. Turning/repositioning program**
☐	**D. Nutrition or hydration intervention** to manage skin problems
☒	**E. Ulcer care**
☐	**F. Surgical wound care**
☐	**G. Application of nonsurgical dressings** (with or without topical medications) other than to feet
☐	**H. Applications of ointments/medications** other than to feet
☐	**I. Application of dressings to feet** (with or without topical medications)
☐	**Z. None of the above** were provided

Scenarios for Pressure Ulcer Coding (cont.)

Discharge Assessment:

Coding:

— **M0100A** (Resident has a Stage 1 or greater, a scar over bony prominence, or a non-removable dressing/device), Check box.

— **M0100B** (Formal assessment instrument), Check box.

— **M0100C** (Clinical assessment), Check box.

— **M0150** (Risk of Pressure Ulcers), Code 1.

— **M0210** (One or more unhealed pressure ulcer(s) at Stage 1 or higher), Code 1.

— **M0300A** (Number of Stage 1 pressure ulcers), Code 0.

— **M0300B1** (Number of Stage 2 pressure ulcers), Code 1.

— **M0300B2** (Number of Stage 2 pressure ulcers present on admission/re-entry), Code 0.

— **M0300B3** (Date of the oldest Stage 2 pressure ulcer), Enter 11-01-2010.

— **M0300C1** (Number of Stage 3 pressure ulcers), Code 0 and skip to **M0300D** (Stage 4).

— **M0300D1** (Number of Stage 4 pressure ulcers), Code 0 and skip to **M0300E** (Unstageable: Non-removable dressing).

— **M0300E1** (Unstageable: Non-removable dressing), Code 0 and skip to **M0300F** (Unstageable: Slough and/or eschar).

— **M0300F1** (Unstageable: Slough and/or eschar), Code 0 and skip to **M0300G** (Unstageable: Deep tissue).

— **M0300G1** (Unstageable: Deep tissue), Code 0 and skip to **M0610** (Dimension of Unhealed Stage 3 or 4 Pressure Ulcers or Eschar).

— **M0610** (Dimension of Unhealed Stage 3 or 4 Pressure Ulcers or Eschar), is NOT completed, as the resident has a Stage 2 pressure ulcer.

— **M0700** (Most severe tissue type for any pressure ulcer), Code 1 (Epithelial tissue).

— **M0800** (Worsening in pressure ulcer status since prior assessment (OBRA, PPS, or Discharge)), **M0800A**, Code 0; **M0800B**, Code 0; **M0800C**, Code 0. This item is completed because the Discharge assessment is NOT the first assessment since the most recent entry of any kind (admission or reentry). Therefore, **A0310E**=0. **M0800A** is coded 0 because the Stage 2 pressure ulcer has not worsened since the prior assessment (14-Day PPS).

— **M0900A** (Were pressure ulcers present on the prior assessment (OBRA, PPS, or Discharge?)), Code 1. This item is completed because the Discharge assessment is NOT the first assessment since the most recent entry of any kind (admission or reentry). Therefore, **A0310E=0**. **M0900A** is coded 1 because there was a Stage 2 pressure ulcer present on the prior assessment (14-Day PPS). **M0900B** (Stage 2), **M0900C** (Stage 3), and **M0900D** (Stage 4) are all Coded 0 because the Stage 2 pressure ulcer is not completely resurfaced with epithelial tissue and there are no healed pressure ulcers at any other Stage.

— **M1030** (Number of Venous and Arterial ulcers), Code 0.

Scenarios for Pressure Ulcer Coding (cont.)

— **M1040** (Other ulcers, wounds and skin problems), Check Z (None of the above).

— **M1200A** (Pressure reducing device for chair), **M1200B** (Pressure reducing device for bed), **M1200C** (Turning/repositioning program), and **M1200E** (Ulcer care) are all checked.

Rationale: On Discharge, the resident's assessment was still that the Stage 2 pressure ulcer was present, all supportive care was being provided, there were no new pressure ulcers, wound had not yet healed, and there were no new skin problems or treatments.

M0800A (Stage 2) is coded as 0 on the Discharge Assessment because the Stage 2 pressure ulcer that is present at the time of this assessment was not at a lesser stage on the prior assessment (14-Day PPS). **M0900A** (Were pressure ulcers present on the prior assessment (OBRA, PPS, or Discharge?)) is coded as a 1 because the Stage 2 pressure ulcer was present on the prior assessment (14-Day PPS).

Scenarios for Pressure Ulcer Coding (cont.)

M0100. Determination of Pressure Ulcer Risk

↓ Check all that apply

☒	A. Resident has a stage 1 or greater, a scar over bony prominence, or a non-removable dressing/device
☒	B. Formal assessment instrument/tool (e.g., Braden, Norton, or other)
☒	C. Clinical assessment
☐	Z. None of the above

M0150. Risk of Pressure Ulcers

Enter Code **1**

Is this resident at risk of developing pressure ulcers?
- 0. No
- 1. Yes

M0210. Unhealed Pressure Ulcer(s)

Enter Code **1**

Does this resident have one or more unhealed pressure ulcer(s) at Stage 1 or higher?
- 0. No → Skip to M0900, Healed Pressure Ulcers
- 1. Yes → Continue to M0300, Current Number of Unhealed (non-epithelialized) Pressure Ulcers at Each Stage

M0300. Current Number of Unhealed (non-epithelialized) Pressure Ulcers at Each Stage

A. Number of Stage 1 pressure ulcers
Stage 1: Intact skin with non-blanchable redness of a localized area usually over a bony prominence. Darkly pigmented skin may not have a visible blanching; in dark skin tones only it may appear with persistent blue or purple hues

Enter Number **0**

B. Stage 2: Partial thickness loss of dermis presenting as a shallow open ulcer with a red or pink wound bed, without slough. May also present as an intact or open/ruptured blister

Enter Number **1**
1. **Number of Stage 2 pressure ulcers** - If 0 → Skip to M0300C, Stage 3

Enter Number **0**
2. **Number of these Stage 2 pressure ulcers that were present upon admission/reentry** - enter how many were noted at the time of admission

3. **Date of oldest Stage 2 pressure ulcer** - Enter dashes if date is unknown:

1	1	–	0	1	–	2	0	1	0
Month			Day			Year			

C. Stage 3: Full thickness tissue loss. Subcutaneous fat may be visible but bone, tendon or muscle is not exposed. Slough may be present but does not obscure the depth of tissue loss. May include undermining and tunneling

Enter Number **0**
1. **Number of Stage 3 pressure ulcers** - If 0 → Skip to M0300D, Stage 4

Enter Number ☐
2. **Number of these Stage 3 pressure ulcers that were present upon admission/reentry** - enter how many were noted at the time of admission

D. Stage 4: Full thickness tissue loss with exposed bone, tendon or muscle. Slough or eschar may be present on some parts of the wound bed. Often includes undermining and tunneling

Enter Number **0**
1. **Number of Stage 4 pressure ulcers** - If 0 → Skip to M0300E, Unstageable: Non-removable dressing

Enter Number ☐
2. **Number of these Stage 4 pressure ulcers that were present upon admission/reentry** - enter how many were noted at the time of admission

M0300 continued on next page

287

Scenarios for Pressure Ulcer Coding (cont.)

M0300. Current Number of Unhealed (non-epithelialized) Pressure Ulcers at Each Stage - Continued

E. Unstageable - Non-removable dressing: Known but not stageable due to non-removable dressing/device

Enter Number
`0`
1. **Number of unstageable pressure ulcers due to non-removable dressing/device** - If 0 → Skip to M0300F, Unstageable: Slough and/or eschar

Enter Number
`[ ]`
2. **Number of these unstageable pressure ulcers that were present upon admission/reentry** - enter how many were noted at the time of admission

F. Unstageable - Slough and/or eschar: Known but not stageable due to coverage of wound bed by slough and/or eschar

Enter Number
`0`
1. **Number of unstageable pressure ulcers due to coverage of wound bed by slough and/or eschar** - If 0→ Skip to M0300G, Unstageable: Deep tissue

Enter Number
`[ ]`
2. **Number of these unstageable pressure ulcers that were present upon admission/reentry** - enter how many were noted at the time of admission

G. Unstageable - Deep tissue: Suspected deep tissue injury in evolution

Enter Number
`0`
1. **Number of unstageable pressure ulcers with suspected deep tissue injury in evolution** - If 0 → Skip to M0610, Dimension of Unhealed Stage 3 or 4 Pressure Ulcers or Eschar

Enter Number
`[ ]`
2. **Number of these unstageable pressure ulcers that were present upon admission/reentry** - enter how many were noted at the time of admission

M0700. Most Severe Tissue Type for Any Pressure Ulcer

Enter Code
`1`

Select the best description of the most severe type of tissue present in any pressure ulcer bed
1. **Epithelial tissue** - new skin growing in superficial ulcer. It can be light pink and shiny, even in persons with darkly pigmented skin
2. **Granulation tissue** - pink or red tissue with shiny, moist, granular appearance
3. **Slough** - yellow or white tissue that adheres to the ulcer bed in strings or thick clumps, or is mucinous
4. **Necrotic tissue (Eschar)** - black, brown, or tan tissue that adheres firmly to the wound bed or ulcer edges, may be softer or harder than surrounding skin

M0800. Worsening in Pressure Ulcer Status Since Prior Assessment (OBRA, PPS, or Discharge)
Complete only if A0310E = 0

Indicate the number of current pressure ulcers that were **not present or were at a lesser stage** on prior assessment (OBRA, PPS, or Discharge). If no current pressure ulcer at a given stage, enter 0

Enter Number
`0`
A. Stage 2

Enter Number
`0`
B. Stage 3

Enter Number
`0`
C. Stage 4

M0900. Healed Pressure Ulcers
Complete only if A0310E = 0

Enter Code
`1`
A. Were pressure ulcers present on the prior assessment (OBRA, PPS, or Discharge)?
   0. **No** → Skip to M1030, Number of Venous and Arterial Ulcers
   1. **Yes** → Continue to M0900B, Stage 2

Indicate the number of pressure ulcers that were noted on the prior assessment (OBRA, PPS, or Discharge) that have completely closed (resurfaced with epithelium). If no healed pressure ulcer at a given stage since the prior assessment (OBRA, PPS, or Discharge), enter 0

Enter Number
`0`
B. Stage 2

Enter Number
`0`
C. Stage 3

Enter Number
`0`
D. Stage 4

Scenarios for Pressure Ulcer Coding (cont.)

M1030. Number of Venous and Arterial Ulcers	
Enter Number `0`	Enter the total number of venous and arterial ulcers present

M1040. Other Ulcers, Wounds and Skin Problems

↓ Check all that apply

Foot Problems

☐	A. **Infection of the foot** (e.g., cellulitis, purulent drainage)
☐	B. **Diabetic foot ulcer(s)**
☐	C. **Other open lesion(s) on the foot**

Other Problems

☐	D. **Open lesion(s) other than ulcers, rashes, cuts** (e.g., cancer lesion)
☐	E. **Surgical wound(s)**
☐	F. **Burn(s)** (second or third degree)

None of the Above

☒	Z. **None of the above** were present

M1200. Skin and Ulcer Treatments

↓ Check all that apply

☒	A. **Pressure reducing device for chair**
☒	B. **Pressure reducing device for bed**
☒	C. **Turning/repositioning program**
☐	D. **Nutrition or hydration intervention** to manage skin problems
☒	E. **Ulcer care**
☐	F. **Surgical wound care**
☐	G. **Application of nonsurgical dressings** (with or without topical medications) other than to feet
☐	H. **Applications of ointments/medications** other than to feet
☐	I. **Application of dressings to feet** (with or without topical medications)
☐	Z. **None of the above** were provided

SECTION N: MEDICATIONS

Intent: The intent of the items in this section is to record the number of days, during the last 7 days (or since admission/reentry if less than 7 days) that any type of injection, insulin, and/or select oral medications were received by the resident.

N0300: Injections

N0300. Injections	
Enter Days ☐	**Record the number of days that injections of any type** were received during the last 7 days or since admission/reentry if less than 7 days. If 0 → Skip to N0400, Medications Received

Item Rationale

Health-related Quality of Life

- Frequency of administration of medication via injection can be an indication of stability of a resident's health status and/or complexity of care needs.

Planning for Care

- Monitor for adverse effects of injected medications.
- Although antigens and vaccines are not considered to be medications per se, it is important to track when they are given to monitor for localized or systemic reactions.

Steps for Assessment

1. Review the resident's medication administration records for the 7-day look-back period (or since admission/reentry if less than 7 days).
2. Review documentation from other health care locations where the resident may have received injections while a resident of the nursing home (e.g., flu vaccine in a physician's office, in the emergency room – as long as the resident was not admitted).
3. Determine if any medications were received by the resident via injection. If received, determine the number of days during the look-back period they were received.

Coding Instructions

Record the number of days during the 7-day look-back period (or since admission/reentry if less than 7 days) that the resident received any type of medication, antigen, vaccine, etc., by subcutaneous, intramuscular, or intradermal injection.

Insulin injections are counted in this item as well as in Item N0350.

- Count the number of days that the resident received any type of injection while a resident of the nursing home.
- Record the number of days that any type of injection was received in Item N0300.

N0300: Injections (cont.)

Coding Tips and Special Populations

- For subcutaneous pumps, code only the number of days that the resident actually required a subcutaneous injection to restart the pump.

- If an antigen or vaccination is provided on 1 day, and another vaccine provided on the next day, the number of days the resident received injections would be **coded 2 days.**

- If two injections were administered on the same day, the number of days the resident received injections would be **coded 1 day.**

Examples

1. During the 7-day look-back period, Mr. T. received an influenza shot on Monday, a PPD test (for tuberculosis) on Tuesday, and a Vitamin B_{12} injection on Wednesday.

   Coding: N0300 would be **coded 3.**
   Rationale: The resident received injections on 3 days during the 7-day look-back period.

2. During the 7-day look-back period, Miss C. received both a influenza shot and her vitamin B_{12} injection on Thursday.

   Coding: N0300 would be **coded 1.**
   Rationale: The resident received injections on 1 day during the 7-day look-back period.

N0350: Insulin

N0350. Insulin	
Enter Days ☐	**A. Insulin injections - Record the number of days that insulin injections** were received during the last 7 days or since admission/reentry if less than 7 days
Enter Days ☐	**B. Orders for insulin - Record the number of days the physician (or authorized assistant or practitioner) changed the resident's insulin orders** during the last 7 days or since admission/reentry if less than 7 days

Item Rationale

Health-related Quality of Life

- Insulin is a medication used to treat diabetes mellitus (DM).

- Individualized meal plans should be created with the resident's input to ensure appropriate meal intake. Residents are more likely to be compliant with their DM diet if they have input related to food choices.

N0350: Insulin (cont.)

Planning for Care

- Orders for insulin may have to change depending on the resident's condition (e.g., fever or other illness) and/or laboratory results.

- Ensure that dosage and time of injections take into account meals, activity, etc., based on individualized resident assessment.

- Monitor for adverse effects of insulin injections (e.g., hypoglycemia).

- Monitor HbA1c and blood glucose levels to ensure appropriate amounts of insulin are being administered.

Steps for Assessment

1. Review the resident's medication administration records for the 7-day look-back period (or since admission/reentry if less than 7 days).
2. Determine if the resident received insulin injections during the look-back period.
3. Determine if the physician (or nurse practitioner, physician assistant, or clinical nurse specialist if allowable under state licensure laws and Medicare) changed the resident's insulin orders during the look-back period.
4. Count the number of days insulin injections were received and/or changed.

Coding Instructions for N0350A

- Enter in Item N0350A, the number of days during the look-back period that insulin injections were received.

Coding Instructions for N0350B

- Enter in Item N0350B, the number of days during the look-back period that the physician (nurse practitioner, physician assistant, or clinical nurse specialist if allowable under state licensure laws and Medicare) changed the resident's insulin orders.

Coding Tips and Special Populations

- A sliding scale dosage schedule that is written to cover different dosages depending on lab values does not count as an order change simply because a different dose is administered based on the sliding scale guidelines.

- If the sliding scale order is new, discontinued, or is the first sliding scale order for the resident, these days **can** be counted and coded.

- For subcutaneous insulin pumps, code only the number of days that the resident actually required a subcutaneous injection to restart the pump.

N0400: Medications Received

N0400. Medications Received	
↓ Check all medications the resident received at any time during the last 7 days or since admission/reentry if less than 7 days	
☐	A. Antipsychotic
☐	B. Antianxiety
☐	C. Antidepressant
☐	D. Hypnotic
☐	E. Anticoagulant (warfarin, heparin, or low-molecular weight heparin)
☐	F. Antibiotic
☐	G. Diuretic
☐	Z. None of the above were received

Item Rationale

Health-related Quality of Life

- Medications are an integral part of the care provided to residents of nursing homes. They are administered to try to achieve various outcomes, such as curing an illness, diagnosing a disease or condition, arresting or slowing a disease's progress, reducing or eliminating symptoms, or preventing a disease or symptom.

- Residents taking medications in these drug classes are at risk of side effects that can adversely affect health, safety, and quality of life.

- While assuring that only those medications required to treat the resident's assessed condition are being used, it is important to reduce the need for or maximize the effectiveness of medications for all residents. Therefore, as part of all medication management, it is important for the interdisciplinary team to consider non-pharmacological approaches. Educating the nursing home staff and providers about non-pharmacological approaches in addition to and/or in conjunction with the use of medication may minimize the need for medications or reduce the dose and duration of those medications.

Planning for Care

- The indications for initiating, withdrawing, or withholding medication(s), as well as the use of non-pharmacological interventions, are determined by assessing the resident's underlying condition, current signs and symptoms, and preferences and goals for treatment. This includes, where possible, the identification of the underlying cause(s), since a diagnosis alone may not warrant treatment with medication.

> ## DEFINITIONS
>
> **ADVERSE CONSEQUENCE**
> An unpleasant symptom or event that is due to or associated with a medication, such as impairment or decline in an individual's mental or physical condition or functional or psycho-social status. It may include various types of adverse drug reactions and interactions (e.g., medication-medication, medication-food, and medication-disease).
>
> **NON-PHARMACOLOGICAL INTERVENTION**
> Approaches to care that do not involve medication, generally directed towards stabilizing or improving a resident's mental, physical and/or psychosocial well-being.

N0400: Medications Received (cont.)

- Target symptoms and goals for use of these medications should be established for each resident. Progress toward meeting the goals should be evaluated routinely.
- Possible adverse effects of drugs in each of these drug groups should be well understood by nursing staff. Educate nursing home staff to be observant for these adverse effects.
- Implement systematic monitoring of each resident taking any of these medications to identify adverse consequences early.

Steps for Assessment

1. Review the resident's medical record for documentation that any of these medications were received by the resident during the 7-day look-back period (or since admission/reentry if less than 7 days).
2. Review documentation from other health care settings where the resident may have received any of these medications while a resident of the nursing home (e.g., valium given in the emergency room).

Coding Instructions

- **Check A, antipsychotic:** if antipsychotic medication was received by the resident at any time during the 7-day look-back period (or since admission/reentry if less than 7 days)
- **Check B, antianxiety:** if anxiolytic medication was received by the resident at any time during the 7-day look-back period (or since admission/reentry if less than 7 days).
- **Check C, antidepressant:** if antidepressant medication was received by the resident at any time during the 7-day look-back period (or since admission/reentry if less than 7 days).
- **Check D, hypnotic:** if hypnotic medication was received by the resident at any time during the 7-day look-back period (or since admission/reentry if less than 7 days).
- **Check E, anticoagulant (e.g., warfarin, heparin, or low- molecular weight heparin):** if anticoagulant medication was received by the resident at any time during the 7-day look-back period (or since admission/reentry if less than 7 days). Do not code antiplatelet medications such as aspirin/extended release, dipyridamole, or clopidogrel here.
- **Check F, antibiotic:** if antibiotics were received by the resident at any time during the 7-day look-back period (or since admission/reentry if less than 7 days).

DEFINITIONS

DOSE
The total amount/ strength/ concentration of a medication given at one time or over a period of time. The individual dose is the amount/strength/ concentration received at each administration. The amount received over a 24-hour period may be referred to as the "daily dose."

MONITORING
The ongoing collection and analysis of information (such as observations and diagnostic test results) and comparison to baseline data in order to ascertain the individual's response to treatment and care, including progress or lack of progress toward a therapeutic goal. Monitoring can detect any complications or adverse consequences of the condition or of the treatments; and support decisions about modifying, discontinuing, or continuing any interventions.

- **Check G, diuretic:** if diuretics were received by the resident at any time during the 7-day look-back period (or since admission/reentry if less than 7 days).
- **Check Z, none of the above were received:** if none of the medications in Item N0400 were received during the 7-day look-back period (or since admission/reentry if less than 7 days).

Coding Tips and Special Populations

- Code medications according to a drug's pharmacological classification, not how it is used. For example, oxazepam may be used as a hypnotic, but it is classified as an antianxicty medication. It would be coded as an antianxiety medication.
- Include any of these medications given to the resident by any route (e.g., PO, IM, or IV) in any setting (e.g., at the nursing home, in a hospital emergency room) while a resident of the nursing home.
- Code a medication even if it was given only once during the look-back period.
- Count long-acting medications, such as fluphenazine decanoate or haloperidol decanoate, that are given every few weeks or monthly **only** if they are given during the 7-day look-back period (or since admission/reentry if less than 7 days).
- Combination medications should be coded in all categories that constitute the combination. For example, if the resident receives a single tablet that combines an antipsychotic and an antidepressant, then both antipsychotic and antidepressant should be coded.
- Over-the-counter sleeping medications are not coded as hypnotics, as they are not classified as hypnotic drugs.
- When residents are having difficulty sleeping, nursing home staff should explore non-pharmacological interventions (e.g., sleep hygiene approaches that individualize the sleep and wake times to accommodate the person's wishes and prior customary routine) to try to improve sleep prior to initiating pharmacologic interventions. If residents are currently on sleep-enhancing medications, nursing home staff can try non-pharmacologic interventions to help reduce the need for these medications or eliminate them.

> **DEFINITIONS**
>
> **SLEEP HYGIENE**
> Practices, habits and environmental factors that promote and/or improve sleep patterns.

- Many psychoactive medications increase confusion, sedation, and falls. For those residents who are already at risk for these conditions, nursing home staff should develop plans of care that address these risks.
- Adverse drug reaction (ADR) is a form of adverse consequence. It may be either a secondary effect of a medication that is usually undesirable and different from the therapeutic effect of the medication or any response to a medication that is noxious and unintended and occurs in doses for prophylaxis, diagnosis, or treatment. The term "side effect" is often used interchangeably with ADR; however, side effects are but one of five ADR categories, the others being hypersensitivity, idiosyncratic response, toxic reactions, and adverse medication interactions. A side effect is an expected, well-known reaction that occurs with a predictable frequency and may or may not constitute an adverse consequence.

- Doses of psychopharmacologic drugs differ in acute and long-term treatment. Doses should always be the lowest possible to achieve the desired therapeutic effects and be deemed necessary to maintain or improve the resident's function, well-being, safety, and quality of life. Duration of treatment should also be in accordance with pertinent literature, including clinical practice guidelines.

- Since medication issues continue to evolve and new medications are being approved regularly, it is important to refer to a current authoritative source for detailed medication information, such as indications and precautions, dosage, monitoring, or adverse consequences.

> **DEFINITIONS**
>
> **GRADUAL DOSE REDUCTION (GDR)** The step-wise tapering of a dose to determine if symptoms, conditions, or risks can be managed by a lower dose or if the dose or medication can be discontinued.

- During the first year in which a resident on a psychopharmacological medication is admitted, or after the nursing home has initiated such medication, nursing home staff should attempt to taper the medication or perform gradual dose reduction (GDR) as long as it is not medically contraindicated. Information on GDR and tapering of medications can be found in the **State Operations Manual, Appendix PP, Guidance to Surveyors for Long Term Care Facilities** (the **Operations Manual** can be found at http://www.cms.gov/Manuals/IOM/list.asp).

- Prior to discontinuing a psychoactive drug, residents may need a GDR or tapering to avoid withdrawal syndrome (e.g., selective serotonin reuptake inhibitors [SRIs], tricyclic antidepressants [TCAs]).

- Residents who are on antidepressants should be closely monitored for worsening of depression and/or suicidal ideation/behavior, especially during initiation or change of dosage in therapy. Stopping antidepressants abruptly puts one at higher risk of suicidal ideation and behavior.

> **DEFINITIONS**
>
> **MEDICATION INTERACTION** The impact of another substance (such as another medication, nutritional supplement including herbal products, food, or substances used in diagnostic studies) upon a medication. The interactions may alter absorption, distribution, metabolism, or elimination. These interactions may decrease the effectiveness of the medication or increase the potential for adverse consequences.

- Anticoagulants must be monitored with dosage frequency determined by clinical circumstances, duration of use, and stability of monitoring results (e.g., Prothrombin Time [PT]/International Normalization Ratio [INR]).

  — Multiple medication interactions exist with use of anticoagulants (information on common medication-medication interactions can be found in the **State Operations Manual, Appendix PP, Guidance to Surveyors for Long Term Care Facilities** [the **Operations Manual** can be found at http://www.cms.gov/Manuals/IOM/list.asp]), which may

    o significantly increase PT/INR results to levels associated with life-threatening bleeding, or

    o decrease PT/INR results to ineffective levels, or increase or decrease the serum concentration of the interacting medication.

o   Herbal and alternative medicine products are considered to be dietary supplements by the Food and Drug Administration (FDA). They are not regulated by the FDA (e.g., they are not reviewed for safety and effectiveness like medications) and their composition is not standardized (e.g., the composition varies among manufacturers). Therefore, they should not be counted as medications (e.g. chamomile, valerian root). Keep in mind that, for clinical purposes, it is important to document a resident's intake of such substances elsewhere in the medical record and to monitor their potential effects as they can interact with other medications. For more information consult the FDA website http://www.fda.gov/Food/DietarySupplements/ConsumerInformation/ucm1104 17.htm#what.

Example

1.   The Medication Administration Record for Mrs. P. reflects the following:

-   Resperidone 0.5 mg PO BID PRN: Received once a day on Monday, Wednesday, and Thursday.
-   Lorazepam 1 mg PO QAM: Received every day.
-   Temazepam 15 mg PO QHS PRN: Received at HS on Tuesday and Wednesday only.

   Coding: The following **Medications** item (N0400), would be checked: **A. antipsychotic,** resperidone is an antipsychotic drug, **B. antianxiety,** lorazepam is an antianxiety drug, and **D. hypnotic,** temazepam is a hypnotic drug. Please note: if a resident is receiving drugs in all of these three classes, simultaneously, there must be a clear clinical indication for the use of these drugs. Administration of these types of drugs, particularly in this combination, could be interpreted as chemically restraining the resident. Adequate documentation is essential in justifying their use.

Additional information on psychopharmacologic medications can be found in the **Diagnostic and Statistical Manual of Mental Disorders, Fourth Edition (DSM-IV)** (or subsequent editions) (http://www.psychiatryonline.com/resourceTOC.aspx?resourceID=1), and the **State Operations Manual, Appendix PP, Guidance to Surveyors for Long Term Care Facilities** (http://www.cms.gov/Manuals/IOM/list.asp).

Additional information on medications can be found in:

The Orange Book, http://www.fda.gov/cder/ob/default.htm

The National Drug Code Directory, http://www.fda.gov/cder/ndc/database/Default.htm

SECTION O: SPECIAL TREATMENTS, PROCEDURES, AND PROGRAMS

Intent: The intent of the items in this section is to identify any special treatments, procedures, and programs that the resident received during the specified time periods.

O0100: Special Treatments, Procedures, and Programs

Do not code services that were provided solely in conjunction with a surgical procedure, such as IV medications or ventilators. Surgical procedures include routine pre- and post-operative procedures.

O0100. Special Treatments, Procedures, and Programs	1. While NOT a Resident	2. While a Resident
Check all of the following treatments, procedures, and programs that were performed during the last **14 days**		
1. **While NOT a Resident** Performed *while NOT a resident* of this facility and within the *last 14 days*. Only check column 1 if resident entered (admission or reentry) IN THE LAST 14 DAYS. If resident last entered 14 or more days ago, leave column 1 blank 2. **While a Resident** Performed *while a resident* of this facility and within the *last 14 days*	↓ Check all that apply ↓	
Cancer Treatments		
A. Chemotherapy	☐	☐
B. Radiation	☐	☐
Respiratory Treatments		
C. Oxygen therapy	☐	☐
D. Suctioning	☐	☐
E. Tracheostomy care	☐	☐
F. Ventilator or respirator	☐	☐
G. BiPAP/CPAP	☐	☐
Other		
H. IV medications	☐	☐
I. Transfusions	☐	☐
J. Dialysis	☐	☐
K. Hospice care	☐	☐
L. Respite care	▓▓▓	☐
M. Isolation or quarantine for active infectious disease (does not include standard body/fluid precautions)	☐	☐
None of the Above		
Z. None of the above	☐	☐

Item Rationale

Health-related Quality of Life

- The treatments, procedures, and programs listed in Item O0100, Special Treatments, Procedures, and Programs, can have a profound effect on an individual's health status, self-image, dignity, and quality of life.

O0100: Special Treatments, Procedures, and Programs (cont.)

Planning for Care

- Reevaluation of special treatments and procedures the resident received or programs that the resident was involved in during the 14-day look-back period is important to ensure the continued appropriateness of the treatments, procedures, or programs.

Steps for Assessment

1. Review the resident's medical record to determine whether or not the resident received any of the special treatments, procedures, or programs within the last 14 days.

Coding Instructions for Column 1

Check all treatments, procedures, and programs received by the resident **prior** to admission/reentry to the facility and within the 14-day look-back period. Leave Column 1 blank if the resident was admitted or reentered the facility more than 14 days ago. If no items apply in the last 14 days, **check Z, none of the above**.

Coding Instructions for Column 2

Check all treatments, procedures, and programs received by the resident **after** admission/re-entry to the facility and within the 14-day look-back period.

- **O0100A, chemotherapy**

Code any type of chemotherapy agent administered as an antineoplastic given by any route in this item. Each drug should be evaluated to determine its reason for use before coding it here. The drugs coded here are those actually used for cancer treatment. For example, megestrol acetate is classified in the **Physician's Desk Reference (PDR)** as an anti-neoplastic drug. One of its side effects is appetite stimulation and weight gain. If megestrol acetate is being given only for appetite stimulation, do **not** code it as chemotherapy in this item, as the resident is not receiving the medication for chemotherapy purposes in this situation. IV's, IV medication, and blood transfusions administered during chemotherapy are **not** recorded under items K0500A (Parenteral/IV), O0100H (IV Medications), or O01001 (Transfusions).

- **O0100B, radiation**

Code intermittent radiation therapy, as well as, radiation administered via radiation implant in this item.

- **O0100C, oxygen therapy**

Code continuous or intermittent oxygen administered via mask, cannula, etc., delivered to a resident to relieve hypoxia in this item. Code oxygen used in Bi-level Positive Airway Pressure/Continuous Positive Airway Pressure (BiPAP/CPAP) here. Do not code hyperbaric oxygen for wound therapy in this item.

- **O0100D, suctioning**

Code only tracheal and/or nasopharyngeal suctioning in this item. Do not code oral suctioning here.

- **O0100E, tracheostomy care**

Code cleansing of the tracheostomy and/or cannula in this item.

O0100: Special Treatments, Procedures, and Programs (cont.)

- **O0100F, ventilator or respirator**

Code any type of electrically or pneumatically powered closed-system mechanical ventilator support devices that ensure adequate ventilation in the resident who is, or who may become, unable to support his or her own respiration in this item. A resident who is being weaned off of a respirator or ventilator in the last 14 days should also be coded here. Do not code this item when the ventilator or respirator is used only as a substitute for BiPAP or CPAP.

- **O0100G, BiPAP/CPAP**

Code any type of CPAP or BiPAP respiratory support devices that prevent the airways from closing by delivering slightly pressurized air through a mask continuously or via electronic cycling throughout the breathing cycle. The BiPAP/CPAP mask enables the individual to support his or her own respiration by providing enough pressure when the individual inhales to keep his or her airways open, unlike ventilators that "breathe" for the individual. If a ventilator or respirator is being used as a substitute for BiPAP/CPAP, code here.

- **O0100H, IV medications**

Code any drug or biological (e.g., contrast material) given by intravenous push, epidural pump, or drip through a central or peripheral port in this item. Do **not** code flushes to keep an IV access port patent, or IV fluids without medication here. Epidural, intrathecal, and baclofen pumps may be coded here, as they are similar to IV medications in that they must be monitored frequently and they involve continuous administration of a substance. Subcutaneous pumps are **not** coded in this item. Do **not** include IV medications of any kind that were administered during dialysis or chemotherapy. Dextrose 50% and/or Lactated Ringers given IV are not considered medications, and should not be coded here. To determine what products are considered medications or for more information consult the FDA website:

The Orange Book, http://www.fda.gov/cder/ob/default.htm

The National Drug Code Directory, http://www.fda.gov/cder/ndc/database/Default.htm

- **O0100I, transfusions**

Code transfusions of blood or any blood products (e.g., platelets, synthetic blood products), which are administered directly into the bloodstream in this item. Do **not** include transfusions that were administered during dialysis or chemotherapy.

- **O0100J, dialysis**

Code peritoneal or renal dialysis that occurs at the nursing home or at another facility in this item. Record treatments of hemofiltration, Slow Continuous Ultrafiltration (SCUF), Continuous Arteriovenous Hemofiltration (CAVH), and Continuous Ambulatory Peritoneal Dialysis (CAPD) in this item. IVs, IV medication, and blood transfusions administered during dialysis are considered part of the dialysis procedure and are **not** to be coded under items K0500A (Parenteral/IV), O0100H (IV medications), or O0100I (transfusions).

O0100: Special Treatments, Procedures, and Programs (cont.)

- **O0100K, hospice care**

Code residents identified as being in a hospice program for terminally ill persons where an array of services is provided for the palliation and management of terminal illness and related conditions. The hospice must be licensed by the state as a hospice provider and/or certified under the Medicare program as a hospice provider.

- **O0100L, respite care**

Code only when the resident's care program involves a short-term stay in the facility for the purpose of providing relief to a primary home-based caregiver(s) in this item.

- **O0100M, isolation or quarantine for active infectious disease (does not include standard body/fluid precautions)**

Code only when the resident requires strict isolation or quarantine in a separate room because of active infection (i.e., symptomatic and/or have a positive test and are in the contagious stage) with a communicable disease, in an attempt to prevent spread of illness. Do not code this item if the resident only has a **history** of infectious disease (e.g., MRSA or C-Diff with no active symptoms), but facility policy requires cohorting of similar infectious disease conditions. Do not code this item if the "isolation" primarily consists of body/fluid precautions, because these types of precautions apply to everyone.

Additional information related to types of precautions: Transmission-Based Precautions must be considered regarding the type and clinical presentation related to the specific communicable disease. The three types of transmission-based precautions are contact, droplet, and airborne. More information related to the types of transmission-based precautions can be found in the **2007 Guideline for Isolation Precautions: Preventing Transmission of Infectious Agents in Healthcare Settings** http://www.cdc.gov/ncidod/dhqp/pdf/guidelines/Isolation2007.pdf.

- **O0100Z, none of the above**

Code if none of the above treatments, procedures, or programs were received.

O0250: Influenza Vaccine

O0250. Influenza Vaccine - Refer to current version of RAI manual for current flu season and reporting period	

Enter Code ☐	**A.** Did the **resident receive the Influenza vaccine in this facility** for this year's Influenza season?
	     0. **No** → Skip to O0250C, If Influenza vaccine not received, state reason
	     1. **Yes** → Continue to O0250B, Date vaccine received

	B. Date vaccine received → Complete date and skip to O0300A, Is the resident's Pneumococcal vaccination up to date? ☐☐ – ☐☐ – ☐☐☐☐ Month Day Year

Enter Code ☐	**C.** If Influenza vaccine not received, state reason:
	    1. **Resident not in facility** during this year's flu season
	    2. **Received outside of this facility**
	    3. **Not eligible** - medical contraindication
	    4. **Offered and declined**
	    5. **Not offered**
	    6. **Inability to obtain vaccine** due to a declared shortage
	    9. **None of the above**

O0250: Influenza Vaccine (cont.)

Item Rationale

Health-related Quality of Life

- When infected with influenza, older adults and persons with underlying health problems are at increased risk for complications and are more likely than the general population to require hospitalization.

- An institutional Influenza A outbreak can result in up to 60 percent of the population becoming ill, with 25 percent of those affected developing complications severe enough to result in hospitalization or death.

- Influenza-associated mortality results not only from pneumonia, but also from subsequent events arising from cardiovascular, cerebrovascular, and other chronic or immunocompromising diseases that can be exacerbated by influenza.

Planning for Care

- Influenza vaccines have been proven effective in preventing hospitalizations.

- Determining the rate of vaccination and causes for non-vaccination assists nursing homes in reaching the Healthy People 2010 (www.healthypeople.gov) national goal of 90 percent immunization among nursing home residents.

Steps for Assessment

1. Review the resident's medical record to determine whether an Influenza vaccine was received in the facility for this year's Influenza season. If vaccination status is unknown, proceed to the next step.

2. Ask the resident if he or she received an Influenza vaccine outside of the facility for this year's Influenza season. If vaccination status is still unknown, proceed to the next step.

3. If the resident is unable to answer, then ask the same question of the responsible party/legal guardian and/or primary care physician. If vaccination status is still unknown, proceed to the next step.

4. If vaccination status cannot be determined, administer the vaccine to the resident according to standards of clinical practice.

Coding Instructions for O0250A, Did the Resident Receive the Influenza Vaccine in This Facility for This Year's Influenza Season?

- **Code 0, no:** if the resident **did NOT receive the influenza vaccine in this facility** during this year's Influenza season. Proceed to **If Influenza vaccine not received, state reason** (O0250C).

- **Code 1, yes:** if the resident **did receive the influenza vaccine in this facility** during this year's Influenza season. Continue to **Date Vaccine Received** (O0250B).

O0250: Influenza Vaccine (cont.)

Coding Instructions for O0250B, Date Vaccine Received

- Enter date vaccine received. Do not leave any boxes blank. If the month contains only a single digit, fill in the first box of the month with a "0". For example, September January 7, 2010 should be entered as 01-07-2010. If the day only contains a single digit, then fill the first box of the day with the "0". For example, May 6, 2009 should be entered as 05-06-2009. A full 8 character date is required. If the date is unknown or the information is not available, a single dash needs to be entered in the first box.

Coding Instructions for O0250C, If Influenza Vaccine Not Received, State Reason

If the resident has not received the Influenza vaccine in this facility for this year's Influenza season (i.e., 0250A=0), code the reason from the following list:

- **Code 1, resident not in facility during this year's Influenza season:** Resident not in the facility during this year's Influenza season.
- **Code 2, received outside of this facility:** includes influenza vaccinations administered in any other setting (e.g., physician office, health fair, grocery store, hospital, fire station) during this year's Influenza season.
- **Code 3, not eligible—medical contraindication:** if vaccination not received due to medical contraindications, including allergic reaction to eggs or other vaccine component(s), a physician order not to immunize, or an acute febrile illness is present. However, the resident should be vaccinated if contraindications end.
- **Code 4, offered and declined:** resident or responsible party/legal guardian has been informed of what is being offered and chooses not to accept the vaccine.
- **Code 5, not offered:** resident or responsible party/legal guardian not offered the vaccine.
- **Code 6, inability to obtain vaccine due to a declared shortage:** vaccine unavailable at the facility due to declared vaccine shortage. However, the resident should be vaccinated once the facility receives the vaccine. The annual supply of inactivated influenza vaccine and the timing of its distribution cannot be guaranteed in any year.
- **Code 9, none of the above:** if none of the listed reasons describe why the vaccination was not administered. This code is also used if the answer is unknown.

Coding Tips and Special Populations

- The Influenza season varies annually. Information about current Influenza season can be obtained by accessing the CDC Seasonal Influenza (Flu) website: http://www.cdc.gov/flu.

O0250: Influenza Vaccine (cont.)

Examples

1. Mrs. J. received the influenza vaccine in the facility during this year's Influenza season, on January 7, 2010.

   Coding: O0250A would be **coded 1, yes**; O0250B would be **coded 01-07-2010**, and O0250C would be skipped.

   Rationale: Mrs. J. received the vaccine in the facility on January 7, 2010, during this year's Influenza season.

2. Mr. R. did not receive the influenza vaccine in the facility during this year's Influenza season due to his known allergy to egg protein.

   Coding: O0250A would be **coded 0, no**; O0250B is skipped, and O0250C would be **coded 3, not eligible-medical contraindication.**

   Rationale: Allergies to egg protein is a medical contraindication to receiving the influenza vaccine, therefore, Mr. R did not receive the vaccine.

3. Resident Mrs. T. received the influenza vaccine at her doctor's office during this year's Influenza season. Her doctor provided documentation of Mrs. T.'s receipt of the vaccine to the facility to place in Mrs. T.'s medical record. He also provided documentation that Mrs. T. was explained the benefits and risks for the vaccine prior to administration.

   Coding: O0250A would be **coded 1, no**; and O0250C would be **coded 2, received outside of this facility.**

   Rationale: Mrs. T. received the influenza vaccine at her doctor's office during this year's Influenza season.

4. Mr. K. wanted to receive the influenza vaccine if it arrived prior to his scheduled discharge October 5th. Mr. K. was discharged prior to the facility receiving their annual shipment of influenza vaccine, and therefore, Mr. K. did not receive the influenza vaccine in the facility. Mr. K. was encouraged to receive the influenza vaccine at his next scheduled physician visit.

   Coding: O0250A would be **coded 0, no**; O0250B is skipped, and O0250C would be **coded 9, none of the above.**

   Rationale: Mr. K. was unable to receive the influenza vaccine in the facility due to the fact that the facility did not receive its shipment of vaccine until after his discharge. None of the codes in O0250C, **Influenza vaccine not received, state reason**, are applicable.

O0300: Pneumococcal Vaccine

O0300. Pneumococcal Vaccine	
Enter Code ☐	**A. Is the resident's Pneumococcal vaccination up to date?** 0. **No** → Continue to O0300B, If Pneumococcal vaccine not received, state reason 1. **Yes** → Skip to O0400, Therapies
Enter Code ☐	**B. If Pneumococcal vaccine not received, state reason:** 1. **Not eligible** - medical contraindication 2. **Offered and declined** 3. **Not offered**

Item Rationale

Health-related Quality of Life

- Pneumococcal disease accounts for more deaths than any other vaccine-preventable bacterial disease.

- Case fatality rates for pneumococcal bacteremia are approximately 20%; however, they can be as high as 60% in the elderly (CDC, 2009).

Planning for Care

- Early detection of outbreaks is essential to control outbreaks of pneumococcal disease in long-term care facilities.

- Conditions that increase the risk of invasive pneumococcal disease include: decreased immune function, damaged or no spleen, chronic diseases of the heart, lungs, liver and kidneys. Other risk factors include smoking and cerebrospinal fluid (CSF) leak (CDC, 2009).

- Determining the rate of pneumococcal vaccination and causes for non-vaccination assists nursing homes in reaching the Healthy People 2010 (www.healthypeople.gov) national goal of 90% immunization among nursing home residents.

Steps for Assessment

1. Determine whether or not the resident should receive the vaccine.

   - All adults 65 years of age or older should receive the pneumococcal vaccine. However, certain person should be vaccinated before the age of 65, which include but are not limited to the following:

     — Immunocompromised persons 2 years of age and older who are at increased risk of pneumococcal disease should be vaccinated. This group includes those with the risk factors listed under **Planning for Care,** as well as Hodgkin's disease, leukemia, lymphoma, multiple myeloma, nephrotic syndrome, cochlear implant, or those who have had organ transplants and are on immunosuppressive protocols. Those on chemotherapy who are immunosuppressed, or those taking high-dose corticosteriods (14 days or longer) should also be vaccinated.

     — Individuals 2 years of age or older with asymptomatic or symptomatic HIV should be vaccinated.

O0300: Pneumococcal Vaccine (cont.)

— Individuals living in environments or social settings (e.g., nursing homes and other long-term care facilities) with an identified increased risk of invasive pneumococcal disease or its complications should be considered for vaccination populations.

— If vaccination status is unknown or the resident/family is uncertain whether or not the vaccine was received, the resident should be vaccinated.

- Pneumococcal vaccine is given once in a lifetime, with certain exceptions. Revaccination is recommended for the following:

  — Individuals 2 years of age or older who are at highest risk for serious pneumococcal infection and for those who are likely to have a rapid decline in pneumococcal antibody levels. Those at highest risk include individuals with asplenia (functional or anatomic), sickle-cell disease, HIV infections or AIDS, cancer, leukemia, lymphoma, Hodgkin disease, multiple myeloma, generalized malignancy, chronic renal failure, nephrotic syndrome, or other conditions associated with immunosuppression (e.g., organ or bone marrow transplant, medication regimens that lower immunity (such as chemotherapy or long-term steroids).

  — Persons 65 years or older should be administered a second dose of pneumococcal vaccine if they received the first dose of vaccine more than 5 years earlier and were less than 65 years old at the time of the first dose.

- If the resident has had a severe allergic reaction to vaccine components or following a prior dose of the vaccine, they should not be vaccinated.

- If the resident has a moderate to severe acute illness, he or she should not be vaccinated until his or her condition improves. However, someone with a minor illness (e.g., a cold) should be vaccinated since minor illnesses are not a contraindication to receiving the vaccine.

(Centers for Disease Control and Prevention. (2009, May). *The Pink Book: Chapters: Epidemiology and Prevention of Vaccine Preventable Diseases (11th ed.).* Retrieved from http://www.cdc.gov/vaccines/pubs/pinkbook/pink-chapters.htm)

O0300: Pneumococcal Vaccine (cont.)

Note: Please refer to the algorithm below for pneumococcal vaccine administration ONLY.

Figure 1 Adopted from the CDC Recommendations and Reports, Prevention of Pneumococcal Disease: Recommendations of the Advisory Committee on Immunization Practices (ACIP) Recommended Adult Immunization Schedule --- United States. (2009, January 9). *MMWR, 57(53),* Q-1-Q-4.

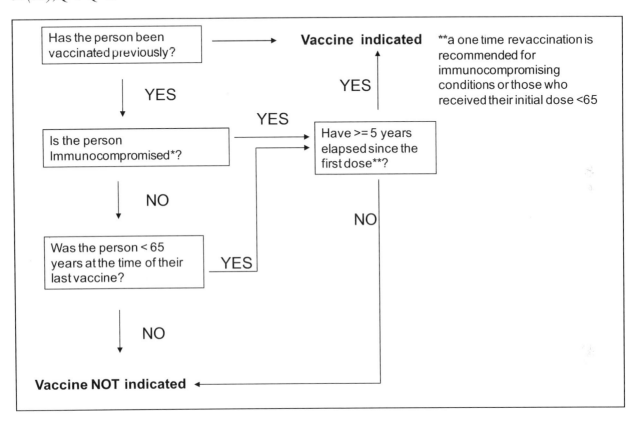

2. Review the resident's medical record and interview resident or responsible party/legal guardian and/or primary care physician to determine pneumococcal vaccination status, using the following steps:

   - Review the resident's medical record to determine whether a pneumococcal vaccine has been received. If vaccination status is unknown, proceed to the next step.

   - Ask the resident if he/she received a pneumococcal vaccine. If vaccination status is still unknown, proceed to the next step.

   - If the resident is unable to answer, ask the same question of a responsible party/legal guardian and/or primary care physician. If vaccination status is still unknown, proceed to the next step.

   - If vaccination status cannot be determined, administer the appropriate vaccine to the resident, according to the standards of clinical practice.

307

O0300: Pneumococcal Vaccine (cont.)

Coding Instructions O0300A, Is the Resident's Pneumococcal Vaccination Up to Date?

- **Code 0, no:** if the resident's pneumococcal vaccination status is not up to date or cannot be determined. Proceed to item O0300B, **If Pneumococcal vaccine not received, state reason**.

- **Code 1, yes:** if the resident's pneumococcal vaccination status is up to date. Skip to O0400, **Therapies**.

Coding Instructions O0300B, If Pneumococcal Vaccine Not Received, State Reason

If the resident has not received a pneumococcal vaccine, code the reason from the following list:

- **Code 1, not eligible:** if the resident is not eligible due to medical contraindications, including a life-threatening allergic reaction to the vaccine or any vaccine component(s) or a physician order not to immunize.

- **Code 2, offered and declined:** resident or responsible party/legal guardian has been informed of what is being offered and chooses not to accept the vaccine.

- **Code 3, not offered:** resident or responsible party/legal guardian not offered the vaccine.

Coding Tips

- The CDC has evaluated inactivated influenza vaccine co-administration with the pneumococcal vaccine systematically among adults. It is safe to give these two vaccinations simultaneously. If the influenza vaccine and pneumococcal vaccine will be given to the resident at the same time, they should be administered at different sites (CDC, 2009). If the resident has had both upper extremities amputated or intramuscular injections are contraindicated in the upper extremities, administer the vaccine(s) according to clinical standards of care.

O0300: Pneumococcal Vaccine (cont.)

Examples

1. Mr. L., who is 72 years old, received the pneumococcal vaccine at his physician's office last year.

   Coding: O0300A would be **coded 1, yes;** skip to O0400, **Therapies.**
   Rationale: Mr. L is over 65 years old and received the pneumococcal vaccine in his physician's office last year at age 71.

2. Mrs. B, who is 95 years old, has never received a pneumococcal vaccine. Her physician has an order stating that she is NOT to be immunized.

   Coding: O0300A would be **coded 0, no;** and O0300B would be **coded 1, not eligible.**
   Rationale: Mrs. B. has never received the pneumococcal vaccine, therefore, her vaccine is not up to date. Her physician has written an order for her not to receive a pneumococcal vaccine, thus she is not eligible for the vaccine

3. Mrs. A. received the pneumococcal vaccine at age 62 when she was hospitalized for a broken hip. She is now 78 and is being admitted to the nursing home for rehabilitation. Her covering physician offered the pneumococcal vaccine to her during his last visit in the nursing home, which she accepted. The facility administered the pneumococcal vaccine to Mrs. A.

   Coding: O0300A would be **coded 1, yes;** skip to O0400, **Therapies.**
   Rationale: Mrs. A. received the pneumococcal vaccine prior to the age of 65. Guidelines suggest that she should be revaccinated since she is over the age of 65 <u>and</u> 5 years have passed since her original vaccination. Mrs. A received the pneumococcal vaccine in the facility.

4. Mr. T. received the pneumococcal vaccine at age 62 when he was living in a congregate care community. He is now 65 years old and is being admitted to the nursing home for chemotherapy and respite care.

   Coding: O0300A would be **coded 1, yes;** skip to O0400, **Therapies.**
   Rationale: Mr. T. received his first dose of pneumococcal vaccine prior to the age of 65 due to him residing in congregate care at the age of 62. Even though Mr. T. is now immune-compromised, less than 5 years have lapsed since he originally received the vaccine. He would be considered up to date with his vaccination.

O0400: Therapies

O0400. Therapies	
A. Speech-Language Pathology and Audiology Services	
Enter Number of Minutes	**1. Individual minutes** - record the total number of minutes this therapy was administered to the resident **individually** in the last 7 days
Enter Number of Minutes	**2. Concurrent minutes** - record the total number of minutes this therapy was administered to the resident **concurrently with one other resident** in the last 7 days
Enter Number of Minutes	**3. Group minutes** - record the total number of minutes this therapy was administered to the resident as **part of a group of residents** in the last 7 days
	If the sum of individual, concurrent, and group minutes is zero, → skip to O0400B, Occupational Therapy
Enter Number of Days	**4. Days** - record the **number of days** this therapy was administered for **at least 15 minutes** a day in the last 7 days
	5. Therapy start date - record the date the most recent therapy regimen (since the most recent entry) started Month Day Year **6. Therapy end date** - record the date the most recent therapy regimen (since the most recent entry) ended - enter dashes if therapy is ongoing Month Day Year
B. Occupational Therapy	
Enter Number of Minutes	**1. Individual minutes** - record the total number of minutes this therapy was administered to the resident **individually** in the last 7 days
Enter Number of Minutes	**2. Concurrent minutes** - record the total number of minutes this therapy was administered to the resident **concurrently with one other resident** in the last 7 days
Enter Number of Minutes	**3. Group minutes** - record the total number of minutes this therapy was administered to the resident as **part of a group of residents** in the last 7 days
	If the sum of individual, concurrent, and group minutes is zero, → skip to O0400C, Physical Therapy
Enter Number of Days	**4. Days** - record the **number of days** this therapy was administered for **at least 15 minutes** a day in the last 7 days
	5. Therapy start date - record the date the most recent therapy regimen (since the most recent entry) started Month Day Year **6. Therapy end date** - record the date the most recent therapy regimen (since the most recent entry) ended - enter dashes if therapy is ongoing Month Day Year
C. Physical Therapy	
Enter Number of Minutes	**1. Individual minutes** - record the total number of minutes this therapy was administered to the resident **individually** in the last 7 days
Enter Number of Minutes	**2. Concurrent minutes** - record the total number of minutes this therapy was administered to the resident **concurrently with one other resident** in the last 7 days
Enter Number of Minutes	**3. Group minutes** - record the total number of minutes this therapy was administered to the resident as **part of a group of residents** in the last 7 days
	If the sum of individual, concurrent, and group minutes is zero, → skip to O0400D, Respiratory Therapy
Enter Number of Days	**4. Days** - record the **number of days** this therapy was administered for **at least 15 minutes** a day in the last 7 days
	5. Therapy start date - record the date the most recent therapy regimen (since the most recent entry) started Month Day Year **6. Therapy end date** - record the date the most recent therapy regimen (since the most recent entry) ended - enter dashes if therapy is ongoing Month Day Year
O0400 continued on next page	

O0400: Therapies (cont.)

O0400. Therapies - Continued	
	D. Respiratory Therapy
Enter Number of Minutes [ ][ ][ ][ ]	**1. Total minutes** - record the total number of minutes this therapy was administered to the resident in the last 7 days If zero, → skip to O0400E, Psychological Therapy
Enter Number of Days [ ]	**2. Days** - record the **number of days** this therapy was administered for **at least 15 minutes** a day in the last 7 days
	E. Psychological Therapy (by any licensed mental health professional)
Enter Number of Minutes [ ][ ][ ][ ]	**1. Total minutes** - record the total number of minutes this therapy was administered to the resident in the last 7 days If zero, → skip to O0400F, Recreational Therapy
Enter Number of Days [ ]	**2. Days** - record the **number of days** this therapy was administered for **at least 15 minutes** a day in the last 7 days
	F. Recreational Therapy (includes recreational and music therapy)
Enter Number of Minutes [ ][ ][ ][ ]	**1. Total minutes** - record the total number of minutes this therapy was administered to the resident in the last 7 days If zero, → skip to O0500, Restorative Nursing Programs
Enter Number of Days [ ]	**2. Days** - record the **number of days** this therapy was administered for **at least 15 minutes** a day in the last 7 days

Item Rationale

Health-related Quality of Life

- Maintaining as much independence as possible in activities of daily living, mobility, and communication is critically important to most people. Functional decline can lead to depression, withdrawal, social isolation, breathing problems, and complications of immobility, such as incontinence and pressure ulcers, which contribute to diminished quality of life. The qualified therapist, in conjunction with the physician and nursing administration, is responsible for determining the necessity for, and the frequency and duration of, the therapy services provided to residents.

- Rehabilitation (i.e., via Speech-Language Pathology Services and Occupational and Physical Therapies) and respiratory, psychological, and recreational therapy can help residents to attain or maintain their highest level of well-being and improve their quality of life.

Planning for Care

- Code only medically necessary therapies that occurred after admission/readmission to the nursing home that were (1) ordered by a physician (physician's assistant, nurse practitioner, and/or clinical nurse specialist) based on a qualified therapist's assessment (i.e., one who meets Medicare requirements or, in some instances, under such a person's direct supervision) and treatment plan, (2) documented in the resident's medical record, and (3) care planned and periodically evaluated to ensure that the resident receives needed therapies and that current treatment plans are effective. Therapy treatment may occur either inside or outside of the facility.

- **For definitions of the types of therapies listed in this section, please refer to the Glossary in Appendix A.**

O0400: Therapies (cont.)

Steps for Assessment

1. Review the resident's medical record (e.g., rehabilitation therapy evaluation and treatment records, recreation therapy notes, mental health professional progress notes), and consult with each of the qualified care providers to collect the information required for this item.

Coding Instructions for Speech-Language Pathology and Audiology Services and Occupational and Physical Therapies

- **Individual minutes**—Enter the total number of minutes of therapy that were provided on an individual basis in the last 7 days. **Enter 0** if none were provided. Individual services are provided by one therapist or assistant to one resident at a time.

- **Concurrent minutes**—Enter the total number of minutes of therapy that were provided on a concurrent basis in the last 7 days. **Enter 0** if none were provided. Concurrent therapy is defined as the treatment of 2 residents at the same time, when the residents are not performing the same or similar activities, regardless of payer source, both of whom must be in line-of-sight of the treating therapist or assistant for Medicare Part A. For Part B, residents may not be treated concurrently: a therapist may treat one resident at a time, and the minutes during the day when the resident is treated individually are added, even if the therapist provides that treatment intermittently (first to one resident and then to another).

- **Group minutes**—Enter the total number of minutes of therapy that were provided in a group in the last 7 days. **Enter 0** if none were provided. Group therapy is defined for Part A as the treatment of 2 to 4 residents, regardless of payer source, who are performing similar activities, and are supervised by a therapist or an assistant who is not supervising any other individuals. For Medicare Part B, treatment of two patients (or more), regardless of payer source, at the same time is documented as group treatment.

- **Days**—Enter the number of days therapy services were provided in the last 7 days. A day of therapy is defined as <u>skilled</u> treatment for 15 minutes or more during the day. **Enter 0** if none were provided **or** if therapy was provided for less than 15 minutes on that day.

- **Therapy Start Date**—Record the date the most recent therapy regimen (since the most recent entry) started. This is the date the initial therapy evaluation is conducted regardless if treatment was rendered or not.

- **Therapy End Date**—Record the date the most recent therapy regimen (since the most recent entry) ended. This is the last date the resident <u>received</u> skilled therapy treatment. Enter dashes if therapy is ongoing.

Coding Instructions for Respiratory, Psychological, and Recreational Therapies

- **Total Minutes**—Enter the actual number of minutes therapy services were provided in the last 7 days. **Enter 0** if none were provided.

O0400: Therapies (cont.)

- **Days**—Enter the number of days therapy services were provided in the last 7 days. A day of therapy is defined as treatment for 15 minutes or more in the day. **Enter 0** if none were provided **or** if therapy was provided for less than 15 minutes in the day.

Coding Tips and Special Populations

Minutes of therapy

- Includes only therapies that were provided once the individual is actually living/being cared for at the long-term care facility. Do **NOT** include therapies that occurred while the person was an inpatient at a hospital or recuperative/rehabilitation center or other long-term care facility, or a recipient of home care or community-based services.
- If a resident returns from a hospital stay, an initial evaluation must be performed after entry to the facility, and only those therapies that occurred since admission/reentry to the facility and after the initial evaluation shall be counted.
- The therapist's time spent on documentation or on initial evaluation is not included.
- The therapist's time spent on subsequent reevaluations, conducted as part of the treatment process, should be counted.
- The resident's treatment time starts when he or she begins the first treatment activity or task and ends when he or she finishes with the last apparatus or intervention/task and the treatment is ended, as long as the services were not interrupted (for example, by a bathroom break or a nontherapeutic rest). The time for the interruption is not considered treatment time and shall not be coded as therapy minutes.
- The time required to adjust equipment or otherwise prepare for the individualized therapy of a particular resident, is the set-up time and may be included in the count of minutes of therapy delivered to the resident.
- For Speech-Language Pathology Services (SLP) and Physical (PT) and Occupational Therapies (OT) include only skilled therapy services. Skilled therapy services **must** meet **all** of the following conditions (Refer to Medicare Benefit Policy Manual, Chapters 8 and 15, for detailed requirements and policies):
  — for Part A, services must be ordered by a physician. For Part B the plan of care must be certified by a physician following the therapy evaluation;
  — the services must be directly and specifically related to an active written treatment plan that is approved by the physician after any needed consultation with the qualified therapist and is based on an initial evaluation performed by a qualified therapist prior to the start of therapy services in the facility;
  — the services must be of a level of complexity and sophistication, or the condition of the resident must be of a nature that requires the judgment, knowledge, and skills of a therapist;

O0400: Therapies (cont.)

- the services must be provided with the expectation, based on the assessment of the resident's restoration potential made by the physician, that the condition of the patient will improve materially in a reasonable and generally predictable period of time, or the services must be necessary for the establishment of a safe and effective maintenance program;

- the services must be considered under accepted standards of medical practice to be specific and effective treatment for the resident's condition; and,

- the services must be reasonable and necessary for the treatment of the resident's condition; this includes the requirement that the amount, frequency, and duration of the services must be reasonable and they must be furnished by qualified personnel.

- Include services provided by a qualified occupational/physical therapy assistant who is employed by (or under contract with) the long-term care facility only if he or she is under the direction of a qualified occupational/physical therapist. Medicare does not recognize speech-language pathology assistants; therefore, services provided by these individuals are not to be coded on the MDS.

- Record only the actual minutes of therapy. The conversion of units to minutes or minutes to units is not appropriate. **Do not round to the nearest 5th minute**. Please note that therapy logs are not an MDS requirement but reflect a standard clinical practice expected of all therapy professionals. These therapy logs may be used to verify the provision of therapy services in accordance with the plan of care and to validate information reported on the MDS assessment.

- Minutes reported on the MDS may not match the time reported on a claim. For example, therapy aide set-up time is recorded on the MDS when it precedes skilled individual therapy; however, the therapy aide time is not included for billing purposes on a therapy Part B claim.

- For purposes of the MDS, providers should record services for respiratory, psychological, and recreational therapies (Item O0400D, E, and F) when the following criteria are met:

  - the physician orders the therapy;

  - the physician's order includes a statement of frequency, duration, and scope of treatment;

  - the services must be directly and specifically related to an active written treatment plan that is based on an initial evaluation performed by qualified personnel (See Glossary in Appendix A for definitions of respiratory, psychological and recreational therapies);

  - the services are required and provided by qualified personnel (See Glossary in Appendix A for definitions of respiratory, psychological and recreational therapies);

  - the services must be reasonable and necessary for treatment of the resident's condition.

O0400: Therapies (cont.)

Non-Skilled Services

- Services provided, at the request of the resident or family, that are not medically necessary (sometimes referred to as family-funded services) shall **not** be counted in item O0400 **Therapies**, even when performed by a therapist or an assistant.

- Nursing homes may elect to have licensed professionals perform repetitive exercises and other maintenance treatments or to supervise aides performing these maintenance services. In these situations, the services shall **not** be coded as therapy in item O0400 **Minutes**, since the specific interventions would be considered restorative nursing care when performed by nurses or aides. Therapeutic services provided by specialists, licensed or not, that are not specifically listed in this manual or on the MDS item set shall **not** be coded as therapy in Item 0400. These services should be documented in the resident's medical record.

- Once the qualified therapist has designed a maintenance program and discharged the resident from a rehabilitation (i.e., skilled) therapy program, the services performed by the therapist and the assistant are **not** to be reported in item O0400A, B, or C **Therapies**. The services may be reported on the MDS assessment in item O0500 **Restorative Nursing Care**, provided the requirements for restorative nursing program are met.

- Services provided by therapy aides are **not** skilled services.

- When a resident refuses to participate in therapy, it is important for care planning purposes to identify why the resident is refusing therapy. However, the time spent investigating the refusal or trying to persuade the resident to participate in treatment is not a skilled service and shall not be included in the therapy minutes.

Co-treatment

When two clinicians, each from a different discipline, treat one resident at the same time. The clinicians must split the time between the two disciplines as they deem appropriate. Each discipline may **not** count the treatment session in full, and the time that was split between the two disciplines, when added together, may not exceed the actual total amount of the treatment session.

Therapy Aides and Students

Therapy Aides

Therapy Aides cannot provide skilled services. Only the time a therapy aide spends on set-up for skilled services preceding individual therapy may be coded on the MDS (e.g., set up the treatment area for wound therapy) and should be coded under individual minutes in O0400 Column 1. The therapy aide must be under direct supervision of the therapist or assistant.

O0400: Therapies (cont.)

Therapy Students

- Medicare Part A—Therapy students must be in line-of-sight supervision of the professional therapist (**Federal Register**, July 30, 1999). Time may be coded on the MDS when the therapist provides skilled services and direction to a student who is participating in the service under line-of-sight supervision.
- Medicare Part B—The following criteria must be met in order for services provided by a student to be billed by the long-term care facility:
  — The qualified professional is present and in the room for the entire session. The student participates in the delivery of services when the qualified practitioner is directing the service, making the skilled judgment, and is responsible for the assessment and treatment.
  — The practitioner is not engaged in treating another patient or doing other tasks at the same time.
  — The qualified professional is the person responsible for the services and, as such, signs all documentation. (A student may, of course, also sign but it is not necessary because the Part B payment is for the clinician's service, not for the student's services.)
  — Physical therapy assistants and occupational therapy assistants are not precluded from serving as clinical instructors for therapy assistant students while providing services within their scope of work and performed under the direction and supervision of a qualified physical or occupational therapist.

Modes of Therapy

A resident may receive therapy via different modes during the same day or even treatment session. The therapist and assistant must determine which mode(s) of therapy and the amount of time the resident receives for each mode and code the MDS appropriately.

Individual Therapy

The treatment of one resident at a time. The resident is receiving the therapist's or the assistant's full attention. Treatment of a resident individually at intermittent times during the day is individual treatment, and the minutes of individual treatment are added for the daily count. For example, the speech-language pathologist treats the resident individually during breakfast for 8 minutes and again at lunch for 13 minutes. The total of individual time for this day would be 21 minutes.

When a therapy student is involved with the treatment of a resident the minutes may be coded as individual therapy when only one resident is being treated by the therapy student and supervising therapist/assistant (Medicare A and Medicare B). The supervising therapist/assistant shall not be engaged in any other activity or treatment.

O0400: Therapies (cont.)

Concurrent Therapy

Medicare Part A

The treatment of 2 residents, who are not performing the same or similar activities, at the same time, regardless of payer source, both of whom must be in line-of-sight of the treating therapist or assistant.

When a therapy student is involved with the treatment, and one of the following occurs, the minutes may be coded as concurrent therapy:

- The therapy student is treating one resident and the supervising therapist/assistant is treating another resident and the therapy student is in line-of-sight; or
- The therapy student is treating 2 residents, both of whom are in line-of-sight of the therapy student and the supervising therapist/assistant; or
- The therapy student is not treating any residents and the supervising therapist/assistant is treating 2 residents at the same time, regardless of payer source, both of whom are in line-of-sight.

Medicare Part B

The treatment of two or more residents, regardless of payer source, at the same time is documented as group treatment.

Group Therapy

Medicare Part A

The treatment of 2 to 4 residents, regardless of payer source, who are performing similar activities, and are supervised by a therapist or assistant who is not supervising any other individuals.

When a therapy student is involved with group therapy treatment, and one of the following occurs, the minutes may be coded as group therapy:

- The therapy student is providing the group treatment and all the residents participating in the group (see definition above) and the therapy student are in line-of-sight of the supervising therapist/assistant who is not supervising other individuals (students or residents); or
- The supervising therapist/assistant is providing the group treatment and the therapy student is not providing treatment to any resident.

Medicare Part B

The treatment of 2 or more individuals simultaneously who may or may not be performing the same activity.

O0400: Therapies (cont.)

When a therapy student is involved with group therapy treatment, and one of the following occurs, the minutes may be coded as group therapy:

- The therapy student is providing group treatment and the supervising therapist/assistant is present and in the room and is not engaged in any other activity or treatment; or
- The supervising therapist/assistant is providing group treatment and the therapy student is not providing treatment to any resident.

Therapy Modalities

Only skilled therapy time (i.e., require the skills, knowledge and judgment of a qualified therapist and all the requirements for skilled therapy are met, see page O-17) shall be recorded on the MDS. In some instances, the time a resident receives certain modalities is partly skilled and partly unskilled time; only the time that is skilled may be recorded on the MDS. For example, a resident is receiving TENS (transcutaneous electrical nerve stimulation) for pain management. The portion of the treatment that is skilled, such as proper electrode placement, establishing proper pulse frequency and duration, and determining appropriate stimulation mode, shall be recorded on the MDS. In other instances, some modalities only meet the requirements of skilled therapy in certain situations. For example, the application of a hot pack is often not a skilled intervention. However, when the resident's condition is complicated and the skills, knowledge, and judgment of the therapist are required for treatment, then those minutes associated with skilled therapy time may be recorded on the MDS.

Dates of Therapy

A resident may have more than one regimen of therapy treatment during an episode of a stay. When this situation occurs the Therapy Start Date for the most recent episode of treatment for the particular therapy (SLP, PT, or OT) should be coded. When a resident's episode of treatment for a given type of therapy extends beyond the ARD, enter dashes in the appropriate Therapy End Date.

For example, Mr. N. was admitted to the nursing home following a fall that resulted in a hip fracture in November 2010. Occupational and Physical therapy started December 3, 2010. His physical therapy ended January 27, 2011 and occupational therapy ended February 11, 2011. Later on during his stay at the nursing home, due to the progressive nature of his Parkinson's disease, he was referred to SLP and OT May 18, 2011 (he remained in the facility the entire time). The speech-language pathologist evaluated him on that day and the occupational therapist evaluated him the next day. The ARD for Mr. N.'s MDS assessment is May 30, 2011. Coding values for his MDS are:

- Item O0400A5 (SLP start date) is 05182011,
- O0400A6 (SLP end date) is dash filled,
- O0400B5 (OT start date) is 05192011,
- O0400B6 (OT end date) is dash filled,

O0400: Therapies (cont.)

- O0400C5 (PT start date) is 12032010, and
- O0400C6 (PT end date) is 01272011.

Examples

1. Mrs. V., whose stay is covered by SNF PPS Part A benefit, begins therapy in an individual session. After 13 minutes the therapist begins working with Mr. S., whose therapy is covered by Medicare Part B, while Mrs. V. continues with her skilled intervention and is in line-of-sight of the treating therapist. The therapist provides treatment during the same time period to Mrs. V. and Mr. S. for 24 minutes, at which time Mrs. V.'s therapy session ends. The therapist continues to treat Mr. S. individually for 10 minutes. Based on the information above, the therapist would code each individual's MDS for this day of treatment as follows:

   - Mrs. V. received individual therapy for 13 minutes and concurrent therapy for 24.
   - Mr. S. received group therapy (Medicare Part B definition) for 24 minutes and individual therapy for 10 minutes. (Please refer to the **Medicare Benefit Policy Manual**, Chapter 15, and the **Medicare Claims Processing Manual**, Chapter 5, for coverage and billing requirements under the Medicare Part B benefit.)

2. Following a stroke, Mrs. F. was admitted to the skilled nursing facility in stable condition for rehabilitation therapy on 10/06/08 under Part A skilled nursing facility coverage. She had slurred speech, difficulty swallowing, severe weakness in both her right upper and lower extremities, and a Stage III pressure ulcer on her left lateral malleolus. She was referred to SLP, OT, and PT with the long-term goal of returning home with her daughter and son-in-law. Her initial SLP evaluation was performed on 10/06/08, the PT initial evaluation on 10/07/08, and the OT initial evaluation on 10/09/08. She was also referred to recreational therapy and respiratory therapy. The interdisciplinary team determined that 10/17/08 was an appropriate ARD for her Medicare-required 14-day MDS. During the look-back period she received the following:

   Speech-language pathology services that were provided over the 7-day look-back period:

   - Individual dysphagia treatments; Monday-Friday for 30 minute sessions each day.
   - Cognitive training; Monday and Thursday for 35 minute concurrent therapy sessions and Tuesday, Wednesday and Friday 25 minute group sessions.
   - Individual speech techniques; Tuesday and Thursday for 20-minute sessions each day.

     Coding: O0400A1 would be **coded 190**; O0400A2 would be **coded 70**; O0400A3 would be **coded 75**; O0400A4 would be **coded 5**; O0400A5 would be **coded 10-06-2008**; and O0400A6 would be **coded with dashes**.

     Rationale: Individual minutes totaled 190 over the 7-day look-back period $[(30 \times 5) + (20 \times 2) = 190]$; concurrent minutes totaled 70 over the 7-day look-back period $(35 \times 2 = 70)$; and group minutes totaled 75 over the 7-day look-back period $(25 \times 3 = 75)$. Therapy was provided 5 out of the 7 days of the look-back period. Date speech-language pathology services began was 10-06-2008, and -'s were used as the therapy end date values because the therapy was ongoing.

O0400: Therapies (cont.)

Occupational therapy services that were provided over the 7-day look-back period:

- Individual sitting balance activities; Monday and Wednesday for 30-minute co-treatment sessions with PT each day (OT and PT split the sessions, with OT recording 20 minutes each session and PT recording 10 minutes each session).
- Individual wheelchair seating and positioning; Monday, Wednesday, and Friday for the following times: 23 minutes, 18 minutes, and 12 minutes.
- Balance/coordination activities; Tuesday-Friday for 20 minutes each day in group sessions.

  Coding: O0400B1 would be **coded 93**, O0400B2 would be **coded 0**, O0400B3 would be **coded 80**, O0400B4 would be **coded 5**, O0400B5 would be **coded 10-09-2008**, and O0400B6 would be **coded with dashes**.

  Rationale: Individual minutes totaled 93 over the 7-day look-back period $[(20 \times 2) + 23 + 18 + 12 = 93]$; concurrent minutes totaled 0 over the 7-day look-back period $(0 \times 0 = 0)$; and group minutes totaled 80 over the 7-day look-back period $(20 \times 4 = 80)$. Therapy was provided 5 out of the 7 days of the look-back period. Date occupational therapy services began was 10-09-2008, and -'s were used as the therapy end date values because the therapy was ongoing.

Physical therapy services that were provided over the 7-day look-back period:

- Individual wound debridement followed by application of routine wound dressing; Monday the session lasted 22 minutes, 5 minutes of which were for the application of the dressing. On Thursday the session lasted 27 minutes, 6 minutes of which were for the application of the dressing. For each session the therapy aidespent 7 minutes preparing the debridement area (set-up time) for needed therapy supplies and equipment for the therapist to conduct wound debridement.
- Individual sitting balance activities; on Monday and Wednesday for 30-minute co-treatment sessions with OT (OT and PT split the sessions, with OT recording 20 minutes each session and PT recording 10 minutes each session).
- Individual bed positioning and bed mobility training; Monday-Friday for 35 minutes each day.
- Concurrent therapeutic exercises; Monday-Friday for 20 minutes each day.

  Coding: O0400C1 would be **coded 247**, O0400C2 would be **coded 100**, O0400C3 would be **coded 0**, O0400C4 would be **coded 5**, O0400C5 would be **coded 10-07-2008**, and O0400C6 would be **coded with dashes**.

  Rationale: Individual minutes totaled 247 over the 7-day look-back period $[(10 \times 2) + (35 \times 5) + (22 - 5) + 7 + (27 - 6) + 7 = 247]$; concurrent minutes totaled 100 over the 7-day look-back period $(20 \times 5 = 100)$; and group minutes totaled 0 over the 7-day look-back period $(0 \times 0 = 0)$. Therapy was provided 5 out of the 7 days of the look-back period. Date physical therapy services began was 10-07-2008, and -'s were used as the therapy end date values because the therapy was ongoing.

O0400: Therapies (cont.)

Respiratory therapy services that were provided over the 7-day look-back period:

- Respiratory therapy services; Sunday-Thursday for 10 minutes each day.
  Coding: O0400D1 would be **coded 50,** O0400D2 would be **coded 0**.
  Rationale: Total minutes were 50 over the 7-day look-back period ($10 \times 5 = 50$). Although a total of 50 minutes of respiratory therapy services were provided over the 7-day look-back period, there were not any days that respiratory therapy was provided for 15 minutes or more. Therefore, O0400D equals **zero days**.

Psychological therapy services that were provided over the 7-day look-back period:

- Psychological therapy services were not provided at all over the 7-day look-back period.
  Coding: O0400E1 would be **coded 0,** O0400E2 would be **coded 0**.
  Rationale: There were no minutes or days of psychological therapy services provided over the 7-day look-back period.

Recreational therapy services that were provided over the 7-day look-back period:

- Recreational therapy services; Tuesday, Wednesday, and Friday for 30-minute sessions each day.
  Coding: O0400F1 would be **coded 90,** O0400F2 would be **coded 3**.
  Rationale: Total minutes were 90 over the 7-day look-back period ($30 \times 3 = 90$). Sessions provided were longer than 15 minutes each day, therefore each day recreational therapy was performed can be counted.

O0400: Therapies (cont.)

O0400. Therapies	
	A. Speech-Language Pathology and Audiology Services

Enter Number of Minutes
`1 9 0`

1. **Individual minutes** - record the total number of minutes this therapy was administered to the resident **individually** in the last 7 days

Enter Number of Minutes
`7 0`

2. **Concurrent minutes** - record the total number of minutes this therapy was administered to the resident **concurrently with one other resident** in the last 7 days

Enter Number of Minutes
`7 5`

3. **Group minutes** - record the total number of minutes this therapy was administered to the resident as **part of a group of residents** in the last 7 days

If the sum of individual, concurrent, and group minutes is zero, → skip to O0400B, Occupational Therapy

Enter Number of Days
`5`

4. **Days** - record the **number of days** this therapy was administered for **at least 15 minutes** a day in the last 7 days

5. **Therapy start date** - record the date the most recent therapy regimen (since the most recent entry) started

`1 0` – `0 6` – `2 0 0 8`
Month   Day   Year

6. **Therapy end date** - record the date the most recent therapy regimen (since the most recent entry) ended - enter dashes if therapy is ongoing

`- -` – `- -` – `- - - -`
Month   Day   Year

B. Occupational Therapy

Enter Number of Minutes
`9 3`

1. **Individual minutes** - record the total number of minutes this therapy was administered to the resident **individually** in the last 7 days

Enter Number of Minutes
`0`

2. **Concurrent minutes** - record the total number of minutes this therapy was administered to the resident **concurrently with one other resident** in the last 7 days

Enter Number of Minutes
`8 0`

3. **Group minutes** - record the total number of minutes this therapy was administered to the resident as **part of a group of residents** in the last 7 days

If the sum of individual, concurrent, and group minutes is zero, → skip to O0400C, Physical Therapy

Enter Number of Days
`5`

4. **Days** - record the **number of days** this therapy was administered for **at least 15 minutes** a day in the last 7 days

5. **Therapy start date** - record the date the most recent therapy regimen (since the most recent entry) started

`1 0` – `0 9` – `2 0 0 8`
Month   Day   Year

6. **Therapy end date** - record the date the most recent therapy regimen (since the most recent entry) ended - enter dashes if therapy is ongoing

`- -` – `- -` – `- - - -`
Month   Day   Year

C. Physical Therapy

Enter Number of Minutes
`2 4 7`

1. **Individual minutes** - record the total number of minutes this therapy was administered to the resident **individually** in the last 7 days

Enter Number of Minutes
`1 0 0`

2. **Concurrent minutes** - record the total number of minutes this therapy was administered to the resident **concurrently with one other resident** in the last 7 days

Enter Number of Minutes
`0`

3. **Group minutes** - record the total number of minutes this therapy was administered to the resident as **part of a group of residents** in the last 7 days

If the sum of individual, concurrent, and group minutes is zero, → skip to O0400D, Respiratory Therapy

Enter Number of Days
`5`

4. **Days** - record the **number of days** this therapy was administered for **at least 15 minutes** a day in the last 7 days

5. **Therapy start date** - record the date the most recent therapy regimen (since the most recent entry) started

`1 0` – `0 7` – `2 0 0 8`
Month   Day   Year

6. **Therapy end date** - record the date the most recent therapy regimen (since the most recent entry) ended - enter dashes if therapy is ongoing

`- -` – `- -` – `- - - -`
Month   Day   Year

O0400 continued on next page

O0400: Therapies (cont.)

O0400. Therapies - Continued	
	D. Respiratory Therapy
Enter Number of Minutes [ ][5][0]	**1. Total minutes** - record the total number of minutes this therapy was administered to the resident in the last 7 days If zero, → skip to O0400E, Psychological Therapy
Enter Number of Days [0]	**2. Days** - record the **number of days** this therapy was administered for **at least 15 minutes** a day in the last 7 days
	E. Psychological Therapy (by any licensed mental health professional)
Enter Number of Minutes [ ][ ][0]	**1. Total minutes** - record the total number of minutes this therapy was administered to the resident in the last 7 days If zero, → skip to O0400F, Recreational Therapy
Enter Number of Days [0]	**2. Days** - record the **number of days** this therapy was administered for **at least 15 minutes** a day in the last 7 days
	F. Recreational Therapy (includes recreational and music therapy)
Enter Number of Minutes [ ][9][0]	**1. Total minutes** - record the total number of minutes this therapy was administered to the resident in the last 7 days If zero, → skip to O0500, Restorative Nursing Programs
Enter Number of Days [3]	**2. Days** - record the **number of days** this therapy was administered for **at least 15 minutes** a day in the last 7 days

O0500: Restorative Nursing Programs

O0500. Restorative Nursing Programs	
Record the **number of days** each of the following restorative programs was performed (for at least 15 minutes a day) in the last 7 calendar days (enter 0 if none or less than 15 minutes daily)	
Number of Days	**Technique**
[ ]	**A. Range of motion (passive)**
[ ]	**B. Range of motion (active)**
[ ]	**C. Splint or brace assistance**
Number of Days	**Training and Skill Practice In:**
[ ]	**D. Bed mobility**
[ ]	**E. Transfer**
[ ]	**F. Walking**
[ ]	**G. Dressing and/or grooming**
[ ]	**H. Eating and/or swallowing**
[ ]	**I. Amputation/prostheses care**
[ ]	**J. Communication**

Item Rationale

Health-related Quality of Life

- Maintaining independence in activities of daily living and mobility is critically important to most people.
- Functional decline can lead to depression, withdrawal, social isolation, and complications of immobility, such as incontinence and pressure ulcers.

323

O0500: Restorative Nursing Programs (cont.)

Planning for Care

- Restorative nursing program refers to nursing interventions that promote the resident's ability to adapt and adjust to living as independently and safely as possible. This concept actively focuses on achieving and maintaining optimal physical, mental, and psychosocial functioning.

- A resident may be started on a restorative nursing program when he or she is admitted to the facility with restorative needs, but is not a candidate for formalized rehabilitation therapy, or when restorative needs arise during the course of a longer-term stay, or in conjunction with formalized rehabilitation therapy. Generally, restorative nursing programs are initiated when a resident is discharged from formalized physical, occupational, or speech rehabilitation therapy.

Steps for Assessment

1. Review the restorative nursing program notes and/or flow sheets in the medical record.
2. For the 7-day look-back period, enter the number of days on which the technique, training or skill practice was performed for a total of at least 15 minutes during the 24-hour period.
3. The following criteria for restorative nursing programs must be met in order to code O0500:

   - Measureable objective and interventions must be documented in the care plan and in the medical record. If a restorative nursing program is in place when a care plan is being revised, it is appropriate to reassess progress, goals, and duration/frequency as part of the care planning process. Good clinical practice would indicate that the results of this reassessment should be documented in the resident's medical record.

   - Evidence of periodic evaluation by the licensed nurse must be present in the resident's medical record. When not contraindicated by state practice act provisions, a progress note written by the restorative aide and countersigned by a licensed nurse is sufficient to document the restorative nursing program once the purpose and objectives of treatment have been established.

   - Nursing assistants/aides must be trained in the techniques that promote resident involvement in the activity.

   - A registered nurse or a licensed practical (vocational) nurse must supervise the activities in a restorative nursing program. Sometimes, under licensed nurse supervision, other staff and volunteers will be assigned to work with specific residents. Restorative nursing does not require a physician's order. Nursing homes may elect to have licensed rehabilitation professionals perform repetitive exercises and other maintenance treatments or to supervise aides performing these maintenance services. In these situations, the services may not be coded as therapy in item O0400, **Therapies,** because the specific interventions are considered restorative nursing services. The therapist's time actually providing the maintenance service can be included when counting restorative nursing minutes. Although therapists may participate, members of the nursing staff are still responsible for overall coordination and supervision of restorative nursing programs.

   - This category does not include groups with more than four residents per supervising helper or caregiver.

O0500: Restorative Nursing Programs (cont.)

Coding Instructions

- This item does not include procedures or techniques carried out by or under the direction of qualified therapists, as identified in **Speech-Language Pathology and Audiology Services** item O0400A, **Occupational Therapy** item O0400B, and **Physical Therapy** O0400C.

- The time provided for items O0500A-J must be coded separately, in time blocks of 15 minutes or more. For example, to check **Technique—Range of Motion [Passive]** item O0500A, 15 or more minutes of passive range of motion (PROM) must have been provided during a 24-hour period in the last 7 days. The 15 minutes of time in a day may be totaled across 24 hours (e.g., 10 minutes on the day shift plus 5 minutes on the evening shift). However, 15-minute time increments cannot be obtained by combining 5 minutes of **Technique—Range of Motion [Passive]** item O0500A, 5 minutes of **Technique—Range of Motion [Active]** item O0500B, and 5 minutes of **Splint or Brace Assistance** item O0500C, over 2 days in the last 7 days.

- Review for each activity throughout the 24-hour period. **Enter 0**, if none.

Technique

Activities provided by restorative nursing staff.

- **O0500A, Range of Motion (Passive)**

  Code provision of passive movements in order to maintain flexibility and useful motion in the joints of the body. These exercises must be individualized to the resident's needs, planned, monitored, evaluated and documented in the resident's medical record.

- **O0500B, Range of Motion (Active)**

  Code exercises performed by the resident, with cueing, supervision, or physical assist by staff that are individualized to the resident's needs, planned, monitored, evaluated , and documented in the resident's medical record. Include active ROM and active-assisted ROM.

- **O0500C, Splint or Brace Assistance**

  Code provision of (1) verbal and physical guidance and direction that teaches the resident how to apply, manipulate, and care for a brace or splint; or (2) a scheduled program of applying and removing a splint or brace. These sessions are individualized to the resident's needs, planned, monitored, evaluated , and documented in the resident's medical record.

O0500: Restorative Nursing Programs (cont.)

Training and Skill Practice

Activities including repetition, physical or verbal cueing, and/or task segmentation provided by any staff member under the supervision of a licensed nurse.

- **O0500D, Bed Mobility**

  Code activities provided to improve or maintain the resident's self-performance in moving to and from a lying position, turning side to side and positioning himself or herself in bed. These activities are individualized to the resident's needs, planned, monitored, evaluated, and documented in the resident's medical record.

- **O0500E, Transfer**

  Code activities provided to improve or maintain the resident's self-performance in moving between surfaces or planes either with or without assistive devices. These activities are individualized to the resident's needs, planned, monitored, evaluated, and documented in the resident's medical record.

- **O0500F, Walking**

  Code activities provided to improve or maintain the resident's self-performance in walking, with or without assistive devices. These activities are individualized to the resident's needs, planned, monitored, evaluated, and documented in the resident's medical record.

- **O0500G, Dressing and/or Grooming**

  Code activities provided to improve or maintain the resident's self-performance in dressing and undressing, bathing and washing, and performing other personal hygiene tasks. These activities are individualized to the resident's needs, planned, monitored, evaluated, and documented in the resident's medical record.

- **O0500H, Eating and/or Swallowing**

  Code activities provided to improve or maintain the resident's self-performance in feeding oneself food and fluids, or activities used to improve or maintain the resident's ability to ingest nutrition and hydration by mouth. These activities are individualized to the resident's needs, planned, monitored, evaluated, and documented in the resident's medical record.

- **O0500I, Amputation/ Prosthesis Care**

  Code activities provided to improve or maintain the resident's self-performance in putting on and removing a prosthesis, caring for the prosthesis, and providing appropriate hygiene at the site where the prosthesis attaches to the body (e.g., leg stump or eye socket). Dentures are not considered to be prostheses for coding this item. These activities are individualized to the resident's needs, planned, monitored, evaluated, and documented in the resident's medical record.

O0500: Restorative Nursing Programs (cont.)

- **O0500J, Communication**

  Code activities provided to improve or maintain the resident's self-performance in functional communication skills or assisting the resident in using residual communication skills and adaptive devices. These activities are individualized to the resident's needs, planned, monitored, evaluated, and documented in the resident's medical record.

Coding Tips and Special Populations

- For range of motion (passive): the caregiver moves the body part around a fixed point or joint through the resident's available range of motion. The resident provides no assistance.

- For range of motion (active): any participation by the resident in the ROM activity should be coded here.

- For both active and passive range of motion: movement by a resident that is incidental to dressing, bathing, etc., does not count as part of a formal restorative nursing program. For inclusion in this section, active or passive range of motion must be a component of an individualized program that is planned, monitored evaluated, and documented in the resident's medical record. Range of motion should be delivered by staff who are trained in the procedures.

- For splint or brace assistance: assess the resident's skin and circulation under the device, and reposition the limb in correct alignment.

- The use of continuous passive motion (CPM) devices in a restorative nursing program is coded when the following criteria are met: (1) ordered by a physician, (2) nursing staff have been trained in technique (e.g., properly aligning resident's limb in device, adjusting available range of motion), and (3) monitoring of the device. Nursing staff should document the application of the device and the effects on the resident. Do **not** include the time the resident is receiving treatment in the device. Include only the actual time staff were engaged in applying and monitoring the device.

- Remember that persons with dementia learn skills best through repetition that occurs multiple times per day.

- Grooming programs, including programs to help residents learn to apply make-up, may be considered restorative nursing programs when conducted by a member of the activity staff. These grooming programs would need to be individualized to the resident's needs, planned, monitored, evaluated, and documented in the resident's medical record.

O0500: Restorative Nursing Programs (cont.)

Examples

1. Mr. V. has lost range of motion in his right arm, wrist, and hand due to a cerebrovascular accident (CVA) experienced several years ago. He has moderate to severe loss of cognitive decision-making skills and memory. To avoid further ROM loss and contractures to his right arm, the occupational therapist fabricated a right resting hand splint and instructions for its application and removal. The nursing coordinator developed instructions for providing passive range of motion exercises to his right arm, wrist, and hand three times per day. The nurse's aides and Mr. V.'s wife have been instructed in how and when to apply and remove the hand splint and how to do the passive ROM exercises. These plans are documented in Mr. V.'s care plan. The total amount of time involved each day in removing and applying the hand splint and completing the ROM exercises is 30 minutes (15 minutes to perform ROM exercises and 15 minutes to apply/remove the splint). The nurse's aides report that there is less resistance in Mr. V.'s affected extremity when bathing and dressing him.

   Coding: Both **Splint or Brace Assistance** item (O0500C), and **Range of Motion (Passive)** item (O0500A), would be **coded 7.**

   Rationale: Because this was the number of days these restorative nursing techniques were provided.

2. Mrs. R.'s right shoulder ROM has decreased slightly over the past week. Upon examination and X-ray, her physician diagnosed her with right shoulder impingement syndrome. Mrs. R. was given exercises to perform on a daily basis to help improve her right shoulder ROM. After initial training in these exercises by the physical therapist, Mrs. R. and the nursing staff were provided with instructions on how to cue and sometimes actively assist Mrs. R. when she cannot make the full ROM required by the exercises on her own. Her exercises are to be performed for 15 minutes, two times per day at change of shift in the morning and afternoon. This information is documented in Mrs. R.'s medical record. The nursing staff cued and sometimes actively assisted Mrs. R. two times daily over the past 7 days.

   Coding: **Range of motion (active)** item (O0500B), would be **coded 7.**

   Rationale: Because this was the number of days restorative nursing training and skill practice for active ROM were provided.

O0500: Restorative Nursing Programs (cont.)

3. Mrs. K. was admitted to the nursing facility 7 days ago following repair to a fractured hip. Physical therapy was delayed due to complications and a weakened condition. Upon admission, she had difficulty moving herself in bed and required total assistance for transfers. To prevent further deterioration and increase her independence, the nursing staff implemented a plan on the second day following admission to teach her how to move herself in bed and transfer from bed to chair using a trapeze, the bed rails, and a transfer board. The plan was documented in Mrs. K.'s medical record and communicated to all staff at the change of shift. The charge nurse documented in the nurse's notes that in the 5 days Mrs. K. has been receiving training and skill practice for bed mobility for 20 minutes a day and transferring for 25 minutes a day, her endurance and strength have improved, and she requires only extensive assistance for transferring. Each day the amount of time to provide this nursing restorative intervention has been decreasing, so that for the past 5 days, the average time is 45 minutes.

   Coding: Both **Bed Mobility** item (O0500D), **Transfer** item (O0500E), would be **coded 5.**

   Rationale: Because this was the number of days that restorative nursing training and skill practice for bed mobility and transfer were provided.

4. Mrs. D. is receiving training and skill practice in walking using a quad cane. Together, Mrs. D. and the nursing staff have set progressive walking distance goals. The nursing staff has received instruction on how to provide Mrs. D. with the instruction and guidance she needs to achieve the goals. She has three scheduled times each day where she learns how to walk with her quad cane. Each teaching and practice episode for walking, supervised by a nursing assistant, takes approximately 15 minutes.

   Coding: Walking item (O0500F), would be **coded 7.**

   Rationale: Because this was the number of days that restorative nursing skill and practice training for walking was provided.

5. Mrs. J. had a CVA less than a year ago resulting in left-sided hemiplegia. Mrs. J. has a strong desire to participate in her own care. Although she cannot dress herself independently, she is capable of participating in this activity of daily living. Mrs. J.'s overall care plan goal is to maximize her independence in ADL's. A plan, documented on the care plan, has been developed to assist Mrs. J. in how to maintain the ability to put on and take off her blouse with no physical assistance from the staff. All of her blouses have been adapted for front closure with velcro. The nursing assistants have been instructed in how to verbally guide Mrs. J. as she puts on and takes off her blouse to enhance her efficiency and maintain her level of function. It takes approximately 20 minutes per day for Mrs. J. to complete this task (dressing and undressing).

   Coding: Dressing or Grooming item (O0500G), would be **coded 7.**

   Rationale: Because this was the number of days that restorative nursing training and skill practice for dressing and grooming were provided.

O0500: Restorative Nursing Programs (cont.)

6. Mr. W.'s cognitive status has been deteriorating progressively over the past several months. Despite deliberate nursing restoration, attempts to promote his independence in feeding himself, he will not eat unless he is fed.

   Coding: **Eating and/or Swallowing** item (O0500H), would be **coded 0.**

   Rationale: Because restorative nursing skill and practice training for eating and/or swallowing were not provided over the last 7 days.

7. Mrs. E. has Amyotrophic Lateral Sclerosis. She no longer has the ability to speak or even to nod her head "yes" or "no." Her cognitive skills remain intact, she can spell, and she can move her eyes in all directions. The speech-language pathologist taught both Mrs. E. and the nursing staff to use a communication board so that Mrs. E. could communicate with staff. The communication board has been in use over the past 2 weeks and has proven very successful. The nursing staff, volunteers, and family members are reminded by a sign over Mrs. E.'s bed that they are to provide her with the board to enable her to communicate with them. This is also documented in Mrs. E.'s care plan. Because the teaching and practice using the communication board had been completed 2 weeks ago and Mrs. E. is able to use the board to communicate successfully, she no longer receives skill and practice training in communication.

   Coding: **Communication** item (O0500J), would be **coded 0.**

   Rationale: Because the resident has mastered the skill of communication, restorative nursing skill and practice training for communication was no longer needed or provided over the last 7 days.

O0600: Physician Examinations

O0600. Physician Examinations	
Enter Days ☐☐	Over the last 14 days, **on how many days did the physician (or authorized assistant or practitioner) examine the resident?**

Item Rationale

Health-related Quality of Life

- Health status that requires frequent physician examinations can adversely affect an individual's sense of well-being and functional status and can limit social activities.

Planning for Care

- Frequency of physician examinations can be an indication of medical complexity and stability of the resident's health status.

O0600: Physician Examinations (cont.)

Steps for Assessment

1. Review the physician progress notes for evidence of examinations of the resident by the physician or other authorized practitioners.

Coding Instructions

- Record the **number of days** that physician progress notes reflect that a physician examined the resident (or since admission if less than 14 days ago).

Coding Tips and Special Populations

- Includes medical doctors, doctors of osteopathy, podiatrists, dentists, and authorized physician assistants, nurse practitioners, or clinical nurse specialists working in collaboration with the physician as allowable by state law.
- Examination (partial or full) can occur in the facility or in the physician's office.
- Do not include physician examinations that occurred prior to admission or readmission to the facility (e.g., during the resident's acute care stay).
- Do not include physician examinations that occurred during an emergency room visit or hospital observation stay.
- If a resident is evaluated by a physician off-site (e.g., while undergoing dialysis or radiation therapy), it can be coded as a physician examination as long as documentation of the physician's evaluation is included in the medical record. The physician's evaluation can include partial or complete examination of the resident, monitoring the resident for response to the treatment, or adjusting the treatment as a result of the examination.
- The licensed psychological therapy by a Psychologist (PhD) should be recorded in O0400E, **Psychological Therapy**.
- Does not include visits made by Medicine Men.

O0700: Physician Orders

O0700. Physician Orders	
Enter Days ☐☐	Over the last 14 days, **on how many days did the physician (or authorized assistant or practitioner) change the resident's orders?**

Item Rationale

Health-related Quality of Life

- Health status that requires frequent physician order changes can adversely affect an individual's sense of well-being and functional status and can limit social activities.

Planning for Care

- Frequency of physician order changes can be an indication of medical complexity and stability of the resident's health status.

O0700: Physician Orders (cont.)

Steps for Assessment

1. Review the physician order sheets in the medical record.
2. Determine the number of days during the 14-day look-back period that a physician changed the resident's orders.

Coding Instructions

- Enter the **number of days** during 14-day look-back period (or since admission, if less than 14 days ago) in which a physician changed the resident's orders.

Coding Tips and Special Populations

- Includes orders written by medical doctors, doctors of osteopathy, podiatrists, dentists, and physician assistants, nurse practitioners, or clinical nurse specialists working in collaboration with the physician as allowable by state law.

- Includes written, telephone, fax, or consultation orders for new or altered treatment. Does **not** include standard admission orders, return admission orders, renewal orders, or clarifying orders without changes. Orders written on the day of admission as a result for an unexpected change/deterioration in condition or injury are considered as new or altered treatment orders and should be counted as a day with order changes.

- The prohibition against counting standard admission or readmission orders applies regardless of whether or not the orders are given at one time or are received at different times on the date of admission or readmission.

- Do not count orders prior to the date of admission or re-entry.

- A sliding scale dosage schedule that is written to cover different dosages depending on lab values, does **not** count as an order change simply because a different dose is administered based on the sliding scale guidelines.

- When a PRN (as needed) order was already on file, the potential need for the service had already been identified. Notification of the physician that the PRN order was activated does **not** constitute a new or changed order and may **not** be counted when coding this item.

- A monthly Medicare Certification is a renewal of an existing order and should **not** be included when coding this item.

- If a resident has multiple physicians (e.g., surgeon, cardiologist, internal medicine), and they all visit and write orders on the same day, the MDS must be coded as 1 day during which a physician visited, and 1 day in which orders were changed.

- Orders requesting a consultation by another physician may be counted. However, the order must be reasonable (e.g., for a new or altered treatment).

- An order written on the last day of the MDS observation period for a consultation planned 3-6 months in the future should be carefully reviewed.

- Orders written to increase the resident's RUG classification and facility payment are **not** acceptable.

- Orders for transfer of care to another physician may **not** be counted.

- Do **not** count orders written by a pharmacist.

SECTION P: RESTRAINTS

Intent: The intent of this section is to record the frequency over the 7-day look-back period that the resident was restrained by any of the listed devices at any time during the day or night. Assessors will evaluate whether or not a device meets the definition of a physical restraint and code only the devices that meet the definition in the appropriate categories of Item P0100.

CMS is committed to reducing unnecessary physical restraint in nursing homes and ensuring that residents are free of physical restraints unless deemed necessary and appropriate as permitted by regulation. Proper interpretation of the physical restraint definition is necessary to understand if nursing homes are accurately assessing devices as physical restraints and meeting the federal requirement for restraint use (see Centers for Medicare & Medicaid Services. [2007, June 22]. Memorandum to State Survey Agency Directors from CMS Director, Survey and Certification Group: Clarification of Terms Used in the Definition of Physical Restraints as Applied to the Requirements for Long Term Care Facilities. Retrieved October 16, 2009, from http://www.cms.gov/SurveyCertificationGenInfo/downloads/SCLetter07-22.pdf).

Are Restraints Prohibited by CMS?

Federal regulations and CMS guidelines do not prohibit use of restraints in nursing homes, except when they are imposed for discipline or convenience and are not required to treat the resident's medical symptoms. The regulation specifically states, "The resident has the right to be free from any physical or chemical restraints imposed for the purposes of discipline or convenience and not required to treat the resident's medical symptoms" (42 CFR 483.13(a)). Research and standards of practice show that restraints have many negative side effects and risks that far outweigh any benefit from their use.

Prior to using any restraint, the nursing home must assess the resident to properly identify the resident's needs and the medical symptom(s) that the restraint is being employed to address. If a restraint is needed to treat the resident's medical symptom, the nursing home is responsible for assessing the appropriateness of that restraint. When the decision is made to use a restraint, CMS encourages, to the extent possible, gradual restraint reduction because there are many negative outcomes associated with restraint use.

> **DEFINITIONS**
>
> **PHYSICAL RESTRAINTS**
> Any manual method or physical or mechanical device, material or equipment attached or adjacent to the resident's body that the individual cannot remove easily, which restricts freedom of movement or normal access to one's body (State Operations Manual, Appendix PP).

While a restraint-free environment is not a federal requirement, the use of restraints should be the exception, not the rule.

P0100: Physical Restraints

P0100. Physical Restraints	
Physical restraints are any manual method or physical or mechanical device, material or equipment attached or adjacent to the resident's body that the individual cannot remove easily which restricts freedom of movement or normal access to one's body	

↓ Enter Codes in Boxes

Coding:
0. **Not used**
1. **Used less than daily**
2. **Used daily**

Used in Bed

☐	A. Bed rail
☐	B. Trunk restraint
☐	C. Limb restraint
☐	D. Other

Used in Chair or Out of Bed

☐	E. Trunk restraint
☐	F. Limb restraint
☐	G. Chair prevents rising
☐	H. Other

Item Rationale

Health-related Quality of Life

- Although the requirements describe the narrow instances when physical restraints may be used, growing evidence supports that physical restraints have a limited role in medical care. Restraints limit mobility and increase the risk for a number of adverse outcomes, such as functional decline, agitation, diminished sense of dignity, depression, and pressure ulcers.
- Residents who are cognitively impaired are at a higher risk of entrapment and injury or death caused by restraints. It is vital that restraints used on this population be carefully considered and monitored. In many cases, the risk of using the device may be greater than the risk of not using the device.
- The risk of restraint-related injury and death is significant.

Planning for Care

- When the use of restraints is considered, thorough assessment of problems to be addressed by restraint use is necessary to determine reversible causes and contributing factors and to identify alternative methods of treating non-reversible issues.
- When the interdisciplinary team determines that the use of restraints is the appropriate course of action, and there is a signed physician order that gives the medical symptom supporting the use of the restraint, the least restrictive device that will meet the resident's needs must be selected.
- Care planning must focus on preventing the adverse effects of restraint use.

P0100: Physical Restraints (cont.)

Steps for Assessment

1. Review the resident's medical record (e.g., physician orders, nurses' notes, nursing assistant documentation) to determine if physical restraints were used during the 7-day look-back period.
2. Consult the nursing staff to determine the resident's cognitive and physical status/limitations.
3. Considering the physical restraint definition as well as the clarifications listed below, observe the resident to determine the effect the restraint has on the resident's normal function. Do not focus on the type of device, intent, or reason behind the use of the device.
4. Evaluate whether the resident can easily and voluntarily remove the device, material, or equipment. If the resident cannot easily and voluntarily remove the restraint, continue with the assessment to determine whether the device restricts freedom of movement or the resident's access to his or her own body.
5. A device should be classified as a restraint only when it meets the criteria of the restraint definition. This can only be determined on a case-by-case basis by individually assessing each and every device (whether or not it is listed specifically on the MDS) and its effect on the resident.
6. Determine if the device, material, or equipment meets the definition of a physical restraint as clarified below. Remember, the decision about coding any device, material, equipment, or physical or manual method as a restraint depends on the effect the device has on the resident.
7. Any device, material, or equipment that meets the definition of a physical restraint must have:

   - physician documentation of a medical symptom that supports the use of the restraint,
   - a physician's order for the type of restraint and parameters of use, and
   - a care plan and a process in place for systematic and gradual restraint reduction (and/or elimination, if possible), as appropriate.

Clarifications

- **"Remove easily"** means that the manual method, device, material, or equipment can be removed intentionally by the resident in the same manner as it was applied by the staff (e.g., side rails are put down or not climbed over, buckles are intentionally unbuckled, ties or knots are intentionally untied), considering the resident's physical condition and ability to accomplish his or her objective (e.g., transfer to a chair, get to the bathroom in time).
- **"Freedom of movement"** means any change in place or position for the body or any part of the body that the person is physically able to control or access.
- **"Medical symptoms/diagnoses"** are defined as an indication or characteristic of a physical or psychological condition. Objective findings derived from clinical evaluation of the resident's medical diagnoses and subjective symptoms should be considered when determining the presence of medical symptom(s) that might support restraint use. **The resident's subjective symptoms may not be used as the sole basis for using a restraint. In addition, the resident's medical symptoms/diagnoses should not be viewed in isolation; rather, the medical symptoms identified should become the context in which to determine the most appropriate method of treatment related to the resident's condition, circumstances, and environment, and not a way to justify restraint use.**

P0100: Physical Restraints (cont.)

- The identification of medical symptoms should assist the nursing home in determining if the specific medical symptom can be improved or addressed by using other, less restrictive interventions. The nursing home should perform all due diligence and document this process to ensure that they have exhausted alternative treatments and less restrictive measures before a restraint is employed to treat the medical symptom, protect the resident's safety, help the resident attain or maintain his or her highest level of physical or psychological well-being and support the resident's goals, wishes, independence, and self-direction.

- **Physical restraints as an intervention do not treat the underlying causes of medical symptoms. Therefore, as with other interventions, physical restraints should not be used without also seeking to identify and address the physical or psychological condition causing the medical symptom**. Restraints may be used, if warranted, as a temporary symptomatic intervention while the actual cause of the medical symptom is being evaluated and managed. Additionally, physical restraints may be used as a symptomatic intervention when they are immediately necessary to prevent a resident from injuring himself/herself or others and/or to prevent the resident from interfering with life-sustaining treatment when no other less restrictive or less risky interventions exist.

Therefore, a clear link must exist between the restraint use and how it benefits the resident by addressing the specific medical symptom. If it is determined, after thorough evaluation and attempts at using alternative treatments and less restrictive methods, that a restraint must still be employed, the medical symptoms that support the use of restraints must be documented in the resident's medical record, ongoing assessments, and care plans. There also must be a physician's order reflecting the use of the restraint and the specific medical symptom being treated by its use. The physician's order alone is not sufficient to employ the use of a restraint. CMS will hold the nursing home ultimately accountable for the appropriateness of that determination.

Coding Instructions

Identify all restraints that were used at anytime (day or night) during the 7-day look-back period.

After determining whether or not a device listed in (P0100) is a restraint and was used during the 7-day look-back period, code the frequency of use:

- **Code 0, not used:** if the device was not used during the 7-day look-back **or** it was used but did not meet the definition.

- **Code 1, used less than daily:** if the device met the definition and was used less than daily.

- **Code 2, used daily:** if the device met the definition and was used on a daily basis during the look-back period.

P0100: Physical Restraints (cont.)

Coding Tips and Special Populations

- Any device that does not fit into the listed categories but that meets the definition of a restraint and has not been excluded from this section should be coded in items P0100D or P0100H, Other. These devices must be care-planned and monitored.

- In classifying any device as a restraint, the assessor must consider the effect the device has on the resident, not the purpose or intent of its use. It is possible for a device to improve the resident's mobility and also have the effect of restraining him or her.

- Exclude from this section items that are typically used in the provision of medical care, such as catheters, drainage tubes, casts, traction, leg, arm, neck, or back braces, abdominal binders, and bandages that are serving in their usual capacity to meet medical need(s).

- **Bed rails** include any combination of partial or full rails (e.g., one-side half-rail, one-side full rail, two-sided half-rails or quarter-rails, rails along the side of the bed that block three-quarters to the whole length of the mattress from top to bottom, etc.). Include in this category enclosed bed systems.

  — Bed rails used as positioning devices. If the use of bed rails (quarter-, half- or three-quarter, one or both, etc.) meets the definition of a physical restraint even though they may improve the resident's mobility in bed, the nursing home must code their use as a restraint at P0100A.

  — Bed rails used with residents who are immobile. If the resident is immobile and cannot voluntarily get out of bed because of a physical limitation and not due to a restraining device or because proper assistive devices were not present, the bed rails do not meet the definition of a restraint.

  For residents who have no voluntary movement, the staff need to determine if there is an appropriate use of bed rails. Bed rails may create a visual barrier and deter physical contact from others. Some residents have no ability to carry out voluntary movements, yet they exhibit involuntary movements. Involuntary movements, resident weight, and gravity's effects may lead to the resident's body shifting toward the edge of the bed. When bed rails are used in these cases, the resident could be at risk for entrapment. For this type of resident, clinical evaluation of alternatives (e.g., a concave mattress to keep the resident from going over the edge of the bed), coupled with frequent monitoring of the resident's position, should be considered. While the bed rails may not constitute a restraint, they may affect the resident's quality of life and create an accident hazard.

- **Trunk restraints** include any device or equipment or material that the resident cannot easily remove such as, but not limited to, vest or waist restraints or belts used in a wheelchair.

- **Limb restraints** include any device or equipment or material that the resident cannot easily remove, that restricts movement of any part of an upper extremity (i.e., hand, arm, wrist) or lower extremity (i.e., foot, leg). Included in this category are mittens.

P0100: Physical Restraints (cont.)

- **Trunk or limb restraints**, if used in both bed and chair, should be marked in both sections.

- **Chairs that prevent rising** include any type of chair with a locked lap board, that places the resident in a recumbent position that restricts rising, or a chair that is soft and low to the floor. Included here are chairs that have a cushion placed in the seat that prohibit the resident from rising.

  — For residents who have the ability to transfer from other chairs, but cannot transfer from a geriatric chair, the geriatric chair <u>would be considered a restraint</u> to that individual, and should be coded as P0100G–Chair Prevents Rising.

  — For residents who have no ability to transfer independently, the geriatric chair <u>does not</u> meet the definition of a restraint, and should not be coded at P0100H–Other.

  — Geriatric chairs used for residents who are immobile. For residents who have no voluntary or involuntary movement, the geriatric chair <u>does not</u> meet the definition of a restraint.

  — Enclosed-frame wheeled walkers, with or without a posterior seat, and other devices like it should not automatically be classified as a restraint. These types of walkers are only classified as a restraint if the resident cannot exit the gate. When deemed a restraint, these walkers should be coded at P0100G–Chair Prevents Rising.

- **Restraints used in emergency situations.** If the resident needs emergency care, restraints may be used for brief periods to permit medical treatment to proceed, unless the resident or legal representative has previously made a valid refusal of the treatment in question. The resident's right to participate in care planning and the right to refuse treatment are addressed at 42 CFR §§483.10(b)(4) and 483.20(k)(2)(ii) respectively. The use of physical restraints in this instance should be limited to preventing the resident from interfering with life-sustaining procedures only and not for routine care.

  — A resident who is injuring himself/herself or is threatening physical harm to others may be restrained in an emergency to safeguard the resident and others. A resident whose unanticipated violent or aggressive behavior places him/her or others in imminent danger does not have the right to refuse the use of restraints, as long as those restraints are used as a last resort to protect the safety of the resident or others and use is limited to the immediate episode.

Additional Information

- **Restraint reduction/elimination.** It is further expected, for residents whose care plan indicates the need for restraints, that the nursing home engages in a systematic and gradual process towards reducing (or eliminating, if possible) the restraints (e.g., gradually increasing the time for ambulation and strengthening activities). This systematic process also applies to recently -admitted residents for whom restraints were used in the previous setting.

P0100: Physical Restraints (cont.)

- **Restraints as a fall prevention approach.** Although restraints have been traditionally used as a fall prevention approach, they have major drawbacks and can contribute to serious injuries. Falls do not constitute self-injurious behavior nor a medical symptom supporting the use of physical restraints. There is no evidence that the use of physical restraints, including but not limited to side rails, will prevent, reduce, or eliminate falls. In fact, in some instances, reducing the use of physical restraints may actually **decrease** the risk of falling. Additionally, falls that occur while a person is physically restrained often result in more severe injuries.

- **Request for restraints.** While a resident, family member, legal representative, or surrogate may request use of a restraint, the nursing home is responsible for evaluating the appropriateness of that request, just as they would for any medical treatment. As with other medical treatments, such as the use of prescription drugs, a resident, family member, legal representative, or surrogate has the right to refuse treatment, but not to demand its use when it is not deemed medically necessary.

  According to 42 CFR 483.13(a), "The resident has the right to be free from any physical or chemical restraints imposed for the purposes of discipline or convenience and not required to treat the resident's medical symptoms." CMS expects that no resident will be restrained for discipline or convenience. Prior to employing any restraint, the nursing home must perform a prescribed resident assessment to properly identify the resident's needs and the medical symptom the restraint is being employed to address. The guidelines in the State Operations Manual (SOM) state, "...the legal surrogate or representative cannot give permission to use restraints for the sake of discipline or staff convenience or when the restraint is not necessary to treat the resident's medical symptoms. That is, the facility may not use restraints in violation of regulation solely based on a resident, legal surrogate or representative's request or approval." The SOM goes on to state, "While Federal regulations affirm the resident's right to participate in care planning and to refuse treatment, the regulations do not create the right for a resident, legal surrogate or representative to demand that the facility use specific medical interventions or treatment that the facility deems inappropriate. Statutory requirements hold the facility ultimately accountable for the resident's care and safety, including clinical decisions."

SECTION Q: PARTICIPATION IN ASSESSMENT AND GOAL SETTING

Intent: The items in this section are intended to record the participation and expectations of the resident, family members, or significant other(s) in the assessment, and to understand the resident's overall goals.

Q0100: Participation in Assessment

Q0100. Participation in Assessment	
Enter Code ☐	**A. Resident participated in assessment** 0. No 1. Yes
Enter Code ☐	**B. Family or significant other participated in assessment** 0. No 1. Yes 9. No family or significant other
Enter Code ☐	**C. Guardian or legally authorized representative participated in assessment** 0. No 1. Yes 9. No guardian or legally authorized representative

Item Rationale

Health-related Quality of Life

- Residents who actively participate in the assessment process through interview and conversation often experience improved quality of life and higher quality care based on their needs, goals, and priorities.

Planning for Care

- The care plan should be individualized and resident-driven.

- During care planning meetings, if the resident is present, he or she should be made comfortable and verbal communication should be directly with him or her.

- Many residents want their family or significant other(s) to be involved in the assessment process.

- When the resident is unable to participate in the assessment process, a family member or significant other, and guardian or legally authorized representatives can provide valuable information about the resident's needs, goals, and priorities.

> **DEFINITIONS**
>
> **RESIDENT'S PARTICIPATION IN ASSESSMENT**
> The resident actively engages in interviews and conversations as necessary to meaningfully contribute to the completion of the MDS 3.0. Interdisciplinary team members should engage the resident during assessment in order to determine the resident's expectations and perspective during assessment.

Q0100: Participation in Assessment (cont.)

Steps for Assessment

1. Review the medical record for documentation that the resident, family or significant other, and guardian or legally authorized representative participated in the assessment process.
2. Ask the resident, the family or significant other (when applicable), and the guardian or legally authorized representative (when applicable) if he or she actively participated in the assessment process.
3. Ask staff members who completed the assessment whether or not the resident, family or significant other, or guardian or legally authorized representative participated in the assessment process.

Coding Instructions for Q0100A, Resident Participated in Assessment

Record the participation of the resident in the assessment process.

- **Code 0, no:** if the resident did not actively participate in the assessment process.
- **Code 1, yes:** if the resident actively and meaningfully participated in the assessment process.

Coding Instructions for Q0100B, Family or Significant Other Participated in Assessment

Record the participation of the family or significant other in the assessment process.

- **Code 0, no:** if the family or significant other did not participate in the assessment process.
- **Code 1, yes:** if the family or significant other(s) did participate in the assessment process.
- **Code 9, no family or significant other:** if there is no family or significant other.

Coding Tips

- Significant other does not include nursing home staff.

> **DEFINITIONS**
>
> **FAMILY OR SIGNIFICANT OTHER**
> A spousal, kinship (e.g., sibling, child, parent, nephew), or in-law relationship; a partner, housemate, primary community caregiver or close friend. Significant other does not, however, include staff at the nursing home.
>
> **GUARDIAN/LEGALLY AUTHORIZED REPRESENTATIVE**
> A person who is authorized, under applicable law, to make decisions for the resident, including giving and withholding consent for medical treatment.

Q0100: Participation in Assessment (cont.)

Coding Instructions for Q0100C, **Guardian or Legally Authorized Representative Participated in Assessment**

Record the participation of the guardian or legally authorized representative in the assessment process.

- **Code 0, no:** if guardian or legally authorized representative did not participate in the assessment process.
- **Code 1, yes:** if guardian or legally authorized representative did participate in the assessment process.
- **Code 9, no guardian or legally authorized representative:** if there is no guardian or legally authorized representative.

Q0300: Resident's Overall Expectation

Complete only on admission assessment.

Q0300. Resident's Overall Expectation	
Complete only if A0310E = 1	
Enter Code ☐	**A. Resident's overall goal established during assessment process** 1. Expects to be **discharged to the community** 2. Expects to **remain in this facility** 3. Expects to be **discharged to another facility/institution** 9. **Unknown or uncertain**
Enter Code ☐	**B. Indicate information source for Q0300A** 1. **Resident** 2. If not resident, then **family or significant other** 3. If not resident, family, or significant other, then **guardian or legally authorized representative** 9. **None of the above**

Item Rationale

This item identifies the resident's general expectations and goals for nursing home stay. The resident should be asked about his or her own expectations regarding return to the community and goals for care. The resident may not be aware of the option of returning to the community and that services and supports may be available in the community to meet long-term care needs.

Some residents have very clear and directed expectations that will change little prior to discharge. Other residents may be unsure or may be experiencing an evolution in their thinking as their clinical condition changes or stabilizes.

Health-related Quality of Life

- Unless the resident's goals for care are understood, his or her needs, goals, and priorities are not likely to be met.

Planning for Care

- The resident's goals should be the basis for care planning.

> **DEFINITIONS**
>
> **DISCHARGE**
> To release from nursing home care. Can be to home, another community setting, or healthcare setting.

Q0300: Resident's Overall Expectation (cont.)

Steps for Assessment

1. Ask the resident about his or her overall expectations after he or she has participated in the assessment process and has a better understanding of his or her current situation and the implications of alternative choices.
2. Ask the resident to consider current clinical status, expectations regarding improvement or worsening, and social supports.
3. Because of a temporary (e.g., delirium) or permanent (e.g., profound dementia) condition, some residents may be unable to provide a clear response. If the resident is unable to communicate his or her preference either verbally or nonverbally, the information can be obtained from the family or significant other, as designated by the individual. If family or the significant other is not available, the information should be obtained from the guardian or legally authorized representative.
4. If goals have not already been stated directly by the resident and documented since admission, ask the resident directly about what his or her expectation is regarding the outcome of this nursing home admission and expectations about returning to the community.
5. The resident's goals—as perceived by the family, significant other, guardian, or legally authorized representative—should be recorded here only if the resident is unable to discuss his or her goals.
6. Encourage the involvement of family or significant others in the discussion if the resident consents. While family, significant others, or, if necessary, the guardian or legally authorized representative can be involved if the resident is uncertain about his or her goals, the response selected must reflect the resident's perspective if he or she is able to express it.

Coding Instructions for Q0300A, Resident's Overall Goals Established during Assessment Process

Record the resident's expectations as expressed, whether they are realistic or not realistic.

- **Code 1, expects to be discharged to the community:** if the resident is in the nursing home for rehabilitation, skilled nursing care, or respite care and indicates an expectation to return home, to assisted living, or to another community setting.

- **Code 2, expects to remain in this facility:** if the resident is in the nursing home for rehabilitation or skilled nursing care and indicates that after this care is complete, he or she expects to remain in the nursing home.

- **Code 3, expects to be discharged to another facility/institution:** if the resident expects to be discharged to another nursing home, rehabilitation facility, or another institution.

- **Code 9, unknown or uncertain:** if the resident is uncertain or if the resident is not able to participate in the discussion or indicate a goal, and family, significant other, or guardian or legally authorized representative are not available to participate in the discussion.

Q0300: Resident's Overall Expectation (cont.)

Coding Tips

- This item is individualized and resident-driven rather than what the nursing home staff judge to be in the best interest of the resident. This item focuses on exploring the resident's options; not whether or not the staff considers them to be good or poor options.
- Avoid trying to guess what the resident might identify as a goal or to judge the resident's goal. Do not infer based on a specific advance care order, such as "do not resuscitate" (DNR).
- The resident should be provided options, as well as, access to information that allows him or her to make the decision and to be supported in directing his or her care planning.

Coding Instructions for Q0300B, Indicate Information Source for Q0300A

- **Code 1, resident:** if the resident is the source for completing this item.
- **Code 2, if not resident, then family or significant other:** if the resident is unable to respond and a family member or significant other is the source for completing this item.
- **Code 3, if not resident, family or significant other, then guardian or legally authorized representative:** if the guardian or legally authorized representative is the source for completing this item because the resident is unable to respond and a family member or significant other is not available to respond.
- **Code 9, none of the above:** if the resident cannot respond and the family or significant other, or guardian or legally authorized representative cannot be contacted or is unable to respond (Q0300A = 9).

Examples

1. Mrs. F. is a 55-year-old married woman who had a cerebrovascular accident (CVA, also known as stroke) 2 weeks ago. She was admitted to the nursing home 1 week ago for rehabilitation, particularly for transfer, gait training, and wheelchair mobility training. Mrs. F. is extremely motivated to return home. Her husband is supportive and has been busy adapting their home to promote her independence. Her goal is to return home once she has completed rehabilitation.

   Coding: Q0300A would be **coded 1, expects to be discharged to the community**.

   Q0300B would be **coded 1, resident**.

   Rationale: Mrs. F. has clear expectations and a goal to return home.

Q0300: Resident's Overall Expectation (cont.)

2. Mr. W. is a 73-year-old man who has severe heart failure and renal dysfunction. He also has a new diagnosis of metastatic colorectal cancer and was readmitted to the nursing home after a prolonged hospitalization for lower gastrointestinal (GI) bleeding. He relies on nursing staff for all activities of daily living (ADLs). He indicates that he is "strongly optimistic" about his future and only wants to think "positive thoughts" about what is going to happen and needs to believe that he will return home.

    Coding: Q0300A would be **coded 1, expects to be discharged to the community**.

    Q0300B would be **coded 1, resident**.

    Rationale: Mr. W has a clear goal to return home. Even if the staff believe this is unlikely based on available social supports and past nursing home residence, this item should be coded based on the resident's expressed goals.

3. Ms. T. is a 93-year-old woman with chronic renal failure, oxygen dependent chronic obstructive pulmonary disease (COPD), severe osteoporosis, and moderate dementia. When queried about her care preferences, she is unable to voice consistent preferences for her own care, simply stating that "It's such a nice day. Now let's talk about it more." When her daughter is asked about goals for her mother's care, she states that "We know her time is coming. The most important thing now is for her to be comfortable. Because of monetary constraints and the level of care that she needs, we feel that we cannot adequately meet her needs. Other than treating simple things, what we really want most is for her to live out whatever time she has in comfort." The assessor confirms that the daughter wants care oriented toward making her mother comfortable in her final days.

    Coding: Q0300A would be **coded 2, expects to remain in this facility**.

    Q0300B would be **coded 2, family or significant other**.

    Rationale: Ms. T is not able to respond, but her daughter has clear expectations that her mother will remain in the nursing home where she will be made comfortable for her remaining days.

4. Mrs. G., an 84-year-old female with severe dementia, is admitted by her daughter for a 7-day period. Her daughter stated that she "just needs to have a break." Her mother has been wandering at times and has little interactive capacity. The daughter is planning to take her mother back home at the end of the week.

    Coding: Q0300A would be **coded 1, expects to be discharged to the community**.

    Q0300B would be **coded 2, family or significant other**.

    Rationale: Mrs. G. is not able to respond but her daughter has clear expectations that her mother will return home at the end of the 7-day respite visit.

Q0300: Resident's Overall Expectation (cont.)

5. Mrs. C. is a 72-year-old woman who had been living alone and was admitted to the nursing home for rehabilitation after a severe fall. Upon admission, she was diagnosed with moderate dementia and was unable to voice consistent preferences for her own care. She has no living relatives and no significant other who is willing to participate in her care decisions. The court appointed a legal guardian to oversee her care. Community-based services, including assisted living and other residential care situations, were discussed with the guardian. The guardian decided that it is in Mrs. C.'s best interest that she be discharged to a nursing home that has a specialized dementia care unit once rehabilitation was complete.

    Coding: Q0300A would be **coded 3, expects to be discharged to another facility/institution**.

    Q0300B would be **coded 3, guardian or legally authorized representative**.

    Rationale: Mrs. C. is not able to respond and has no family or significant other available to participate in her care decisions. A court-appointed legal guardian determined that it is in Mrs. C.'s best interest to be discharged to a nursing home that could provide dementia care once rehabilitation was complete.

6. Ms. K. is a 40-year-old with cerebral palsy and a learning disability. She lived in a group home 5 years ago, but after a hospitalization for pneumonia she was admitted to the nursing home for respiratory therapy. Although her group home bed is no longer available, she is now medically stable and there is no medical reason why she could not transition back to the community. Ms. K. states she wants to return to the group home. Her legal guardian agrees that she should return to the community to a small group home.

    Coding: Q0300A would be **coded 1, expects to be discharged to the community (small group homes are considered to be community setting)**.

    Q0300B would be **coded 3, guardian or legally authorized representative**.

    Rationale: Ms. K. is able to respond and says she would like to go back to the group home but is unable to make decisions about her medical and other care needs. When the legal guardian was told that Ms. K. is medically stable and would like to go back to the community, she decided that it is in Ms. K.'s best interest to be transferred to a group home.

Q0400: Discharge Plan

Q0400. Discharge Plan	
Enter Code ⬜	**A. Is there an active discharge plan in place for the resident to return to the community?** 0. **No** 1. **Yes** → Skip to Q0600, Referral
Enter Code ⬜	**B. What determination was made by the resident and the care planning team regarding discharge to the community?** 0. **Determination not made** 1. **Discharge to community determined to be feasible** → Skip to Q0600, Referral 2. **Discharge to community determined to be not feasible** → Skip to next active section (V or X)

Q0400: Discharge Plan (cont.)

Item Rationale

Health-related Quality of Life

- Returning home or to a noninstitutional setting can be very important to the resident's health and quality of life.

- For residents that have been in the facility for a long time, it is important to discuss with them their interest in talking with local contact agency (LCA) experts about returning to the community. There are improved community resources and supports that may benefit these residents and allow them to return to a community setting.

- Being discharged from the nursing home without an adequate discharge plan could result in the resident's decline and increase the chances for rehospitalization and aftercare, so a thorough examination of the options with the resident and local community experts is imperative.

Planning for Care

- Some nursing home residents may be able to return to the community if they are provided appropriate assistance and referral to community resources.

- Important progress has been made so that individuals have more choices, care options, and available supports to meet care preferences and needs in the least restrictive setting possible. This progress resulted from the U. S. Supreme Court Olmstead ruling, which states that residents needing long-term care services have a right to receive services in the least restrictive and most integrated setting.

- The care plan should include the name and contact information of a primary care provider chosen by the resident, family, significant other, guardian or legally authorized representative, arrangements for the durable medical equipment (if needed), formal and informal supports that will be available, the persons and provider(s) in the community who will meet the resident's needs, and the place the resident is going to be living.

- Discharge instructions should include at a minimum:
  — the individuals preferences and needs for care and supports;
    o personal identification and contact information, including Advance Directives;
    o provider contact information of primary care physician, pharmacy, and community care agency including personal care services (if applicable) etc.;
    o brief medical history;
    o current medications, treatments, therapies, and allergies;
    o arrangements for durable medical equipment;
    o arrangements for housing; and
    o contact information at the nursing home if a problem arises during discharge
  — A follow-up appointment with the designated primary care provider in the community and other specialists (as appropriate).
  — Medication education.

347

Q0400: Discharge Plan (cont.)

— Prevention and disease management education, focusing especially on warning symptoms for when to call the doctor.

— Who to call in case of an emergency or if symptoms of decline occur.

— Nursing facility procedures and discharge planning for subacute and rehabilitation community discharges are most often well defined and efficient.

— Section Q has been broadened beyond the traditional definition of discharge planning for sub-acute residents to encompass long stay residents including the elderly, disabled, intellectually challenged, and younger nursing home residents. In addition to home health and other medical services, discharge planning may include expanded resources such as assistance with locating housing, employment, and social engagement opportunities.

    o   Asking the resident and family about whether they want to talk to someone about a return to the community gives the resident voice and respects his or her wishes. This step in no way guarantees discharge but provides an opportunity for the resident to interact with LCA experts.

    o   The nursing home staff must not make an interdisciplinary determination that discharge is not feasible without consulting the resident if the resident can be interviewed.

    o   Each NH needs to develop relationships with their LCAs to work with them to contact the resident and their family concerning a potential return to the community. A thorough review of medical, psychological, functional, and financial information is necessary in order to assess what each individual resident needs and whether or not there are sufficient community resources and finances to support a transition to the community.

    o   Enriched transition resources including housing, in-home caretaking services and meals, home modifications, etc. are now more readily available and will grow over time. Resource availability and eligibility coverage varies across local communities and States, and may be barriers to some residents being able to return to the community.

    o   Should it occur, an unsuccessful transition may create stress and disappointment for the resident and family that will require support and nursing home care planning interventions.

- Involve community mental health resources (as appropriate) to ensure that the resident has support and active coping skills that will help him or her to readjust to community living.

- Use teach-back methods to ensure that the resident understands all of the factors associated with his or her discharge.

- For additional guidance, see CMS' **Planning for Your Discharge: A checklist for patients and caregivers preparing to leave a hospital, nursing home, or other health care setting**. Available at http://www.medicare.gov/Publications/Pubs/pdf/11376.pdf

Q0400: Discharge Plan (cont.)

Steps for Assessment

1. A review should be conducted of the care plan, the medical record, and clinician progress notes, including but not limited to nursing, physician, social services and therapy.
2. If the resident is being discharged, an evaluation of the site should be conducted to determine the safety of the resident's surroundings and the need for assistive/adaptive devices, medical supplies, and equipment.
3. The resident, interdisciplinary team, and local contact agency (when a referral has been made to a local community contact agency) should determine the services and assistance that the resident will need post discharge (e.g., homemaker, meal preparation, ADL assistance, transportation, prescription assistance) and make appropriate referrals.
4. Eligibility for financial assistance through various funding sources (e.g., private funds, family assistance, Medicaid, long-term care insurance) should be assessed prior to discharge to determine where the resident will be discharged (e.g., home, assisted living, board and care, group living).
5. Determine if there will be family involvement and support after discharge.

Coding Instructions for Q0400A, Is There an Active Discharge plan in Place for the Resident to Return to the Community?

- **Code 0, no:** if there is not an active discharge plan in place for the resident to return to the community.
- **Code 1, yes:** if there is an active discharge plan in place for the resident to return to the community; skip to **Referral** item (Q0600).

Coding Instructions for Q0400B, What Determination Was Made by the Resident and the Care Planning Team Regarding Discharge to the Community?

- **Code 0:** if a determination is not made by the resident and the care planning team regarding discharge to the community.
- **Code 1:** if discharge to the community is determined to be feasible; skip to item Q0600 (Referral).
- **Code 2:** if discharge to the community is determined to be not feasible; skip to the next active assessment section (Section V or X).

Coding Tips

- This item is individualized and resident-driven, and the interdisciplinary team must interview residents and/or their family members, whenever possible, and determine their preferences and agreement.

Q0400: Discharge Plan (cont.)

- The nursing home interdisciplinary team should not assume that any particular resident is unable to be discharged. The nursing home should code Q0400B as **2 after** they have fully explored the resident's preferences and possible home and community based services/options available to the resident. Most likely, this would require consultation with community resource experts at the LCA.

Examples

1. Ms. G is a 45-year-old woman, 300 lbs., who is cognitively intact. She has CHF and shortness of breath requiring oxygen at night. Ms. G also requires assistance with bathing and transfers to the commode. She has resided at the nursing home for 3 years. Her nursing home admission was a result of the fact that her family and friends, who visited regularly, could not care for her at home. Although she expresses interest in talking to someone about returning to the community, the interdisciplinary team is uncertain whether there would be sufficient community resources available and whether her family would agree to the discharge.

   Coding: Q0400B would be **coded 1, discharge to the community is determined to be feasible; skip to item Q0600 (Referral)**.

   Rationale: Ms. G expresses the desire to talk to someone about the return to the community and the local contact agency representative can help address the interdisciplinary team's legitimate concerns about available and sufficient community resources particularly accessible and affordable housing and to talk to the resident's family.

2. Mrs. R is an 82-year-old widowed woman with advanced Alzheimer's disease. She has no family, and has resided at the nursing home for 4½ years. The resident is not able to be interviewed.

   Coding: Q0400B would be **coded 2, discharge to the community is determined to be not feasible; skip to the next active assessment section (Section V or X)**.

   Rationale: Mrs. R is not able to be interviewed and there is no family or other resources to support her return to the community.

Q0500: Return to Community

For Admission, Quarterly, and Annual Assessments.

Q0500. Return to Community	
Enter Code	**A. Has the resident been asked about returning to the community?** 0. **No** 1. **Yes** - previous response was "**no**" 2. **Yes** - previous response was "**yes**" → Skip to Q0600, Referral 3. **Yes** - previous response was "**unknown**"
Enter Code	**B. Ask the resident** (or family or significant other if resident is unable to respond): "**Do you want to talk to someone about the possibility of returning to the community?**" 0. **No** 1. **Yes** 9. **Unknown or uncertain**

Q0500: Return to Community (cont.)

Item Rationale

The goal of follow-up action is to initiate and maintain collaboration between the nursing home and the local contact agency to support the resident's expressed interest in being transitioned to community living. This includes the nursing home supporting the resident in achieving his or her highest level of functioning and the local contact agency providing informed choices for community living and assisting the resident in transitioning to community living.

Health-related Quality of Life

- Returning home or to a noninstitutional setting can be very important to the resident's health and quality of life.
- This item identifies the resident's desire to speak with someone about returning to community living. Based on the Americans with Disabilities Act and the 1999 U.S. Supreme Court decision in **Olmstead v. L.C.,** residents needing long-term care services have a right to receive services in the least restrictive and most integrated setting.
- Item Q0500B requires that the resident be asked the question directly and formalizes the opportunity for the resident to be informed of and consider his or her options to return to community living. This ensures that the resident's desire to learn about the possibility of returning to the community will be obtained and appropriate follow-up measures will be taken.
- The goal is to obtain the expressed interest of the resident and focus on the resident's preferences.

Planning for Care

- Some nursing home residents may be able to return to the community if they are provided appropriate assistance to facilitate care in a noninstitutional setting.

Steps for Assessment: Interview Instructions

1. At the initial admission assessment and in subsequent follow-up assessments (as applicable), determine if the resident has been asked about returning to the community.
2. If the resident has not been asked about returning to the community or if the resident has been asked and his or her previous response was no or unknown, make the resident comfortable by assuring him or her that this is a routine question that is asked of all residents.
3. Ask the resident if he or she would like to speak with someone about the possibility of returning to live in the community. Inform the resident that answering yes to this item signals the resident's request for more information and will initiate a contact by someone with more information about supports available for living in the community. Answering yes does not commit the resident to leave the nursing home at a specific time; nor does it ensure that the resident will be able to move back to the community. Answering no is also not a permanent commitment. Also inform the resident that he or she can change his or her decision (i.e., whether or not he or she wants to speak with someone) at any time.

351

Q0500: Return to Community (cont.)

4. Explain that this item is meant to explore the possibility of different ways of receiving ongoing care.
5. If the resident is unable to communicate his or her preference either verbally or nonverbally, the information can then be obtained from family or a significant other, as designated by the individual. If family or significant others is not available, a guardian or legally authorized representative can provide the information.
6. Ask the resident if he or she wants information about different kinds of supports that may be available for community living. Responding yes will be a way for the individual—and his or her family, significant other, or guardian or legally authorized representative—to obtain additional information about services and supports that would be available to support community living.

Coding Instructions for Q0500A, Has the Resident Been Asked about Returning to the Community?

- **Code 0, no:** if the resident (or family or significant other, or guardian or legally authorized representative) states that he or she has not been asked about the possibility of returning to the community.
- **Code 1, yes—previous response was no:** if the resident (or family or significant other, or guardian or legally authorized representative) states that he or she was previously asked about the possibility of returning to the community and the previous response was no.
- **Code 2, yes—previous response was yes:** if the resident (or family or significant other, or guardian or legally authorized representative) states that he or she was previously asked about the possibility of returning to the community and the previous response was yes. If Code 2 is entered, skip to Q0600 (Referral).
- **Code 3, yes—previous response was unknown:** if the resident (or family or significant other, or guardian or legally authorized representative) states that he or she was previously asked about the possibility of returning to the community but the previous response is unknown.

Coding Instructions for Q0500B, Ask the Resident (or Family or Significant Other if Resident Is Unable to Respond): "Do You Want to Talk to Someone about the Possibility of Returning to the Community?"

- **Code 0, no:** if the resident (or family or significant other, or guardian or legally authorized representative) states that he or she does not want to talk to someone about the possibility of returning to the community.
- **Code 1, yes:** if the resident (or family- or significant other, or guardian or legally authorized representative) states that he or she does want to talk to someone about the possibility of returning to the community.
- **Code 9, unknown or uncertain:** if the resident cannot respond and the family or significant other is not available to respond on the resident's behalf and a guardian or legally authorized representative is not available or has not been appointed by the court.

Q0500: Return to Community (cont.)

Coding Tips

- A "yes—previous response was yes" response to item Q0500A will trigger follow-up care planning and contact with the designated local contact agency about the resident's request within 10 business days of a yes response being given. This code is intended to initiate contact with the local agency for follow-up as the resident desires.

- Some residents will have a very clear expectation and some may have changed their expectations over time. Other residents may be unsure or unaware of the opportunities available to them for community living with services and supports.

Examples

1. Mr. B. is an 82-year-old male with COPD. He was referred to the nursing home by his physician for end-of-life palliative care. He responded, "I'm afraid I can't" to item Q0500B. The assessor should ask follow-up questions to understand why Mr. B. is afraid and explain that obtaining more information may help overcome some of his fears. He should also be informed that someone from a local agency is available to provide him with more information about receiving services and supports in the community. At the close of this discussion, Mr. B. says that he would like more information on community supports.

   Coding: Q0500A would be **coded 0, no**.
   Q0500B would be **coded 1, yes**.

   Rationale: Q0500A would be coded as no because Mr. B. had not been asked previously about returning to the community. Coding Q0500B as yes should trigger a visit by the nursing home social worker to assess fears and concerns, with any additional follow-up care planning that is needed and to initiate contact with the designated local agency within 10 business days.

2. Ms. C. is a 45-year-old woman with cerebral palsy and a learning disability who has been living in the Hope Nursing Home for the past 20 years. She once lived in a group home but became ill and required hospitalization for pneumonia. After recovering in the hospital, Ms. C. was sent to the nursing home because she now required regular chest physical therapy and was told that she could no longer live in her previous group home because her needs were more intensive. No one had asked her about returning to the community until now. When administered the MDS assessment, she responded yes to item Q0500B.

   Coding: Q0500A would be **coded 0, no**.
   Q0500B would be **coded 1, yes**.

   Rationale: Ms. C.'s discussions with staff in the nursing home should result in a visit by the nursing home social worker or discharge planner. Her response should be noted in her care plan, and care planning should be initiated to assess her preferences and needs for possible transition to the community. Nursing home staff should contact the designated local agency within 10 business days for them to initiate discussions with Ms. C. about returning to community living.

Q0500: Return to Community (cont.)

3. Mr. D. is a 65-year-old man with a severe heart condition and interstitial pulmonary fibrosis. At the last quarterly assessment, Mr. D. had been asked about returning to the community and his response was no. He also responds no to item Q0500B. The assessor should ask why he responded no. Depending on the response, follow-up questions could include, "Is it that you think you cannot get the care you need in the community? Do you have a home to return to? Do you have any family or friends to assist you in any way?" Mr. D. responds no to the follow-up questions and does not want to offer any more information or talk about it.

    Coding: Q0500A would be **coded 1, yes—previous response was no**.
    Q0500B would be **coded 0, no**.

    Rationale: Mr. D. had been previously asked if he wanted to talk to someone about returning to the community. He had responded no. During this assessment, he was asked again about returning to the community and he again responded no.

Q0600: Referral

Q0600. Referral	
Enter Code ☐	**Has a referral been made to the local contact agency?** 0. **No** - determination has been made by the resident and the care planning team that contact is not required 1. **No** - referral not made 2. **Yes**

Item Rationale

Health-related Quality of Life

*   Returning home or to a noninstitutional setting can be very important to the resident's health and quality of life.

Planning for Care

*   Some nursing home residents may be able to return to the community if they are provided appropriate assistance and referral to appropriate community resources to facilitate care in a noninstitutional setting.

Steps for Assessment: Interview Instructions

1. If Item Q0400A is coded 1, yes, then complete this item.
2. If Item Q0400B is coded 1, yes, then complete this item,
3. If Item Q0500A is coded 2, yes-previous response was yes, then complete this item.

> **DEFINITIONS**
>
> **DESIGNATED LOCAL CONTACT AGENCY**
> Each state has community contact agencies that can provide individuals with information about community living options and available supports and services. These local contact agencies may be a single entry point agency, an Aging/Disabled Resource Center (ADRC), an Area Agency on Aging (AAA), a Center for Independent Living (CIL), or other state designated entities. See Appendix C for listings.

Q0600: Referral (cont.)

Coding Instructions

- **Code 0, no:** determination has been made by the resident (or family or significant other, or guardian or legally authorized representative) and the care planning team that the designated local contact agency does not need to be contacted.
- **Code 1, no:** determination has been made by the resident (or family or significant other, or guardian or legally authorized representative) and the care planning team that the designated local contact agency needs to be contacted but the referral has not made.
- **Code 2, yes:** if referral was made to the local contact agency. For example, the resident responded yes to Q0500A. The facility care planning team was notified and initiated contact with the local contact agency.

SECTION V: CARE AREA ASSESSMENT (CAA) SUMMARY

Intent: The MDS does not constitute a comprehensive assessment. Rather, it is a preliminary assessment to identify potential resident problems, strengths, and preferences. Care Areas are triggered by MDS item responses that indicate the need for additional assessment based on problem identification, known as "triggered care areas," which form a critical link between the MDS and decisions about care planning.

There are 20 CAAs in Version 3.0 of the RAI, which includes the addition of "Pain" and "Return to the Community Referral." These CAAs cover the majority of care areas known to be problematic for nursing home residents. The Care Area Assessment (CAA) process provides guidance on how to focus on key issues identified during a comprehensive MDS assessment and directs facility staff and health professionals to evaluate triggered care areas.

The interdisciplinary team (IDT) then identifies relevant assessment information regarding the resident's status. After obtaining input from the resident, the resident's family, significant other, guardian, or legally authorized representative, the IDT decides whether or not to develop a care plan for triggered care areas. Chapter 4 of this manual provides detailed instructions on the CAA process and development of an individualized care plan.

Whereas the MDS identifies actual or potential problem areas, the CAA process provides for further assessment of the triggered areas by guiding staff to look for causal or confounding factors, some of which may be reversible. It is important that the CAA documentation include the causal or unique risk factors for decline or lack of improvement. The plan of care then addresses these factors, with the goal of promoting the resident's highest practicable level of functioning: (1) improvement where possible, or (2) maintenance and prevention of avoidable declines.

V0100: Items From the Most Recent Prior OBRA or PPS Assessment

V0100. Items From the Most Recent Prior OBRA or Scheduled PPS Assessment	
Complete only if A0310E = 0 and if the following is true for the **prior assessment**: A0310A = 01- 06 or A0310B = 01- 06	
Enter Code	**A. Prior Assessment Federal OBRA Reason for Assessment** (A0310A value from prior assessment)
	01. **Admission** assessment (required by day 14)
	02. **Quarterly** review assessment
	03. **Annual** assessment
	04. **Significant change in status** assessment
	05. **Significant correction** to **prior comprehensive** assessment
	06. **Significant correction** to **prior quarterly** assessment
	99. **Not OBRA required** assessment
Enter Code	**B. Prior Assessment PPS Reason for Assessment** (A0310B value from prior assessment)
	01. **5-day** scheduled assessment
	02. **14-day** scheduled assessment
	03. **30-day** scheduled assessment
	04. **60-day** scheduled assessment
	05. **90-day** scheduled assessment
	06. **Readmission/return** assessment
	07. **Unscheduled assessment used for PPS** (OMRA, significant or clinical change, or significant correction assessment)
	99. **Not PPS** assessment
	C. Prior Assessment Reference Date (A2300 value from prior assessment)
	☐☐ - ☐☐ - ☐☐☐☐ Month Day Year
Enter Score	**D. Prior Assessment Brief Interview for Mental Status (BIMS) Summary Score** (C0500 value from prior assessment)
Enter Score	**E. Prior Assessment Resident Mood Interview (PHQ-9©) Total Severity Score** (D0300 value from prior assessment)
Enter Score	**F. Prior Assessment Staff Assessment of Resident Mood (PHQ-9-OV) Total Severity Score** (D0600 value from prior assessment)

Item Rationale

The items in V0100 are used to determine whether to trigger several of the CAAs that compare a resident's current status with their prior status. The values of these items are derived from a prior OBRA or scheduled PPS assessment that was performed since the most recent admission of any kind (i.e., since the most recent entry or reentry), if one is available. Items V0100A, B, C, D, E and F are skipped on the first assessment (OBRA or PPS) following the most recent admission of any kind (i.e., when A0310E = 1, Yes). Complete these items only if a prior assessment has been completed since the most recent admission of any kind to the facility (i.e., when A0310E = 0, No) and if the prior assessment is an OBRA or a scheduled PPS assessment. If such an assessment is available, the values of V0100A, B, C, D, E, and F should be copied from the corresponding items on that prior assessment.

Coding Instructions for V0100A, Prior Assessment Federal OBRA Reason for Assessment (A0310A Value from Prior Assessment)

- Record in V0100A the value for A0310A (Federal OBRA Reason for Assessment) from the most recent prior OBRA or scheduled PPS assessment, if one is available (see "Item Rationale", above, for details). One of the available values (01 through 06 or 99) must be selected.

357

V0100: Items From the Most Recent Prior OBRA or PPS Assessment (cont.)

Coding Instructions for V0100B, Prior Assessment PPS Reason for Assessment (A0310B Value from Prior Assessment)

- Record in V0100B the value for A0310B (PPS Assessment) from the most recent prior OBRA or scheduled PPS assessment, if one is available (see "Item Rationale", above, for details). One of the available values (01 through 07 or 99) must be selected.

  Note: The values for V0100A and V0100B cannot both be 99, indicating that the prior assessment is neither an OBRA nor a PPS assessment. If the value of V0100A is 99 (not an OBRA assessment), then the value for V0100B must be 01 through 07, indicating a PPS assessment. If the value of V0100B is 99 (not a PPS assessment), then the value for V0100A must be 01 through 06, indicating an OBRA assessment.

Coding Instructions for V0100C, Prior Assessment Reference Date (A2300 Value from Prior Assessment)

- Record in V0100C the value of A2300 (Assessment Reference Date) from the most recent prior OBRA or scheduled PPS assessment, if one is available (see "Item Rationale", above, for details).

Coding Instructions for V0100D, Prior Assessment Brief Interview for Mental Status (BIMS) Summary Score (C0500 Value from Prior Assessment)

- Record in V0100D, the value for C0500 Mental Status (BIMS) Summary Score from the most recent prior OBRA or scheduled PPS assessment, if one is available (see "Item Rationale", above, for details). This item will be compared with the corresponding item on the current assessment to evaluate resident improvement or decline in the Delirium care area.

Coding Instructions for V0100E, Prior Assessment Resident Mood Interview (PHQ-9©) Total Severity Score (D0300 Value from Prior Assessment)

- Record in V0100E the value of D0300 (Resident Mood Interview [PHQ-9©] Total Severity Score) from the most recent prior OBRA or scheduled PPS assessment, if one is available (see "Item Rationale," above, for details). This item will be compared with the corresponding item on the current assessment to evaluate resident decline in the Mood State care area.

Coding Instructions for V0100F, Prior Assessment Staff Assessment of Resident Mood (PHQ-9-OV©) Total Severity Score (D0600 Value from Prior Assessment)

- Record in V0100F the value for item D0600 (Staff Assessment of Resident Mood Interview [PHQ-9-OV©] Total Severity Score) from the most recent prior OBRA or scheduled PPS assessment, if one is available (see "Item Rationale", above, for details). This item will be compared with the corresponding item on the current assessment to evaluate resident decline in the Mood State care area.

V0200: CAAs and Care Planning

V0200. CAAs and Care Planning

1. Check column A if Care Area is triggered.
2. For each triggered Care Area, indicate whether a new care plan, care plan revision, or continuation of current care plan is necessary to address the problem(s) identified in your assessment of the care area. The Addressed in Care Plan column must be completed within 7 days of completing the RAI (MDS and CAA(s)). Check column B if the triggered care area is addressed in the care plan.
3. Indicate in the Location and Date of CAA Information column where information related to the CAA can be found. CAA documentation should include information on the complicating factors, risks, and any referrals for this resident for this care area.

A. CAA Results

Care Area	A. Care Area Triggered	B. Addressed in Care Plan	Location and Date of CAA Information
	↓ Check all that apply ↓		
01. Delirium	☐	☐	
02. Cognitive Loss/Dementia	☐	☐	
03. Visual Function	☐	☐	
04. Communication	☐	☐	
05. ADL Functional/Rehabilitation Potential	☐	☐	
06. Urinary Incontinence and Indwelling Catheter	☐	☐	
07. Psychosocial Well-Being	☐	☐	
08. Mood State	☐	☐	
09. Behavioral Symptoms	☐	☐	
10. Activities	☐	☐	
11. Falls	☐	☐	
12. Nutritional Status	☐	☐	
13. Feeding Tube	☐	☐	
14. Dehydration/Fluid Maintenance	☐	☐	
15. Dental Care	☐	☐	
16. Pressure Ulcer	☐	☐	
17. Psychotropic Drug Use	☐	☐	
18. Physical Restraints	☐	☐	
19. Pain	☐	☐	
20. Return to Community Referral	☐	☐	

B. Signature of RN Coordinator for CAA Process and Date Signed

1. Signature

2. Date ☐☐ – ☐☐ – ☐☐☐☐
   Month   Day   Year

C. Signature of Person Completing Care Plan and Date Signed

1. Signature

2. Date ☐☐ – ☐☐ – ☐☐☐☐
   Month   Day   Year

V0200: CAAs and Care Planning (cont.)

Item Rationale

- Items V0200A 01 through 20 document which triggered care areas require further assessment, decision as to whether or not a triggered care area is addressed in the resident care plan, and the location and date of CAA documentation. The CAA Summary documents the interdisciplinary team's and the resident, resident's family or representative's final decision(s) on which triggered care areas will be addressed in the care plan.

Coding Instructions for V0200A, CAAs

- Facility staff are to use the RAI triggering mechanism to determine which care areas require review and additional assessment. The triggered care areas are checked in Column A "Care Area Triggered" in the CAAs section. For each triggered care area, use the CAA process and current standard of practice, evidence-based or expert-endorsed clinical guidelines and resources to conduct further assessment of the care area. Document relevant assessment information regarding the resident's status. Chapter 4 of this manual provides detailed instructions on the CAA process, care planning, and documentation.

- For each triggered care area, Column B "Care Planning Decision -Addressed in Care Plan" is checked to indicate that a new care plan, care plan revision, or continuation of the current care plan is necessary to address the issue(s) identified in the assessment of that care area. The "Care Planning Decision - Addressed in Care Plan" column must be completed within 7 days of completing the RAI, as indicated by the date in V0200C2, which is the date that the care planning decision(s) were completed and that the resident's care plan was completed. For each triggered care area, indicate the date and location of the CAA documentation in the "Location and Date of CAA Documentation" column. Chapter 4 of this manual provides detailed instructions on the CAA process, care planning, and documentation.

Coding Instructions for V0200B, Signature of RN Coordinator for CAA Process and Date Signed

V0200B1, Signature

- Signature of the RN coordinating the CAA process.

V0200B2, Date

- Date that the RN coordinating the CAA process certifies that the CAAs have been completed. The CAA review must be completed no later than the 14th day of admission (admission date + 13 calendar days) for an Admission assessment and within 14 days of the Assessment Reference Date (A2300) for an Annual assessment, Significant Change in Status assessment, or a Significant Correction to Prior Full assessment. This date is considered the date of completion for the RAI.

V0200: CAAs and Care Planning (cont.)

V0200C, Signature of Person Completing Care Plan Decision and Date Signed

V0200C1, Signature

- Signature of the staff person facilitating the care planning decision-making. Person signing does not have to be an RN.

V0200C2, Date

- The date on which a staff member completes the care planning decision column (V0200A, Column B), which is done after the care plan is completed. The care plan must be completed within 7 days of the completion of the comprehensive assessment (MDS and CAAs), as indicated by the date in V0200B2.
- Following completion of the MDS,CAAs (V0200A, Columns A and B) and the care plan, the MDS 3.0 comprehensive assessment record must be transmitted to the QIES Assessment Submission and Processing (ASAP) system within 14 days of the V0200C2 date.

Clarifications:

- The signatures at V0200B1 and V0200C1 can be provided by the same person, if the person actually completed both functions. However, it is not a requirement that the same person complete both functions.
- If a resident is discharged prior to the completion of Section V, a comprehensive assessment may be in progress when a resident is discharged. Although the resident has been discharged, the facility may complete and submit the assessment. **The following guidelines apply to completing a <u>comprehensive assessment*</u> when the resident has been discharged**:
  1. Complete all required MDS items from Section A through Section Z and indicate the date of completion in Z0500B. Encode and verify these items.
  2. Complete the care area triggering process by checking all triggered care areas in V0200A, Column A.
  3. Sign and enter the date the CAAs were completed at V0200B1 and V0200B2.
  4. Dash fill all of the "Care Planning Decision-Addressed in Care Plan" items in V0200A, Column B, which indicates that the decisions are unknown.
  5. Sign and enter the date that care planning decisions were completed at V0200C1 and V0200C2. Use the same date used in V0200B2.
  6. Submit the record.

  *Please see Chapter 2 for additional detailed instructions regarding options for when residents are discharged prior to completion of the RAI.

SECTION X: CORRECTION REQUEST

Intent: The purpose of Section X is to indicate whether an MDS record is a new record to be added to the QIES ASAP system or a request to modify or inactivate a record already present in the database. This information is provided in the first item in the section (X0100). If this is a new record, then all items in this section except the first item are skipped. If this is a request to modify or inactivate an existing record, then the other items in this section must be completed.

A modification request is used to correct a QIES ASAP record containing incorrect MDS item values due to:

- transcription errors,
- data entry errors,
- software product errors,
- item coding errors, and/or
- other error requiring modification

The modification request record contains correct values for all MDS items (not just the values previously in error), including the Section X items. The corrected record will replace the prior erroneous record in the QIES ASAP database.

In some cases, an incorrect MDS record requires a completely new assessment of the resident in addition to a modification request for that incorrect record. Please refer to Chapter 5 of this manual, Submission and Correction of the MDS Assessments, to determine if a new assessment is required in addition to a modification request.

An inactivation request is used to move an existing record in the QIES ASAP database from the active file to an archive (history file) so that it will not be used for reporting purposes. Inactivations should be used when the event did not occur (e.g., a discharge was submitted when the resident was not discharged). The inactivation request only includes the Section X items. All other MDS sections are skipped.

The modification and inactivation processes are automated and neither completely removes the prior erroneous record from the QIES ASAP database. The erroneous record is archived in a history file. In certain cases, it is necessary to delete a record and not retain any information about the record in the QIES ASAP database. This requires a request from the facility to the facility's state agency to manually delete all traces of a record from the QIES ASAP database. The policy and procedures for a Manual Correction/Deletion Request are provided in Chapter 5 of this manual.

A Manual Deletion Request is required **only** in the following three cases:

1. **Item A0410 Submission Requirement is incorrect.** Submission of MDS assessment records to the QIES ASAP system constitutes a release of private information and must conform to privacy laws. Only records required by the State and/or the Federal governments may be stored in the QIES ASAP database. If a record has been submitted with the incorrect Submission Requirement value in Item A0410, then that record must be manually deleted and, in some cases, a new record with a corrected A0410 value submitted. Item A0410 cannot be corrected by modification or inactivation. See Chapter 5 of this manual for details.

2. **Inappropriate submission of a test record as a production record.** Removal of a test record from the QIES ASAP database requires manual deletion. Otherwise information for a "bogus" resident will be retained in the database and this resident will appear on some reports to the facility.
3. **Record was submitted for the wrong facility.** If a QIES ASAP record was submitted for an incorrect facility, the record must be removed manually and then a new record for the correct facility must be submitted to the **QIES ASAP database. Manual deletion of the record for the wrong facility** is necessary to ensure that the resident is not associated with that facility and does not appear on reports to that facility.

X0100: Type of Record

X0100. Type of Record	
Enter Code ☐	1. **Add new record** → Skip to Z0100, Medicare Part A Billing 2. **Modify existing record** → Continue to X0150, Type of Provider 3. **Inactivate existing record** → Continue to X0150, Type of Provider

Coding Instructions for X0100, **Type of Record**

- **Code 1, Add new record:** if this is a **new record** that has not been previously submitted and accepted in the QIES ASAP system. If this item is **coded as 1**, then the remainder of Section X is skipped and the assessor should proceed to Section Z, Assessment Administration.

  If there is an existing database record for the same resident, the same facility, the same reasons for assessment/tracking, and the same date (assessment reference date, entry date, or discharge date), then the current record is a duplicate and not a new record. In this case, the submitted record will be rejected and not accepted in the QIES ASAP system and a "fatal" error will be reported to the facility on the Final Validation Report.

- **Code 2, Modify existing record:** if this is a **request to modify** the MDS items for a record that already has been submitted and accepted in the QIES ASAP system.

  If this item is **coded as 2**, then the remaining items in Section X and the items in all other MDS sections must be completed.

  When a modification request is submitted, the QIES ASAP System will take the following steps:

  1. The system will attempt to locate the existing record in the QIES ASAP database for this facility with the resident, reasons for assessment/tracking, and date (assessment reference date, entry date, or discharge date) indicated in subsequent Section X items.
  2. If the existing record is not found, the submitted modification record will be rejected and not accepted in the QIES ASAP system. A "fatal" error will be reported to the facility on the Final Validation Report.
  3. If the existing record is found, then the items in all sections of the submitted modification record will be edited. If there are any fatal errors, the modification record will be rejected and not accepted in the QIES ASAP system. The "fatal" error(s) will be reported to the facility on the Final Validation Report.

X0100: Type of Record (cont.)

4. If the modification record passes all the edits, it will replace the prior record being modified in the QIES ASAP database. The prior record will be moved to a history file in the QIES ASAP database.

- **Code 3, Inactivate existing record:** if this is a **request to inactivate** a record that already has been submitted and accepted in the QIES ASAP system.

  If this item is **coded as 3**, then the remaining items in Section X must be completed and all other MDS sections are skipped.

  When an inactivation request is submitted, the QIES ASAP system will take the following steps:

  1. The system will attempt to locate the existing record in the QIES ASAP system for this facility with the resident, reasons for assessment/tracking, and date (assessment reference date, entry date, or discharge date) indicated in subsequent Section X items.
  2. If the existing record is not found in the QIES ASAP database, the submitted inactivation request will be rejected and a "fatal" error will be reported to the facility on the Final Validation Report.
  3. All items in Section X of the submitted record will be edited. If there are any fatal errors, the current inactivation request will be rejected and no record will be inactivated in the QIES ASAP system.
  4. If the existing record is found, it will be removed from the active records in the QIES ASAP database and moved to a history file.

Identification of Record to be Modified/Inactivated

The Section X items from X0200 through X0700 identify the existing QIES ASAP database assessment or tracking record that is in error. In this section, reproduce the information **EXACTLY** as it appeared on the existing erroneous record, even if the information is incorrect. This information is necessary to locate the existing record in the database.

Example: A MDS assessment for Joan L. Smith is submitted and accepted by the QIES ASAP system. A data entry error is then identified on the previously submitted and accepted record. When the encoder "data entered" the prior assessment for Joan L Smith, he typed "John" by mistake. To correct this data entry error, the facility will modify the erroneous record and complete the items in Section X including items under Identification of Record to be Modified/Inactivated. When completing X0200A, the Resident First Name, "John" will be entered in this item. This will permit the MDS system to locate the previously submitted assessment that is being corrected. If the correct name "Joan" were entered, the QIES ASAP system would not locate the prior assessment.

The correction to the name from "John" to "Joan" will be made by recording "Joan" in the "normal" A0500A, Resident First Name in the modification record. The modification record must include all items appropriate for that assessment, not just the corrected name. This modification record will then be submitted and accepted to the QIES ASAP system which causes the desired correction to be made.

X0150: Type of Provider

X0150. Type of Provider	
Enter Code ☐	**Type of provider** 1. **Nursing home (SNF/NF)** 2. **Swing Bed**

Coding Instructions for X0150, **Type of Provider**

This item contains the type of provider identified from the prior erroneous record to be modified/ inactivated.

- **Code 1, Nursing home (SNF/NF):** if the facility is a Nursing home (SNF/NF).
- **Code 2, Swing Bed:** if the facility is a Swing Bed facility.

X0200: Name of Resident

These items contain the resident's name from the prior erroneous record to be modified/ inactivated.

X0200. **Name of Resident** on existing record to be modified/inactivated	
	A. **First name:** ☐☐☐☐☐☐☐☐☐☐☐
	C. **Last name:** ☐☐☐☐☐☐☐☐☐☐☐☐☐☐☐☐☐☐

Coding Instructions for X0200A, **First Name**

- Enter the first name of the resident exactly as submitted for item A0500A "Legal Name of Resident—First Name" on the prior erroneous record to be modified/inactivated. Start entry with the leftmost box. If the first name was left blank on the prior record, leave X0200A blank.
- Note that the first name in X0200A does not have to match the current value of A0500A on a modification request. The entries may be different if the modification is correcting the first name.

Coding Instructions for X0200C, **Last Name**

- Enter the last name of the resident exactly as submitted for item A0500C "Legal Name of Resident— Last Name" on the prior erroneous record to be modified/inactivated. Start entry with the leftmost box. The last name in X0200C cannot be blank.
- Note that the last name in X0200C does not have to match the current value of A0500C on a modification request. The entries may be different if the modification is correcting the last name.

X0300: Gender

X0300. Gender on existing record to be modified/inactivated	
Enter Code ☐	1. **Male** 2. **Female**

Coding Instructions for X0300, **Gender**

- Enter the gender code 1 "Male," 2 "Female," or – (dash value indicating unable to determine) exactly as submitted for item A0800 "Gender" on the prior erroneous record to be modified/inactivated.

- Note that the gender in X0300 does not have to match the current value of A0800 on a modification request. The entries may be different if the modification is correcting the gender.

X0400: Birth Date

X0400. **Birth Date** on existing record to be modified/inactivated
☐☐ – ☐☐ – ☐☐☐☐ Month   Day   Year

Coding Instructions for X0400, **Birth Date**

- Fill in the boxes with the birth date exactly as submitted for item A0900 "Birth Date" on the prior erroneous record to be modified/inactivated. If the month or day contains only a single digit, fill in the first box with a 0 For example, January 2, 1918, should be entered as:

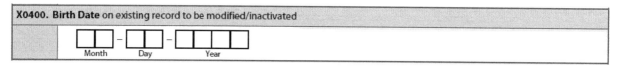

0	1		0	2		1	9	1	8

If the birth date in MDS item A0900 on the prior record was a partial date, with day of the month unknown and the day of the month boxes were left blank, then the day of the month boxes must be blank in X0400. If the birth date in MDS item A0900 on the prior record was a partial date with both month and day of the month unknown and the month and day of the month boxes were left blank, then the month and day of the month boxes must be blank in X0400.

- Note that the birth date in X0400 does not have to match the current value of A0900 on a modification request. The entries may be different if the modification is correcting the birth date.

X0500: Social Security Number

X0500. **Social Security Number** on existing record to be modified/inactivated
☐☐☐ - ☐☐ - ☐☐☐☐

Coding Instructions for X0500, **Social Security Number**

- Fill in the boxes with the Social Security number exactly as submitted for item A0600 "Social Security and Medicare numbers" on the prior erroneous record to be modified/inactivated. If the Social Security number was unknown or unavailable and left blank on the prior record, leave X0500 blank.

- Note that the Social Security number in X0500 does not have to match the current value of A0600 on a modification request. The entries may be different if the modification is correcting the Social Security number.

X0600: Type of Assessment/Tracking

These items contain the reasons for assessment/tracking from the prior erroneous record to be modified/inactivated.

X0600. **Type of Assessment** on existing record to be modified/inactivated	
Enter Code ☐☐	**A. Federal OBRA Reason for Assessment** 01. **Admission** assessment (required by day 14) 02. **Quarterly** review assessment 03. **Annual** assessment 04. **Significant change in status** assessment 05. **Significant correction** to **prior comprehensive** assessment 06. **Significant correction** to **prior quarterly** assessment 99. **Not OBRA required** assessment
Enter Code ☐☐	**B. PPS Assessment** **PPS Scheduled Assessments for a Medicare Part A Stay** 01. **5-day** scheduled assessment 02. **14-day** scheduled assessment 03. **30-day** scheduled assessment 04. **60-day** scheduled assessment 05. **90-day** scheduled assessment 06. **Readmission/return** assessment **PPS Unscheduled Assessments for a Medicare Part A Stay** 07. **Unscheduled assessment** used for PPS (OMRA, significant or clinical change, or significant correction assessment) **Not PPS Assessment** 99. **Not PPS** assessment
Enter Code ☐	**C. PPS Other Medicare Required Assessment - OMRA** 0. **No** 1. **Start of therapy** assessment 2. **End of therapy** assessment 3. **Both Start and End of therapy** assessment
Enter Code ☐	**D. Is this a Swing Bed clinical change assessment?** Complete only if X0150 = 2 0. **No** 1. **Yes**
Enter Code ☐☐	**F. Entry/discharge reporting** 01. **Entry** record 10. **Discharge** assessment-**return not anticipated** 11. **Discharge** assessment-**return anticipated** 12. **Death in facility** record 99. **Not entry/discharge** record

X0600: Type of Assessment/Tracking (cont.)

Coding Instructions for X0600A, Federal OBRA Reason for Assessment

- Fill in the boxes with the Federal OBRA reason for assessment/tracking code exactly as submitted for item A0310A "Federal OBRA Reason for Assessment" on the prior erroneous record to be modified/inactivated.

- Note that the Federal OBRA reason for assessment/tracking code in X0600A does not have to match the current value of A0310A on a modification request. The entries may be different if the modification is correcting the Federal OBRA reason for assessment/tracking code.

Coding Instructions for X0600B, PPS Assessment

- Fill in the boxes with the PPS assessment type code exactly as submitted for item A0310B "PPS Assessment" on the prior erroneous record to be modified/inactivated.

- Note that the PPS assessment code in X0600B does not have to match the current value of A0310B on a modification request. The entries may be different if the modification is correcting the PPS assessment code.

Coding Instructions for X0600C, PPS Other Medicare Required Assessment—OMRA

- Fill in the boxes with the PPS OMRA code exactly as submitted for item A0310C "PPS—OMRA" on the prior erroneous record to be modified/inactivated.

- Note that the PPS OMRA code in X0600C does not have to match the current value of A0310C on a modification request. The entries may be different if the modification is correcting the PPS OMRA code.

Coding Instructions for X0600D, Is this a Swing Bed clinical change assessment? (Complete only if X0150=2)

- Enter the code exactly as submitted for item A0310D "Is this a Swing Bed clinical change assessment?" on the prior erroneous record to be modified/inactivated.

- **Code 0, no:** if the assessment submitted was not coded as a swing bed clinical change assessment.

- **Code 1, yes:** if the assessment submitted was coded as a swing bed clinical change assessment.

- Note that the code in X0600D does not have to match the current value of A0310D on a modification request. The entries may be different if the modification is correcting the Swing Bed clinical change assessment code.

X0600: Type of Assessment/Tracking (cont.)

Coding Instructions for X0600F, Entry/discharge reporting

- Enter the number corresponding to the entry/discharge code exactly as submitted for item A0310F "Entry/discharge reporting" on the prior erroneous record to be modified/inactivated.

  01. Entry record

  10. Discharge assessment-return not anticipated

  11. Discharge assessment-return anticipated

  12. Death in facility record

  99. Not entry/discharge

- Note that the Entry/discharge code in X0600F does not have to match the current value of A0310F on a modification request. The entries may be different if the modification is correcting the Entry/discharge reason for completing the assessment.

X0700: Date on Existing Record to Be Modified/Inactivated – Complete one only

The item that is completed in this section is the event date for the prior erroneous record to be modified/inactivated. The event date is the assessment reference date for an assessment record, the discharge date for a discharge record, or the entry date for an entry record. In the QIES ASAP system, this date is often referred to as the "target date." Enter only one (1) date in X0700

X0700. Date on existing record to be modified/inactivated - Complete one only

A. Assessment Reference Date - Complete only if X0600F = 99
☐☐ - ☐☐ - ☐☐☐☐
Month   Day   Year

B. Discharge Date - Complete only if X0600F = 10, 11, or 12
☐☐ - ☐☐ - ☐☐☐☐
Month   Day   Year

C. Entry Date - Complete only if X0600F = 01
☐☐ - ☐☐ - ☐☐☐☐
Month   Day   Year

Coding Instructions for X0700A, Assessment Reference Date— Complete Only if X0600F = 99

- If the prior erroneous record to be modified/inactivated is an OBRA assessment or a PPS assessment, where X0600F = 99, enter the assessment reference date here exactly as submitted in item A2300 "Assessment Reference Date" on the prior record.

- Note that the assessment reference date in X0700A does not have to match the current value of A2300 on a modification request. The entries may be different if the modification is correcting the assessment reference date. The entries may also be different if the type of assessment/tracking record is being changed.

X0700: Date on Existing Record to Be Modified/Inactivated (cont.)

For example, if the incorrect QIES ASAP database record indicates an admission assessment but the record should have been an entry record, then the assessment reference date for the prior record is entered in Item X0700A (Assessment Reference Date). However, the new assessment reference date in A2300 would be blank. The assessment reference date is not active on an entry record. Instead, the entry date would be entered in item A1600.

Coding Instructions for X0700B, Discharge Date—Complete Only If X0600F = 10, 11, or 12

- If the prior erroneous record to be modified/inactivated is a discharge record (indicated by X0600F = 10, 11, or 12), enter the discharge date here exactly as submitted for item A2000 "Discharge Date" on the prior record. If the prior erroneous record was a discharge combined with an OBRA or PPS assessment, then that prior record will contain both a completed assessment reference date (A2300) and discharge date (A2000) and these two dates will be identical. If such a record is being modified or inactivated, enter the prior discharge date in X0700B and leave the prior assessment reference date in X0700A blank.
- Note that the discharge date in X0700B does not have to match the current value of A2000 on a modification request. The entries may be different if the modification is correcting the discharge date. The entries may also be different if the type of assessment/tracking record is being changed.

Coding Instructions for X0700C, Entry Date—Complete Only If X0600F = 01

- If the prior erroneous record to be modified/inactivated is an entry record (indicated by X0600F = 01), enter the entry date here exactly as submitted for item A1600 "Entry Date [date of admission/reentry into the facility]" on the prior record.
- Note that the entry date in X0700C does not have to match the current value of A1600 on a modification request. The entries may be different if the modification is correcting the entry date. The entries may also be different if the type of assessment/tracking record is being changed.

X0800: Correction Attestation Section

The items in this section indicate the number of times the QIES ASAP database record has been corrected, the reason for the current modification/inactivation request, the person attesting to the modification/inactivation request, and the date of the attestation.

This item may be populated automatically by the nursing home's date entry software, however, if it is not, the nursing home should enter this information.

Correction Attestation Section - Complete this section to explain and attest to the modification/inactivation request
X0800. Correction Number
Enter Number [ ][ ] Enter the number of correction requests to modify/inactivate the existing record, including the present one

X0800: Correction Attestation Section (cont.)

Coding Instructions for X0800, **Correction Number**

- Enter the total number of correction requests to modify/inactivate the QIES ASAP record that is in error. Include the present modification/inactivation request in this number.
- For the first correction request (modification/inactivation) for an MDS record, code a value of 01 (zero-one); for the second correction request, code a value of 02 (zero-two); etc. With each succeeding request, X0800 is incremented by one. For values between one and nine, a leading zero should be used in the first box. For example, enter "01" into the two boxes for X0800.
- This item identifies the total number of correction requests following the original assessment or tracking record, including the present request. Note that Item X0800 is used to track successive correction requests in the QIES ASAP database.

X0900: Reasons for Modification

The items in this section indicate the possible reasons for the modification request of the record in the QIES ASAP database. Check all that apply. These items should only be completed when X0100 = 2, indicating a modification request. If X0100 = 3, indicating an inactivation request, these items should be skipped.

X0900. Reasons for Modification - Complete only if Type of Record is to modify a record in error (X0100 = 2)
↓ Check all that apply
☐ A. Transcription error
☐ B. Data entry error
☐ C. Software product error
☐ D. Item coding error
☐ Z. Other error requiring modification   If "Other" checked, please specify:

Coding Instructions for X0900A, **Transcription Error**

- Check the box if any errors in the prior QIES ASAP record were caused by data transcription errors.
- A transcription error includes any error made recording MDS assessment or tracking form information from other sources. An example is transposing the digits for the resident's weight (e.g., recording "191" rather than the correct weight of "119" that appears in the medical record).

Coding Instructions for X0900B, **Data Entry Error**

- Check the box if any errors in the prior QIES ASAP record were caused by data entry errors.
- A data entry error includes any error made while encoding MDS assessment or tracking form information into the facility's computer system. An example is an error where the response to the individual minutes of physical therapy O0400C1 is incorrectly encoded as "3000" minutes rather than the correct number of "0030" minutes.

X0900: Reasons for Modification (cont.)

Coding Instructions for X0900C, Software Product Error

- Check the box if any errors in the prior QIES ASAP record were caused by software product errors.
- A software product error includes any error created by the encoding software, such as storing an item in the wrong format (e.g., storing weight as "020" instead of "200").

Coding Instructions for X0900D, Item Coding Error

- Check the box if any errors in the prior QIES ASAP record were caused by item coding errors.
- An item coding error includes any error made coding an MDS item, such as choosing an incorrect code for the Activities of Daily Living (ADL) bed mobility self-performance item G0110A1 (e.g., choosing a code of "4" for a resident who requires limited assistance and should be coded as "2"). Item coding errors may result when an assessor makes an incorrect judgment or misunderstands the RAI coding instructions.

Coding Instructions for X0900Z, Other Error Requiring Modification

- Check the box if any errors in the prior QIES ASAP record were caused by other types of errors not included in Items X0900A through X0900D.
- Such an error includes any other type of error that causes a QIES ASAP record to require modification under the Correction Policy. An example would be when a record is prematurely submitted prior to final completion of editing and review. Facility staff should describe the "other error" in the space provided with the item.

X1050: Reasons for Inactivation

The items in this section indicate the possible reasons for the inactivation request. Check all that apply. These items should only be completed when X0100 = 3, indicating an inactivation request. If X0100 = 2, indicating a modification request, these items should be skipped.

X1050. Reasons for Inactivation - Complete only if Type of Record is to inactivate a record in error (X0100 = 3)	
↓ Check all that apply	
☐	A. Event did not occur
☐	Z. Other error requiring inactivation If "Other" checked, please specify:

Coding Instructions for X1050A, Event Did Not Occur

- Check the box if the prior QIES ASAP record does not represent an event that actually occurred.
- An example would be a discharge record submitted for a resident, but there was no actual discharge. There was **no event**.

X1050: Reasons for Inactivation (cont.)

Coding Instructions for X1050Z, **Other Reason Requiring Inactivation**

- Check the box if any errors in the prior QIES ASAP record were caused by other types of errors not included in Item X1050A.
- Facility staff should describe the "other error" in the space provided with the item.

X1100: RN Assessment Coordinator Attestation of Completion

The items in this section identify the RN coordinator attesting to the correction request and the date of the attestation.

X1100. RN Assessment Coordinator Attestation of Completion

A. Attesting individual's first name:

B. Attesting individual's last name:

C. Attesting individual's title:

D. Signature

E. Attestation date

Month — Day — Year

Coding Instructions for X1100A, **Attesting Individual's First Name**

- Enter the first name of the facility staff member attesting to the completion and accuracy of the corrected information. Start entry with the leftmost box.

Coding Instructions for X1100B, **Attesting Individual's Last Name**

- Enter the last name of the facility staff member attesting to the completion and accuracy of the corrected information. Start entry with the leftmost box.

Coding Instructions for X1100C, **Attesting Individual's Title**

- Enter the title of the facility staff member attesting to the completion and accuracy of the corrected information on the line provided.

Coding Instructions for X1100D, **Signature**

- The attesting individual must sign the correction request here, certifying the completion and accuracy. The entire correction request should be completed and signed within 14 days of detecting an error in an QIES ASAP record. The correction request, including the signature of the attesting facility staff, must be kept with the modified or inactivated MDS record and retained in the resident's medical record or electronic record.

X1100: RN Assessment Coordinator Attestation of Completion (cont.)

Coding Instructions for X1100E, Attestation Date

- Enter the date the attesting facility staff member attested to the completion and accuracy of the corrected information.
- Do not leave any boxes blank. For a one-digit month or day, place a zero in the first box. For example, January 2, 2011, should be entered as:

0	1

0	2

2	0	1	1

SECTION Z: ASSESSMENT ADMINISTRATION

Intent: The intent of the items in this section is to provide billing information and signatures of persons completing the assessment.

Z0100: Medicare Part A Billing

Z0100. Medicare Part A Billing	
	A. Medicare Part A HIPPS code (RUG group followed by assessment type indicator):
	☐☐☐☐☐☐☐
	B. RUG version code:
	☐☐☐☐☐☐☐☐☐☐
Enter Code ☐	**C. Is this a Medicare Short Stay assessment?** 0. No 1. Yes

Item Rationale

- Used to capture the Resource Utilization Group (RUG) followed by Health Insurance Prospective Payment System (HIPPS) modifier based on type of assessment.

Coding Instructions for Z0100A, **Medicare Part A HIPPS Code**

> **DEFINITIONS**
>
> **MEDICARE-COVERED STAY** Skilled Nursing Facility stays billable to Medicare Part A. Does not include stays billable to Medicare Advantage HMO plans.

- Typically the software data entry product will calculate this value.
- The HIPPS code is a Skilled Nursing Facility (SNF) Part A billing code and is composed of a five-position code representing the RUG group code, plus a two-position assessment type indicator. For information on HIPPS, access: http://www.cms.gov/ProspMedicareFeeSvcPmtGen/02_HIPPSCodes.asp#TopOfPage.

- If the value for Z0100A is not automatically calculated by the software data entry product, enter the HIPPS code in the spaces provided (see Chapter 6 of this manual, Medicare Skilled Nursing Home Prospective Payment System, for a step-by-step worksheet for manually determining the RUG code and a table that defines the assessment type indicator).

> **DEFINITIONS**
>
> **HIPPS CODE**
> Health Insurance Prospective Payment System code is comprised of the RUG category calculated by the assessment followed by an indicator of the type of assessment that was completed.

- Note that the RUG included in this HIPPS code takes into account all MDS items used in the RUG logic and is the "normal" group since the classification considers the rehabilitation therapy received. This classification uses all reported speech/language pathology and auditory services, occupational therapy, and physical therapy values in Item O0400 (Therapies).
- This HIPPS code is usually used for Medicare SNF Part A billing by the provider.
- Left-justify the 5-character HIPPS code. The extra two spaces are supplied for future use, if necessary.

Z0100: Medicare Part A Billing (cont.)

Coding Instructions for Z0100B, RUG Version Code

- Typically the software data entry product will calculate this value.

- If the value for Z0100B is not automatically calculated by the software data entry product, enter the RUG version code in the spaces provided. This is the version code appropriate to the RUG included in the Medicare Part A HIPPS code in Item Z0100A.

- With MDS 3.0 implementation on October 1, 2010, the initial Medicare RUG-IV Version Code is "1.0066".

Coding Instructions for Z0100C, Is This a Medicare Short Stay Assessment?

- **Code 1, No:** if this is not a Medicare Short Stay Assessment.

- **Code 2, Yes:** if this is a Medicare Short Stay Assessment.

Coding Tip

The CMS standard RUG-IV grouper automatically determines whether or not this is a Medicare Short Stay Assessment. MDS software typically makes this determination automatically. If the value for Z0100C is not automatically calculated by the software data entry product, use the definition found in Chapter 6 to determine the correct response.

> **DEFINITIONS**
>
> **MEDICARE SHORT STAY ASSESSMENT** is a Start of Therapy Other Medicare Required Assessment (OMRA) and is used for a short Medicare Part A stay that was not long enough to allow a complete rehabilitation therapy regimen to be established. This type of assessment allows an alternative Medicare Short Stay assessment RUG rehabilitation therapy classification as described in Chapter 6, Medicare Skilled Nursing Home Prospective Payment System.

Z0150: Medicare Part A Non-Therapy Billing

Z0150. Medicare Part A Non-Therapy Billing
A. Medicare Part A non-therapy HIPPS code (RUG group followed by assessment type indicator):
☐☐☐☐☐
B. RUG version code:
☐☐☐☐☐☐☐☐☐☐

Item Rationale

Used to capture the Resource Utilization Group non-therapy (RUG) followed by Health Insurance Prospective Payment System (HIPPS) modifier based on type of assessment. The non-therapy RUG is the code obtained when all rehabilitation therapy is ignored and will be limited to the Extensive Services, Special Care High, Special Care Low, Clinically Complex, Behavior and Cognitive Performance, and the Physical Function codes.

Z0150: Medicare Part A Non-Therapy Billing (cont.)

Coding Instructions for Z0150A, **Medicare Part A Non-therapy HIPPS Code**

- Typically the software data entry product will calculate this value.
- The HIPPS code is a SNF Part A billing code and is comprised of a five-position code representing the RUG code, plus a two-position assessment type indicator. For information on HIPPS, access http://www.cms.gov/ProspMedicareFeeSvcPmtGen/02_HIPPSCodes.asp#TopOfPage.
- If the value for Z0150A is not automatically calculated by the software data entry product, enter the HIPPS code in the spaces provided (see Chapter 6 of this manual, Medicare Skilled Nursing Home Prospective Payment System, for a step-by-step worksheet for manually determining the RUG-IV group and a table that defines assessment type indicator). Note that the RUG included in this HIPPS code is the "non-therapy" group and classification ignores the rehabilitation therapy received. This classification ignores all reported speech/language pathology and auditory services, occupational therapy, and physical therapy values in Item O0400 (Therapies).
- In some instances, this non-therapy HIPPS code may be required for Medicare SNF Part A billing by the provider.
- Left-justify the 5-character HIPPS code. The extra two spaces are supplied for future use, if necessary.

Coding Instructions for Z0150B, **RUG Version Code**

- Typically the software data entry product will calculate this value.
- If the value for Z0150B is not automatically calculated by the software data entry product, enter the RUG version code in the spaces provided. This is the version code appropriate to the RUG included in the Medicare Part A non-therapy HIPPS code in Item Z0150A.
- With MDS 3.0 implementation on October 1, 2010, the initial Medicare RUG-IV Version Code is "1.0066".

Z0200: State Medicaid Billing (if required by the state)

Z0200. State Medicaid Billing (if required by the state)
A. RUG Case Mix group:
☐☐☐☐☐☐☐☐☐☐
B. RUG version code:
☐☐☐☐☐☐☐☐☐☐

Item Rationale

- Used to capture the payment code in states that employ the MDS for Medicaid case-mix reimbursement.

Z0200: State Medicaid Billing (cont.)

Coding Instructions for Z0200A, RUG Case Mix Group

- If the state has selected a standard RUG model, this item will usually be populated automatically by the software data entry product. Otherwise, enter the case-mix code calculated based on the MDS assessment.

Coding Instructions for Z0200B, RUG Version Code

- If the state has selected a standard RUG model, this item will usually be populated automatically by the software data entry product. Otherwise, enter the case mix version code in the spaces provided. This is the version code appropriate to the code in Item Z0200A.

Z0250: Alternate State Medicaid Billing (if required by state)

Z0250. Alternate State Medicaid Billing (if required by the state)
A. RUG Case Mix group:
[ ][ ][ ][ ][ ][ ][ ][ ][ ]
B. RUG version code:
[ ][ ][ ][ ][ ][ ][ ][ ][ ]

Item Rationale

- Used to capture an alternate payment group in states that employ the MDS for Medicaid case-mix reimbursement. States may want to capture a second payment group for Medicaid purposes to allow evaluation of the fiscal impact of changing to a new payment model or to allow blended payment between two models during a transition period.

Coding Instructions for Z0250A, RUG Case Mix Group

- If the state has selected a standard RUG model, this item will usually be populated automatically by the software data entry product. Otherwise, enter the case-mix code calculated based on the MDS assessment.

Coding Instructions for Z0250B, RUG Version Code

- If the state has selected a standard RUG model, this item will usually be populated automatically by the software data entry product. Otherwise, enter the case mix version code in the spaces provided. This is the version code appropriate to the code in Item Z0250A.

Z0300: Insurance Billing

Z0300. Insurance Billing	
A. RUG Case Mix group:	[ ][ ][ ][ ][ ][ ][ ][ ][ ][ ]
B. RUG version code:	[ ][ ][ ][ ][ ][ ][ ][ ][ ]

Item Rationale

- Allows providers and vendors to capture case-mix codes required by other payers (e.g. private insurance or the Department of Veterans Affairs).

Coding Instructions for Z0300A, **RUG Case Mix Group**

- If the other payer has selected a standard RUG model, this item may be populated automatically by the software data entry product. Otherwise, enter the case-mix code in the space provided. This code is for use by other payment systems such as private insurance or the Department of Veterans Affairs.

Coding Instructions for Z0300B, **RUG Version Code**

- If the other payor has selected a standard RUG model, this item may be populated automatically by the software data entry product. Otherwise, enter an appropriate version code in the spaces provided. This is the version code appropriate to the case-mix code in Item Z0300A.

Z0400: Signatures of Persons Completing the Assessment or Entry/Death Reporting

Z0400. Signature of Persons Completing the Assessment or Entry/Death Reporting			
I certify that the accompanying information accurately reflects resident assessment information for this resident and that I collected or coordinated collection of this information on the dates specified. To the best of my knowledge, this information was collected in accordance with applicable Medicare and Medicaid requirements. I understand that this information is used as a basis for ensuring that residents receive appropriate and quality care, and as a basis for payment from federal funds. I further understand that payment of such federal funds and continued participation in the government-funded health care programs is conditioned on the accuracy and truthfulness of this information, and that I may be personally subject to or may subject my organization to substantial criminal, civil, and/or administrative penalties for submitting false information. I also certify that I am authorized to submit this information by this facility on its behalf.			
Signature	Title	Sections	Date Section Completed
A.			
B.			
C.			
D.			
E.			
F.			
G.			
H.			
I.			
J.			
K.			
L.			

Item Rationale

- To obtain the signature of all persons who completed any part of the MDS. Legally, it is an attestation of accuracy with the primary responsibility for its accuracy with the person selecting the MDS item response. Each person completing a section or portion of a section of the MDS is required to sign the Attestation Statement.

- The importance of accurately completing and submitting the MDS cannot be over-emphasized. The MDS is the basis for the development of:

  — an individualized care plan;

  — the Medicare Prospective Payment System

  — Medicaid reimbursement programs

  — quality monitoring activities, such as the quality indicator/quality measure reports

  — the data-driven survey and certification process

  — the quality measures used for public reporting

  — research and policy development.

Z0400: Signatures of Persons Completing the Assessment (cont.)

Coding Instructions

- All staff who completed any part of the MDS must enter their signatures, titles, sections or portion(s) of section(s) they completed, and the date completed.

- If a staff member cannot sign Z0400 on the same day that he or she completed a section or portion of a section, when the staff member signs, use the date the item originally was completed.

- Read the Attestation Statement carefully. You are certifying that the information you entered on the MDS, to the best of your knowledge, most accurately reflects the resident's status. Penalties may be applied for submitting false information.

Coding Tips and Special Populations

- Two or more staff members can complete items within the same section of the MDS. When filling in the information for Z0400, any staff member who has completed a subset of item within a section should identify which item(s) he/she completed within that section.

- Nursing homes may use electronic signatures for medical record documentation, including the MDS, when permitted to do so by state and local law and when authorized by the nursing home's policy. Nursing homes must have written policies in place that meet any and all state and federal privacy and security requirements to ensure proper security measures to protect the use of an electronic signature by anyone other than the person to whom the electronic signature belongs.

- Although the use of electronic signatures for the MDS does not require that the entire record be maintained electronically, most facilities have the option to maintain a resident's record by computer rather than hard copy.

- Whenever copies of the MDS are printed and dates are automatically encoded, be sure to note that it is a "copy" document and not the original.

Z0500: Signature of RN Assessment Coordinator Verifying Assessment Completion

Z0500. Signature of RN Assessment Coordinator Verifying Assessment Completion	
A. Signature:	B. Date RN Assessment Coordinator signed assessment as complete: ☐☐ - ☐☐ - ☐☐☐☐ Month Day Year

Item Rationale

- Federal regulation requires the RN assessment coordinator to sign and thereby certify that the assessment is complete.

381

Z0500: Signature of RN Assessment Coordinator Verifying Assessment Completion (cont.)

Steps for Assessment

1. Verify that all items on this assessment or tracking record are complete.
2. Verify that Item Z0400 (Signature of Persons Completing the Assessment) contains attestation for all MDS sections.

Coding Instructions

- For Z0500B, use the actual date that the MDS was completed, reviewed, and signed as complete by the RN assessment coordinator. This date will generally be later than the date(s) at Z0400, which documents when portions of the assessment information were completed by assessment team members.

- If for some reason the MDS cannot be signed by the RN assessment coordinator on the date it is completed, the RN assessment coordinator should use the actual date that it is signed.

Coding Tips

- The RN assessment coordinator is not certifying the accuracy of portions of the assessment that were completed by other health professionals.

- Nursing homes may use electronic signatures for medical record documentation, including the MDS, when permitted to do so by state and local law and when authorized by the nursing home's policy. Nursing homes must have written policies in place that meet any and all state and federal privacy and security requirements to ensure proper security measures to protect the use of an electronic signature by anyone other than the person to whom the electronic signature belongs.

- Although the use of electronic signatures for the MDS does not require that the entire record be maintained electronically, most facilities have the option to maintain a resident's record by computer rather than hard copy.

- Whenever copies of the MDS are printed and dates are automatically encoded, be sure to note that it is a "copy" document and not the original.

MINIMUM DATA SET (MDS) - Version 3.0
RESIDENT ASSESSMENT AND CARE SCREENING
ALL ITEM LISTING

Section A	Identification Information

A0100. Facility Provider Numbers

A. National Provider Identifier (NPI):

B. CMS Certification Number (CCN):

C. State Provider Number:

A0200. Type of Provider

Enter Code | **Type of provider**
1. **Nursing home (SNF/NF)**
2. **Swing Bed**

A0310. Type of Assessment

Enter Code | **A. Federal OBRA Reason for Assessment**
01. **Admission** assessment (required by day 14)
02. **Quarterly** review assessment
03. **Annual** assessment
04. **Significant change in status** assessment
05. **Significant correction** to **prior comprehensive** assessment
06. **Significant correction** to **prior quarterly** assessment
99. **Not OBRA required** assessment

Enter Code | **B. PPS Assessment**
PPS Scheduled Assessments for a Medicare Part A Stay
01. **5-day** scheduled assessment
02. **14-day** scheduled assessment
03. **30-day** scheduled assessment
04. **60-day** scheduled assessment
05. **90-day** scheduled assessment
06. **Readmission/return** assessment
PPS Unscheduled Assessments for a Medicare Part A Stay
07. **Unscheduled assessment used for PPS** (OMRA, significant or clinical change, or significant correction assessment)
Not PPS Assessment
99. **Not PPS** assessment

Enter Code | **C. PPS Other Medicare Required Assessment - OMRA**
0. **No**
1. **Start of therapy** assessment
2. **End of therapy** assessment
3. **Both Start and End of therapy** assessment

Enter Code | **D. Is this a Swing Bed clinical change assessment?** Complete only if A0200 = 2
0. **No**
1. **Yes**

Enter Code | **E. Is this assessment the first assessment** (OBRA, PPS, or Discharge) **since the most recent admission?**
0. **No**
1. **Yes**

Enter Code | **F. Entry/discharge reporting**
01. **Entry** record
10. **Discharge** assessment-**return not anticipated**
11. **Discharge** assessment-**return anticipated**
12. **Death in facility** record
99. **Not entry/discharge** record

Section A	Identification Information

A0410. Submission Requirement

<table>
<tr>
<td>Enter Code
☐</td>
<td>1. Neither federal nor state required submission
2. State but not federal required submission (FOR NURSING HOMES ONLY)
3. Federal required submission</td>
</tr>
</table>

A0500. Legal Name of Resident

A. First name:	B. Middle initial:
C. Last name:	D. Suffix:

A0600. Social Security and Medicare Numbers

A. Social Security Number:

___ ___ — ___ ___ — ___ ___ ___ ___

B. Medicare number (or comparable railroad insurance number):

A0700. Medicaid Number - Enter "+" if pending, "N" if not a Medicaid recipient

A0800. Gender

<table>
<tr>
<td>Enter Code
☐</td>
<td>1. Male
2. Female</td>
</tr>
</table>

A0900. Birth Date

___ ___ — ___ ___ — ___ ___ ___ ___

Month   Day   Year

A1000. Race/Ethnicity

↓ Check all that apply

☐	A. American Indian or Alaska Native
☐	B. Asian
☐	C. Black or African American
☐	D. Hispanic or Latino
☐	E. Native Hawaiian or Other Pacific Islander
☐	F. White

A1100. Language

<table>
<tr>
<td>Enter Code
☐</td>
<td>A. Does the resident need or want an interpreter to communicate with a doctor or health care staff?
0. No
1. Yes → Specify in A1100B, Preferred language
9. Unable to determine

B. Preferred language:</td>
</tr>
</table>

Section A Identification Information

A1200. Marital Status

Enter Code	1. **Never married** 2. **Married** 3. **Widowed** 4. **Separated** 5. **Divorced**

A1300. Optional Resident Items

A. **Medical record number:**

B. **Room number:**

C. **Name by which resident prefers to be addressed:**

D. **Lifetime occupation(s)** - put "/" between two occupations**:**

A1500. Preadmission Screening and Resident Review (PASRR)

Complete only if A0310A = 01

Enter Code	**Has the resident been evaluated by Level II PASRR and determined to have a serious mental illness and/or mental retardation or a a related condition?** 0. **No** 1. **Yes** 9. **Not a Medicaid certified unit**

A1550. Conditions Related to MR/DD Status

If the resident is 22 years of age or older, complete only if A0310A = 01
If the resident is 21 years of age or younger, complete only if A0310A = 01, 03, 04, or 05

↓ **Check all conditions that are related to MR/DD status** that were manifested before age 22, and are likely to continue indefinitely

	MR/DD With Organic Condition
☐	A. **Down syndrome**
☐	B. **Autism**
☐	C. **Epilepsy**
☐	D. **Other organic condition related to MR/DD**
	MR/DD Without Organic Condition
☐	E. **MR/DD with no organic condition**
	No MR/DD
☐	Z. **None of the above**

A1600. Entry Date (date of this admission/reentry into the facility)

— —
Month   Day   Year

A1700. Type of Entry

Enter Code	1. **Admission** 2. **Reentry**

Section A — Identification Information

A1800. Entered From

Enter Code [ ]

01. **Community** (private home/apt., board/care, assisted living, group home)
02. **Another nursing home or swing bed**
03. **Acute hospital**
04. **Psychiatric hospital**
05. **Inpatient rehabilitation facility**
06. **MR/DD facility**
07. **Hospice**
99. **Other**

A2000. Discharge Date
Complete only if A0310F = 10, 11, or 12

___ — ___ — _____
Month   Day   Year

A2100. Discharge Status
Complete only if A0310F = 10, 11, or 12

Enter Code [ ]

01. **Community** (private home/apt., board/care, assisted living, group home)
02. **Another nursing home or swing bed**
03. **Acute hospital**
04. **Psychiatric hospital**
05. **Inpatient rehabilitation facility**
06. **MR/DD facility**
07. **Hospice**
08. **Deceased**
99. **Other**

A2200. Previous Assessment Reference Date for Significant Correction
Complete only if A0310A = 05 or 06

___ — ___ — _____
Month   Day   Year

A2300. Assessment Reference Date

Observation end date:

___ — ___ — _____
Month   Day   Year

A2400. Medicare Stay

Enter Code [ ]

A. Has the resident had a Medicare-covered stay since the most recent entry?

0. **No** → Skip to B0100, Comatose
1. **Yes** → Continue to A2400B, Start date of most recent Medicare stay

B. Start date of most recent Medicare stay:

___ — ___ — _____
Month   Day   Year

C. End date of most recent Medicare stay - Enter dashes if stay is ongoing:

___ — ___ — _____
Month   Day   Year

Look back period for all items is 7 days unless another time frame is indicated

Section B	Hearing, Speech, and Vision

B0100. Comatose

Enter Code

Persistent vegetative state/no discernible consciousness
- 0. **No** → Continue to B0200, Hearing
- 1. **Yes** → Skip to G0110, Activities of Daily Living (ADL) Assistance

B0200. Hearing

Enter Code

Ability to hear (with hearing aid or hearing appliances if normally used)
- 0. **Adequate** - no difficulty in normal conversation, social interaction, listening to TV
- 1. **Minimal difficulty** - difficulty in some environments (e.g., when person speaks softly or setting is noisy)
- 2. **Moderate difficulty** - speaker has to increase volume and speak distinctly
- 3. **Highly impaired** - absence of useful hearing

B0300. Hearing Aid

Enter Code

Hearing aid or other hearing appliance used in completing B0200, Hearing
- 0. **No**
- 1. **Yes**

B0600. Speech Clarity

Enter Code

Select best description of speech pattern
- 0. **Clear speech** - distinct intelligible words
- 1. **Unclear speech** - slurred or mumbled words
- 2. **No speech** - absence of spoken words

B0700. Makes Self Understood

Enter Code

Ability to express ideas and wants, consider both verbal and non-verbal expression
- 0. **Understood**
- 1. **Usually understood** - difficulty communicating some words or finishing thoughts **but** is able if prompted or given time
- 2. **Sometimes understood** - ability is limited to making concrete requests
- 3. **Rarely/never understood**

B0800. Ability To Understand Others

Enter Code

Understanding verbal content, however able (with hearing aid or device if used)
- 0. **Understands** - clear comprehension
- 1. **Usually understands** - misses some part/intent of message **but** comprehends most conversation
- 2. **Sometimes understands** - responds adequately to simple, direct communication only
- 3. **Rarely/never understands**

B1000. Vision

Enter Code

Ability to see in adequate light (with glasses or other visual appliances)
- 0. **Adequate** - sees fine detail, including regular print in newspapers/books
- 1. **Impaired** - sees large print, but not regular print in newspapers/books
- 2. **Moderately impaired** - limited vision; not able to see newspaper headlines but can identify objects
- 3. **Highly impaired** - object identification in question, but eyes appear to follow objects
- 4. **Severely impaired** - no vision or sees only light, colors or shapes; eyes do not appear to follow objects

B1200. Corrective Lenses

Enter Code

Corrective lenses (contacts, glasses, or magnifying glass) used in completing B1000, Vision
- 0. **No**
- 1. **Yes**

387

Section C — Cognitive Patterns

C0100. Should Brief Interview for Mental Status (C0200-C0500) be Conducted?

Attempt to conduct interview with all residents

| Enter Code | 0. **No** (resident is rarely/never understood) → Skip to and complete C0700-C1000, Staff Assessment for Mental Status |
| | 1. **Yes** → Continue to C0200, Repetition of Three Words |

Brief Interview for Mental Status (BIMS)

C0200. Repetition of Three Words

Enter Code	Ask resident: "*I am going to say three words for you to remember. Please repeat the words after I have said all three. The words are:* **sock, blue, and bed.** *Now tell me the three words.*"
	Number of words repeated after first attempt
	0. **None**
	1. **One**
	2. **Two**
	3. **Three**
	After the resident's first attempt, repeat the words using cues ("*sock, something to wear; blue, a color; bed, a piece of furniture*"). You may repeat the words up to two more times.

C0300. Temporal Orientation (orientation to year, month, and day)

Enter Code	Ask resident: "*Please tell me what year it is right now.*"
	A. Able to report correct year
	0. **Missed by > 5 years** or no answer
	1. **Missed by 2-5 years**
	2. **Missed by 1 year**
	3. **Correct**

Enter Code	Ask resident: "*What month are we in right now?*"
	B. Able to report correct month
	0. **Missed by > 1 month** or no answer
	1. **Missed by 6 days to 1 month**
	2. **Accurate within 5 days**

Enter Code	Ask resident: "*What day of the week is today?*"
	C. Able to report correct day of the week
	0. **Incorrect** or no answer
	1. **Correct**

C0400. Recall

Enter Code	Ask resident: "*Let's go back to an earlier question. What were those three words that I asked you to repeat?*"
	If unable to remember a word, give cue (something to wear; a color; a piece of furniture) for that word.
	A. Able to recall "sock"
	0. **No** - could not recall
	1. **Yes, after cueing** ("something to wear")
	2. **Yes, no cue required**

Enter Code	**B. Able to recall "blue"**
	0. **No** - could not recall
	1. **Yes, after cueing** ("a color")
	2. **Yes, no cue required**

Enter Code	**C. Able to recall "bed"**
	0. **No** - could not recall
	1. **Yes, after cueing** ("a piece of furniture")
	2. **Yes, no cue required**

C0500. Summary Score

| Enter Score | **Add scores** for questions C0200-C0400 and fill in total score (00-15) |
| | **Enter 99 if unable to complete one or more questions of the interview** |

Section C — Cognitive Patterns

C0600. Should the Staff Assessment for Mental Status (C0700 - C1000) be Conducted?

Enter Code [ ]
- 0. **No** (resident was able to complete interview) → Skip to C1300, Signs and Symptoms of Delirium
- 1. **Yes** (resident was unable to complete interview) → Continue to C0700, Short-term Memory OK

Staff Assessment for Mental Status

Do not conduct if Brief Interview for Mental Status (C0200-C0500) was completed

C0700. Short-term Memory OK

Enter Code [ ] Seems or appears to recall after 5 minutes
- 0. **Memory OK**
- 1. **Memory problem**

C0800. Long-term Memory OK

Enter Code [ ] Seems or appears to recall long past
- 0. **Memory OK**
- 1. **Memory problem**

C0900. Memory/Recall Ability

↓ Check all that the resident was normally able to recall

- [ ] A. **Current season**
- [ ] B. **Location of own room**
- [ ] C. **Staff names and faces**
- [ ] D. **That he or she is in a nursing home**
- [ ] Z. **None of the above** were recalled

C1000. Cognitive Skills for Daily Decision Making

Enter Code [ ] Made decisions regarding tasks of daily life
- 0. **Independent** - decisions consistent/reasonable
- 1. **Modified independence** - some difficulty in new situations only
- 2. **Moderately impaired** - decisions poor; cues/supervision required
- 3. **Severely impaired** - never/rarely made decisions

Delirium

C1300. Signs and Symptoms of Delirium (from CAM©)

Code **after completing** Brief Interview for Mental Status or Staff Assessment, and reviewing medical record

Coding:
- 0. **Behavior not present**
- 1. **Behavior continuously present, does not fluctuate**
- 2. **Behavior present, fluctuates** (comes and goes, changes in severity)

↓ Enter Codes in Boxes

[ ] A. **Inattention** - Did the resident have difficulty focusing attention (easily distracted, out of touch or difficulty following what was said)?

[ ] B. **Disorganized thinking** - Was the resident's thinking disorganized or incoherent (rambling or irrelevant conversation, unclear or illogical flow of ideas, or unpredictable switching from subject to subject)?

[ ] C. **Altered level of consciousness** - Did the resident have altered level of consciousness (e.g., **vigilant** - startled easily to any sound or touch; **lethargic** - repeatedly dozed off when being asked questions, but responded to voice or touch; **stuporous** - very difficult to arouse and keep aroused for the interview; **comatose** - could not be aroused)?

[ ] D. **Psychomotor retardation**- Did the resident have an unusually decreased level of activity such as sluggishness, staring into space, staying in one position, moving very slowly?

C1600. Acute Onset Mental Status Change

Enter Code [ ] Is there evidence of an acute change in mental status from the resident's baseline?
- 0. **No**
- 1. **Yes**

Copyright © 1990 Annals of Internal Medicine. All rights reserved. Adapted with permission.

Section D   Mood

D0100. Should Resident Mood Interview be Conducted? - Attempt to conduct interview with all residents

Enter Code
☐

0. **No** (resident is rarely/never understood) → Skip to and complete D0500-D0600, Staff Assessment of Resident Mood (PHQ-9-OV)
1. **Yes** → Continue to D0200, Resident Mood Interview (PHQ-9©)

D0200. Resident Mood Interview (PHQ-9©)

Say to resident: *"Over the last 2 weeks, have you been bothered by any of the following problems?"*

If symptom is present, enter 1 (yes) in column 1, Symptom Presence.
If yes in column 1, then ask the resident: "About **how often** have you been bothered by this?"
Read and show the resident a card with the symptom frequency choices. Indicate response in column 2, Symptom Frequency.

1. Symptom Presence	**2. Symptom Frequency**
0. **No** (enter 0 in column 2)	0. **Never or 1 day**
1. **Yes** (enter 0-3 in column 2)	1. **2-6 days** (several days)
9. **No response** (leave column 2 blank)	2. **7-11 days** (half or more of the days)
	3. **12-14 days** (nearly every day)

	1. Symptom Presence	2. Symptom Frequency
	↓ Enter Scores in Boxes ↓	
A. Little interest or pleasure in doing things	☐	☐
B. Feeling down, depressed, or hopeless	☐	☐
C. Trouble falling or staying asleep, or sleeping too much	☐	☐
D. Feeling tired or having little energy	☐	☐
E. Poor appetite or overeating	☐	☐
F. Feeling bad about yourself - or that you are a failure or have let yourself or your family down	☐	☐
G. Trouble concentrating on things, such as reading the newspaper or watching television	☐	☐
H. Moving or speaking so slowly that other people could have noticed. Or the opposite - being so fidgety or restless that you have been moving around a lot more than usual	☐	☐
I. Thoughts that you would be better off dead, or of hurting yourself in some way	☐	☐

D0300. Total Severity Score

Enter Score
☐

Add scores for all frequency responses in Column 2, Symptom Frequency. Total score must be between 00 and 27. Enter 99 if unable to complete interview (i.e., Symptom Frequency is blank for 3 or more items).

D0350. Safety Notification - Complete only if D0200I1 = 1 indicating possibility of resident self harm

Enter Code
☐

Was responsible staff or provider informed that there is a potential for resident self harm?
0. **No**
1. **Yes**

Copyright © Pfizer Inc. All rights reserved. Reproduced with permission.

Section D — Mood

D0500. Staff Assessment of Resident Mood (PHQ-9-OV*)
Do not conduct if Resident Mood Interview (D0200-D0300) was completed

Over the last 2 weeks, did the resident have any of the following problems or behaviors?

If symptom is present, enter 1 (yes) in column 1, Symptom Presence.
Then move to column 2, Symptom Frequency, and indicate symptom frequency.

1. Symptom Presence
  0. **No** (enter 0 in column 2)
  1. **Yes** (enter 0-3 in column 2)

2. Symptom Frequency
  0. **Never or 1 day**
  1. **2-6 days** (several days)
  2. **7-11 days** (half or more of the days)
  3. **12-14 days** (nearly every day)

	1. Symptom Presence	2. Symptom Frequency
	↓ Enter Scores in Boxes ↓	
A. Little interest or pleasure in doing things		
B. Feeling or appearing down, depressed, or hopeless		
C. Trouble falling or staying asleep, or sleeping too much		
D. Feeling tired or having little energy		
E. Poor appetite or overeating		
F. Indicating that s/he feels bad about self, is a failure, or has let self or family down		
G. Trouble concentrating on things, such as reading the newspaper or watching television		
H. Moving or speaking so slowly that other people have noticed. Or the opposite - being so fidgety or restless that s/he has been moving around a lot more than usual		
I. States that life isn't worth living, wishes for death, or attempts to harm self		
J. Being short-tempered, easily annoyed		

D0600. Total Severity Score

[Enter Score]   Add scores for all frequency responses in Column 2, Symptom Frequency. Total score must be between 00 and 30.

D0650. Safety Notification - Complete only if D0500I1 = 1 indicating possibility of resident self harm

Enter Code	Was responsible staff or provider informed that there is a potential for resident self harm?
	0. **No**
	1. **Yes**

* Copyright © Pfizer Inc. All rights reserved.

Section E — Behavior

E0100. Psychosis

↓ Check all that apply

☐	**A. Hallucinations** (perceptual experiences in the absence of real external sensory stimuli)
☐	**B. Delusions** (misconceptions or beliefs that are firmly held, contrary to reality)
☐	**Z. None of the above**

Behavioral Symptoms

E0200. Behavioral Symptom - Presence & Frequency

Note presence of symptoms and their frequency

Coding:
0. **Behavior not exhibited**
1. **Behavior of this type occurred 1 to 3 days**
2. **Behavior of this type occurred 4 to 6 days,** but less than daily
3. **Behavior of this type occurred daily**

↓ Enter Codes in Boxes

Code	
☐	**A. Physical behavioral symptoms directed toward others** (e.g., hitting, kicking, pushing, scratching, grabbing, abusing others sexually)
☐	**B. Verbal behavioral symptoms directed toward others** (e.g., threatening others, screaming at others, cursing at others)
☐	**C. Other behavioral symptoms not directed toward others** (e.g., physical symptoms such as hitting or scratching self, pacing, rummaging, public sexual acts, disrobing in public, throwing or smearing food or bodily wastes, or verbal/vocal symptoms like screaming, disruptive sounds)

E0300. Overall Presence of Behavioral Symptoms

Enter Code	Were any behavioral symptoms in questions E0200 coded 1, 2, or 3?
☐	0. **No →** Skip to E0800, Rejection of Care
	1. **Yes →** Considering all of E0200, Behavioral Symptoms, answer E0500 and E0600 below

E0500. Impact on Resident

Did any of the identified symptom(s):

Enter Code	A. **Put the resident at significant risk for physical illness or injury?**
☐	0. **No**
	1. **Yes**

Enter Code	B. **Significantly interfere with the resident's care?**
☐	0. **No**
	1. **Yes**

Enter Code	C. **Significantly interfere with the resident's participation in activities or social interactions?**
☐	0. **No**
	1. **Yes**

E0600. Impact on Others

Did any of the identified symptom(s):

Enter Code	A. **Put others at significant risk for physical injury?**
☐	0. **No**
	1. **Yes**

Enter Code	B. **Significantly intrude on the privacy or activity of others?**
☐	0. **No**
	1. **Yes**

Enter Code	C. **Significantly disrupt care or living environment?**
☐	0. **No**
	1. **Yes**

E0800. Rejection of Care - Presence & Frequency

Enter Code	Did the resident reject evaluation or care (e.g., bloodwork, taking medications, ADL assistance) **that is necessary to achieve the resident's goals for health and well-being?** Do not include behaviors that have already been addressed (e.g., by discussion or care planning with the resident or family), and/or determined to be consistent with resident values, preferences, or goals.
☐	0. **Behavior not exhibited**
	1. **Behavior of this type occurred 1 to 3 days**
	2. **Behavior of this type occurred 4 to 6 days,** but less than daily
	3. **Behavior of this type occurred daily**

Section E — Behavior

E0900. Wandering - Presence & Frequency

Enter Code	Has the resident wandered?
☐	0. **Behavior not exhibited** → Skip to E1100, Change in Behavioral or Other Symptoms
	1. **Behavior of this type occurred 1 to 3 days**
	2. **Behavior of this type occurred 4 to 6 days**, but less than daily
	3. **Behavior of this type occurred daily**

E1000. Wandering - Impact

Enter Code	A. **Does the wandering place the resident at significant risk of getting to a potentially dangerous place** (e.g., stairs, outside of the facility)?
☐	0. **No**
	1. **Yes**

Enter Code	B. **Does the wandering significantly intrude on the privacy of activities of others?**
☐	0. **No**
	1. **Yes**

E1100. Change in Behavior or Other Symptoms

Consider all of the symptoms assessed in items E0100 through E1000

Enter Code	How does resident's current behavior status, care rejection, or wandering **compare to prior assessment (OBRA or PPS)?**
☐	0. **Same**
	1. **Improved**
	2. **Worse**
	3. **N/A** because no prior MDS assessment

Section F — Preferences for Customary Routine and Activities

F0300. Should Interview for Daily and Activity Preferences be Conducted? - Attempt to interview all residents able to communicate. If resident is unable to complete, attempt to complete interview with family member or significant other

Enter Code	
	0. **No** (resident is rarely/never understood <u>and</u> family/significant other not available) → Skip to and complete F0800, Staff Assessment of Daily and Activity Preferences
	1. **Yes** → Continue to F0400, Interview for Daily Preferences

F0400. Interview for Daily Preferences

Show resident the response options and say: **"While you are in this facility..."**

↓ Enter Codes in Boxes

Coding:
1. **Very important**
2. **Somewhat important**
3. **Not very important**
4. **Not important at all**
5. **Important, but can't do or no choice**
9. **No response or non-responsive**

A.	how important is it to you to **choose what clothes to wear?**
B.	how important is it to you to **take care of your personal belongings or things?**
C.	how important is it to you to **choose between a tub bath, shower, bed bath, or sponge bath?**
D.	how important is it to you to **have snacks available between meals?**
E.	how important is it to you to **choose your own bedtime?**
F.	how important is it to you to **have your family or a close friend involved in discussions about your care?**
G.	how important is it to you to **be able to use the phone in private?**
H.	how important is it to you to **have a place to lock your things to keep them safe?**

F0500. Interview for Activity Preferences

Show resident the response options and say: **"While you are in this facility..."**

↓ Enter Codes in Boxes

Coding:
1. **Very important**
2. **Somewhat important**
3. **Not very important**
4. **Not important at all**
5. **Important, but can't do or no choice**
9. **No response or non-responsive**

A.	how important is it to you to **have books, newspapers, and magazines to read?**
B.	how important is it to you to **listen to music you like?**
C.	how important is it to you to **be around animals such as pets?**
D.	how important is it to you to **keep up with the news?**
E.	how important is it to you to **do things with groups of people?**
F.	how important is it to you to **do your favorite activities?**
G.	how important is it to you to **go outside to get fresh air when the weather is good?**
H.	how important is it to you to **participate in religious services or practices?**

F0600. Daily and Activity Preferences Primary Respondent

Enter Code	
	Indicate primary respondent for Daily and Activity Preferences (F0400 and F0500)
	1. **Resident**
	2. **Family or significant other** (close friend or other representative)
	9. **Interview could not be completed** by resident or family/significant other ("No response" to 3 or more items")

Section F — Preferences for Customary Routine and Activities

F0700. Should the Staff Assessment of Daily and Activity Preferences be Conducted?

Enter Code		
☐	0.	**No** (because Interview for Daily and Activity Preferences (F0400 and F0500) was completed by resident or family/significant other) → Skip to and complete G0110, Activities of Daily Living (ADL) Assistance
	1.	**Yes** (because 3 or more items in Interview for Daily and Activity Preferences (F0400 and F0500) were not completed by resident or family/significant other) → Continue to F0800, Staff Assessment of Daily and Activity Preferences

F0800. Staff Assessment of Daily and Activity Preferences

Do not conduct if Interview for Daily and Activity Preferences (F0400-F0500) was completed

Resident Prefers:

↓ Check all that apply

☐	A. Choosing clothes to wear
☐	B. Caring for personal belongings
☐	C. Receiving tub bath
☐	D. Receiving shower
☐	E. Receiving bed bath
☐	F. Receiving sponge bath
☐	G. Snacks between meals
☐	H. Staying up past 8:00 p.m.
☐	I. Family or significant other involvement in care discussions
☐	J. Use of phone in private
☐	K. Place to lock personal belongings
☐	L. Reading books, newspapers, or magazines
☐	M. Listening to music
☐	N. Being around animals such as pets
☐	O. Keeping up with the news
☐	P. Doing things with groups of people
☐	Q. Participating in favorite activities
☐	R. Spending time away from the nursing home
☐	S. Spending time outdoors
☐	T. Participating in religious activities or practices
☐	Z. None of the above

Section G   Functional Status

G0110. Activities of Daily Living (ADL) Assistance
Refer to the ADL flow chart in the RAI manual to facilitate accurate coding

Instructions for Rule of 3
- When an activity occurs three times at any one given level, code that level.
- When an activity occurs three times at multiple levels, code the most dependent, exceptions are total dependence (4), activity must require full assist every time, and activity did not occur (8), activity must not have occurred at all. Example, three times extensive assistance (3) and three times limited assistance (2), code extensive assistance (3).
- When an activity occurs at various levels, but not three times at any given level, apply the following:
  - When there is a combination of full staff performance, and extensive assistance, code extensive assistance.
  - When there is a combination of full staff performance, weight bearing assistance and/or non-weight bearing assistance code limited assistance (2).

If none of the above are met, code supervision.

1. ADL Self-Performance
Code for **resident's performance** over all shifts - not including setup. If the ADL activity occurred 3 or more times at various levels of assistance, code the most dependent - except for total dependence, which requires full staff performance every time

Coding:

Activity Occurred 3 or More Times
0. **Independent** - no help or staff oversight at any time
1. **Supervision** - oversight, encouragement or cueing
2. **Limited assistance** - resident highly involved in activity; staff provide guided maneuvering of limbs or other non-weight-bearing assistance
3. **Extensive assistance** - resident involved in activity, staff provide weight-bearing support
4. **Total dependence** - full staff performance every time during 7-day period

Activity Occurred 2 or Fewer Times
7. **Activity occurred only once or twice** - activity did occur but only once or twice
8. **Activity did not occur** - activity (or any part of the ADL) was not performed by resident or staff at all over the entire 7-day period

2. ADL Support Provided
Code for **most support provided** over all shifts; code regardless of resident's self-performance classification

Coding:
0. **No** setup or physical help from staff
1. **Setup** help only
2. **One** person physical assist
3. **Two+** persons physical assist
8. ADL activity itself **did not occur** during entire period

	1. Self-Performance	2. Support
	↓ Enter Codes in Boxes ↓	
A. Bed mobility - how resident moves to and from lying position, turns side to side, and positions body while in bed or alternate sleep furniture		
B. Transfer - how resident moves between surfaces including to or from: bed, chair, wheelchair, standing position (**excludes** to/from bath/toilet)		
C. Walk in room - how resident walks between locations in his/her room		
D. Walk in corridor - how resident walks in corridor on unit		
E. Locomotion on unit - how resident moves between locations in his/her room and adjacent corridor on same floor. If in wheelchair, self-sufficiency once in chair		
F. Locomotion off unit - how resident moves to and returns from off-unit locations (e.g., areas set aside for dining, activities or treatments). **If facility has only one floor**, how resident moves to and from distant areas on the floor. If in wheelchair, self-sufficiency once in chair		
G. Dressing - how resident puts on, fastens and takes off all items of clothing, including donning/removing a prosthesis or TED hose. Dressing includes putting on and changing pajamas and housedresses		
H. Eating - how resident eats and drinks, regardless of skill. Do not include eating/drinking during medication pass. Includes intake of nourishment by other means (e.g., tube feeding, total parenteral nutrition, IV fluids administered for nutrition or hydration)		
I. Toilet use - how resident uses the toilet room, commode, bedpan, or urinal; transfers on/off toilet; cleanses self after elimination; changes pad; manages ostomy or catheter; and adjusts clothes. Do not include emptying of bedpan, urinal, bedside commode, catheter bag or ostomy bag		
J. Personal hygiene - how resident maintains personal hygiene, including combing hair, brushing teeth, shaving, applying makeup, washing/drying face and hands (**excludes** baths and showers)		

Section G	Functional Status

G0120. Bathing

How resident takes full-body bath/shower, sponge bath, and transfers in/out of tub/shower (**excludes** washing of back and hair). Code for **most dependent** in self-performance and support

Enter Code	**A. Self-performance**
☐	0. **Independent** - no help provided
	1. **Supervision** - oversight help only
	2. **Physical help limited to transfer only**
	3. **Physical help in part of bathing activity**
	4. **Total dependence**
	8. **Activity itself did not occur** during the entire period

Enter Code	**B. Support provided**
☐	(Bathing support codes are as defined in item **G0110 column 2, ADL Support Provided**, above)

G0300. Balance During Transitions and Walking

After observing the resident, **code the following walking and transition items for most dependent**

Coding:
0. **Steady at all times**
1. **Not steady, but able to stabilize without human assistance**
2. **Not steady, only able to stabilize with human assistance**
8. **Activity did not occur**

↓ **Enter Codes in Boxes**

☐	**A. Moving from seated to standing position**
☐	**B. Walking** (with assistive device if used)
☐	**C. Turning around** and facing the opposite direction while walking
☐	**D. Moving on and off toilet**
☐	**E. Surface-to-surface transfer** (transfer between bed and chair or wheelchair)

G0400. Functional Limitation in Range of Motion

Code for limitation that interfered with daily functions or placed resident at risk of injury

Coding:
0. **No impairment**
1. **Impairment on one side**
2. **Impairment on both sides**

↓ **Enter Codes in Boxes**

☐	**A. Upper extremity** (shoulder, elbow, wrist, hand)
☐	**B. Lower extremity** (hip, knee, ankle, foot)

G0600. Mobility Devices

↓ **Check all that were normally used**

☐	**A. Cane/crutch**
☐	**B. Walker**
☐	**C. Wheelchair** (manual or electric)
☐	**D. Limb prosthesis**
☐	**Z. None of the above** were used

G0900. Functional Rehabilitation Potential

Complete only if A0310A = 01

Enter Code	A. Resident believes he or she is **capable of increased independence** in at least some ADLs
☐	0. **No**
	1. **Yes**
	2. **Unable to determine**

Enter Code	B. Direct care staff believe resident is **capable of increased independence** in at least some ADLs
☐	0. **No**
	1. **Yes**

397

Section H — Bladder and Bowel

H0100. Appliances

↓ Check all that apply

☐	**A. Indwelling catheter** (including suprapubic catheter and nephrostomy tube)
☐	**B. External catheter**
☐	**C. Ostomy** (including urostomy, ileostomy, and colostomy)
☐	**D. Intermittent catheterization**
☐	**Z. None of the above**

H0200. Urinary Toileting Program

Enter Code ☐
A. Has a trial of a toileting program (e.g., scheduled toileting, prompted voiding, or bladder training) been attempted on admission/reentry or since urinary incontinence was noted in this facility?
- 0. **No** → Skip to H0300, Urinary Continence
- 1. **Yes** → Continue to H0200B, Response
- 9. **Unable to determine** → Skip to H0200C, Current toileting program or trial

Enter Code ☐
B. Response - What was the resident's response to the trial program?
- 0. **No improvement**
- 1. **Decreased wetness**
- 2. **Completely dry** (continent)
- 9. **Unable to determine** or trial in progress

Enter Code ☐
C. Current toileting program or trial - Is a toileting program (e.g., scheduled toileting, prompted voiding, or bladder training) currently being used to manage the resident's urinary continence?
- 0. **No**
- 1. **Yes**

H0300. Urinary Continence

Enter Code ☐
Urinary continence - Select the one category that best describes the resident
- 0. **Always continent**
- 1. **Occasionally incontinent** (less than 7 episodes of incontinence)
- 2. **Frequently incontinent** (7 or more episodes of urinary incontinence, but at least one episode of continent voiding)
- 3. **Always incontinent** (no episodes of continent voiding)
- 9. **Not rated,** resident had a catheter (indwelling, condom), urinary ostomy, or no urine output for the entire 7 days

H0400. Bowel Continence

Enter Code ☐
Bowel continence - Select the one category that best describes the resident
- 0. **Always continent**
- 1. **Occasionally incontinent** (one episode of bowel incontinence)
- 2. **Frequently incontinent** (2 or more episodes of bowel incontinence, but at least one continent bowel movement)
- 3. **Always incontinent** (no episodes of continent bowel movements)
- 9. **Not rated,** resident had an ostomy or did not have a bowel movement for the entire 7 days

H0500. Bowel Toileting Program

Enter Code ☐
Is a toileting program currently being used to manage the resident's bowel continence?
- 0. **No**
- 1. **Yes**

H0600. Bowel Patterns

Enter Code ☐
Constipation present?
- 0. **No**
- 1. **Yes**

Section I	Active Diagnoses

Active Diagnoses in the last 7 days - Check all that apply

Diagnoses listed in parentheses are provided as examples and should not be considered as all-inclusive lists

Cancer

☐ **I0100. Cancer** (with or without metastasis)

Heart/Circulation

☐ **I0200. Anemia** (e.g., aplastic, iron deficiency, pernicious, and sickle cell)

☐ **I0300. Atrial Fibrillation or Other Dysrhythmias** (e.g., bradycardias and tachycardias)

☐ **I0400. Coronary Artery Disease (CAD)** (e.g., angina, myocardial infarction, and atherosclerotic heart disease (ASHD))

☐ **I0500. Deep Venous Thrombosis (DVT), Pulmonary Embolus (PE), or Pulmonary Thrombo-Embolism (PTE)**

☐ **I0600. Heart Failure** (e.g., congestive heart failure (CHF) and pulmonary edema)

☐ **I0700. Hypertension**

☐ **I0800. Orthostatic Hypotension**

☐ **I0900. Peripheral Vascular Disease (PVD) or Peripheral Arterial Disease (PAD)**

Gastrointestinal

☐ **I1100. Cirrhosis**

☐ **I1200. Gastroesophageal Reflux Disease (GERD) or Ulcer** (e.g., esophageal, gastric, and peptic ulcers)

☐ **I1300. Ulcerative Colitis, Crohn's Disease, or Inflammatory Bowel Disease**

Genitourinary

☐ **I1400. Benign Prostatic Hyperplasia (BPH)**

☐ **I1500. Renal Insufficiency, Renal Failure, or End-Stage Renal Disease (ESRD)**

☐ **I1550. Neurogenic Bladder**

☐ **I1650. Obstructive Uropathy**

Infections

☐ **I1700. Multidrug-Resistant Organism (MDRO)**

☐ **I2000. Pneumonia**

☐ **I2100. Septicemia**

☐ **I2200. Tuberculosis**

☐ **I2300. Urinary Tract Infection (UTI) (LAST 30 DAYS)**

☐ **I2400. Viral Hepatitis** (e.g., Hepatitis A, B, C, D, and E)

☐ **I2500. Wound Infection** (other than foot)

Metabolic

☐ **I2900. Diabetes Mellitus (DM)** (e.g., diabetic retinopathy, nephropathy, and neuropathy)

☐ **I3100. Hyponatremia**

☐ **I3200. Hyperkalemia**

☐ **I3300. Hyperlipidemia** (e.g., hypercholesterolemia)

☐ **I3400. Thyroid Disorder** (e.g., hypothyroidism, hyperthyroidism, and Hashimoto's thyroiditis)

Musculoskeletal

☐ **I3700. Arthritis** (e.g., degenerative joint disease (DJD), osteoarthritis, and rheumatoid arthritis (RA))

☐ **I3800. Osteoporosis**

☐ **I3900. Hip Fracture** - any hip fracture that has a relationship to current status, treatments, monitoring (e.g., sub-capital fractures, and fractures of the trochanter and femoral neck)

☐ **I4000. Other Fracture**

Neurological

☐ **I4200. Alzheimer's Disease**

☐ **I4300. Aphasia**

☐ **I4400. Cerebral Palsy**

☐ **I4500. Cerebrovascular Accident (CVA), Transient Ischemic Attack (TIA), or Stroke**

☐ **I4800. Dementia** (e.g. Non-Alzheimer's dementia such as vascular or multi-infarct dementia; mixed dementia; frontotemporal dementia such as Pick's disease; and dementia related to stroke, Parkinson's or Creutzfeldt-Jakob diseases)

Neurological Diagnoses continued on next page

Section I — Active Diagnoses

Active Diagnoses in the last 7 days - Check all that apply

Diagnoses listed in parentheses are provided as examples and should not be considered as all-inclusive lists

Neurological - Continued

- ☐ I4900. **Hemiplegia or Hemiparesis**
- ☐ I5000. **Paraplegia**
- ☐ I5100. **Quadriplegia**
- ☐ I5200. **Multiple Sclerosis (MS)**
- ☐ I5250. **Huntington's Disease**
- ☐ I5300. **Parkinson's Disease**
- ☐ I5350. **Tourette's Syndrome**
- ☐ I5400. **Seizure Disorder or Epilepsy**
- ☐ I5500. **Traumatic Brain Injury (TBI)**

Nutritional

- ☐ I5600. **Malnutrition** (protein or calorie) or at risk for malnutrition

Psychiatric/Mood Disorder

- ☐ I5700. **Anxiety Disorder**
- ☐ I5800. **Depression** (other than bipolar)
- ☐ I5900. **Manic Depression** (bipolar disease)
- ☐ I5950. **Psychotic Disorder** (other than schizophrenia)
- ☐ I6000. **Schizophrenia** (e.g., schizoaffective and schizophreniform disorders)
- ☐ I6100. **Post Traumatic Stress Disorder (PTSD)**

Pulmonary

- ☐ I6200. **Asthma, Chronic Obstructive Pulmonary Disease (COPD), or Chronic Lung Disease** (e.g., chronic bronchitis and restrictive lung diseases such as asbestosis)
- ☐ I6300. **Respiratory Failure**

Vision

- ☐ I6500. **Cataracts, Glaucoma, or Macular Degeneration**

None of Above

- ☐ I7900. **None of the above active diagnoses** within the last 7 days

Other

- ☐ I8000. **Additional active diagnoses**
  Enter diagnosis on line and ICD code in boxes. Include the decimal for the code in the appropriate box.

  A. _____

  B. _____

  C. _____

  D. _____

  E. _____

  F. _____

  G. _____

  H. _____

  I. _____

  J. _____

Section J — Health Conditions

J0100. Pain Management - Complete for all residents, regardless of current pain level

At any time in the last **5** days, has the resident:

Enter Code		
	A.	**Been on a scheduled pain medication regimen?** 0. **No** 1. **Yes**
	B.	**Received PRN pain medications?** 0. **No** 1. **Yes**
	C.	**Received non-medication intervention for pain?** 0. **No** 1. **Yes**

J0200. Should Pain Assessment Interview be Conducted?

Attempt to conduct interview with all residents. If resident is comatose, skip to J1100, Shortness of Breath (dyspnea)

Enter Code
- 0. **No** (resident is rarely/never understood) ➞ Skip to and complete J0800, Indicators of Pain or Possible Pain
- 1. **Yes** ➞ Continue to J0300, Pain Presence

Pain Assessment Interview

J0300. Pain Presence

Enter Code

Ask resident: "***Have you had pain or hurting at any time*** in the last 5 days?"
- 0. **No** ➞ Skip to J1100, Shortness of Breath
- 1. **Yes** ➞ Continue to J0400, Pain Frequency
- 9. **Unable to answer** ➞ Skip to J0800, Indicators of Pain or Possible Pain

J0400. Pain Frequency

Enter Code

Ask resident: "***How much of the time have you experienced pain or hurting*** over the last 5 days?"
- 1. **Almost constantly**
- 2. **Frequently**
- 3. **Occasionally**
- 4. **Rarely**
- 9. **Unable to answer**

J0500. Pain Effect on Function

Enter Code		
	A.	Ask resident: "*Over the past 5 days,* ***has pain made it hard for you to sleep at night?***" 0. **No** 1. **Yes** 9. **Unable to answer**
	B.	Ask resident: "*Over the past 5 days,* ***have you limited your day-to-day activities because of pain?***" 0. **No** 1. **Yes** 9. **Unable to answer**

J0600. Pain Intensity - Administer **ONLY ONE** of the following pain intensity questions (A or B)

Enter Rating		
	A.	**Numeric Rating Scale (00-10)** Ask resident: "*Please rate your worst pain over the last 5 days on a zero to ten scale, with zero being no pain and ten as the worst pain you can imagine.*" (Show resident 00 -10 pain scale) **Enter two-digit response. Enter 99 if unable to answer.**
Enter Code	**B.**	**Verbal Descriptor Scale** Ask resident: "*Please rate the intensity of your worst pain over the last 5 days.*" (Show resident verbal scale) 1. **Mild** 2. **Moderate** 3. **Severe** 4. **Very severe, horrible** 9. **Unable to answer**

Section J — Health Conditions

J0700. Should the Staff Assessment for Pain be Conducted?

Enter Code	0. **No** (J0400 = 1 thru 4) → Skip to J1100, Shortness of Breath (dyspnea) 1. **Yes** (J0400 = 9) → Continue to J0800, Indicators of Pain or Possible Pain

Staff Assessment for Pain

J0800. Indicators of Pain or Possible Pain in the last 5 days

↓ **Check all that apply**

☐	**A. Non-verbal sounds** (crying, whining, gasping, moaning, or groaning)
☐	**B. Vocal complaints of pain** (that hurts, ouch, stop)
☐	**C. Facial expressions** (grimaces, winces, wrinkled forehead, furrowed brow, clenched teeth or jaw)
☐	**D. Protective body movements or postures** (bracing, guarding, rubbing or massaging a body part/area, clutching or holding a body part during movement)
☐	**Z. None of these signs observed or documented** → If checked, skip to J1100, Shortness of Breath (dyspnea)

J0850. Frequency of Indicator of Pain or Possible Pain in the last 5 days

Enter Code	Frequency with which resident complains or shows evidence of pain or possible pain 1. **Indicators of pain** or possible pain observed **1 to 2 days** 2. **Indicators of pain** or possible pain observed **3 to 4 days** 3. **Indicators of pain** or possible pain observed **daily**

Other Health Conditions

J1100. Shortness of Breath (dyspnea)

↓ **Check all that apply**

☐	**A. Shortness of breath** or trouble breathing **with exertion** (e.g., walking, bathing, transferring)
☐	**B. Shortness of breath** or trouble breathing **when sitting at rest**
☐	**C. Shortness of breath** or trouble breathing **when lying flat**
☐	**Z. None of the above**

J1300. Current Tobacco Use

Enter Code	**Tobacco use** 0. **No** 1. **Yes**

J1400. Prognosis

Enter Code	Does the resident have a condition or chronic disease that may result in a **life expectancy of less than 6 months?** (Requires physician documentation) 0. **No** 1. **Yes**

J1550. Problem Conditions

↓ **Check all that apply**

☐	**A. Fever**
☐	**B. Vomiting**
☐	**C. Dehydrated**
☐	**D. Internal bleeding**
☐	**Z. None of the above**

Section J — Health Conditions

J1700. Fall History on Admission
Complete only if A0310A = 01 or A0310E = 1

Enter Code	
[ ]	**A.** Did the resident have a fall any time in the **last month** prior to admission? 0. **No** 1. **Yes** 9. **Unable to determine**
[ ]	**B.** Did the resident have a fall any time in the **last 2-6 months** prior to admission? 0. **No** 1. **Yes** 9. **Unable to determine**
[ ]	**C.** Did the resident have any **fracture related to a fall in the 6 months** prior to admission? 0. **No** 1. **Yes** 9. **Unable to determine**

J1800. Any Falls Since Admission or Prior Assessment (OBRA, PPS, or Discharge), whichever is more recent

Enter Code	
[ ]	Has the resident **had any falls since admission or the prior assessment** (OBRA, PPS, or Discharge), whichever is more recent? 0. **No** → Skip to K0100, Swallowing Disorder 1. **Yes** → Continue to J1900, Number of Falls Since Admission or Prior Assessment (OBRA, PPS, or Discharge)

J1900. Number of Falls Since Admission or Prior Assessment (OBRA, PPS, or Discharge), whichever is more recent

↓ Enter Codes in Boxes

Coding:		
0. **None** 1. **One** 2. **Two or more**	[ ]	**A.** **No injury** - no evidence of any injury is noted on physical assessment by the nurse or primary care clinician; no complaints of pain or injury by the resident; no change in the resident's behavior is noted after the fall
	[ ]	**B.** **Injury (except major)** - skin tears, abrasions, lacerations, superficial bruises, hematomas and sprains; or any fall-related injury that causes the resident to complain of pain
	[ ]	**C.** **Major injury** - bone fractures, joint dislocations, closed head injuries with altered consciousness, subdural hematoma

Section K — Swallowing/Nutritional Status

K0100. Swallowing Disorder

Signs and symptoms of possible swallowing disorder

↓ Check all that apply

☐	A. Loss of liquids/solids from mouth when eating or drinking
☐	B. Holding food in mouth/cheeks or residual food in mouth after meals
☐	C. Coughing or choking during meals or when swallowing medications
☐	D. Complaints of difficulty or pain with swallowing
☐	Z. None of the above

K0200. Height and Weight - While measuring, if the number is X.1 - X.4 round down; X.5 or greater round up

☐ inches	A. Height (in inches). Record most recent height measure since admission
☐ pounds	B. Weight (in pounds). Base weight on most recent measure in last 30 days; measure weight consistently, according to standard facility practice (e.g., in a.m. after voiding, before meal, with shoes off, etc.)

K0300. Weight Loss

Enter Code ☐	Loss of 5% or more in the last month or loss of 10% or more in last 6 months 0. **No** or unknown 1. **Yes, on** physician-prescribed weight-loss regimen 2. **Yes, not on** physician-prescribed weight-loss regimen

K0500. Nutritional Approaches

↓ Check all that apply

☐	A. Parenteral/IV feeding
☐	B. Feeding tube - nasogastric or abdominal (PEG)
☐	C. Mechanically altered diet - require change in texture of food or liquids (e.g., pureed food, thickened liquids)
☐	D. Therapeutic diet (e.g., low salt, diabetic, low cholesterol)
☐	Z. None of the above

K0700. Percent Intake by Artificial Route - Complete K0700 only if K0500A or K0500B is checked

Enter Code ☐	A. Proportion of total calories the resident received through parenteral or tube feeding 1. **25% or less** 2. **26-50%** 3. **51% or more**
Enter Code ☐	B. Average fluid intake per day by IV or tube feeding 1. **500 cc/day or less** 2. **501 cc/day or more**

Section L — Oral/Dental Status

L0200. Dental

↓ Check all that apply

☐	A. Broken or loosely fitting full or partial denture (chipped, cracked, uncleanable, or loose)
☐	B. No natural teeth or tooth fragment(s) (edentulous)
☐	C. Abnormal mouth tissue (ulcers, masses, oral lesions, including under denture or partial if one is worn)
☐	D. Obvious or likely cavity or broken natural teeth
☐	E. Inflamed or bleeding gums or loose natural teeth
☐	F. Mouth or facial pain, discomfort or difficulty with chewing
☐	G. Unable to examine
☐	Z. None of the above were present

Section M — Skin Conditions

Report based on highest stage of existing ulcer(s) at its worst; do not "reverse" stage

M0100. Determination of Pressure Ulcer Risk

↓ Check all that apply

☐	**A. Resident has a stage 1 or greater, a scar over bony prominence, or a non-removable dressing/device**
☐	**B. Formal assessment instrument/tool** (e.g., Braden, Norton, or other)
☐	**C. Clinical assessment**
☐	**Z. None of the above**

M0150. Risk of Pressure Ulcers

Enter Code	**Is this resident at risk of developing pressure ulcers?** 0. **No** 1. **Yes**
☐	

M0210. Unhealed Pressure Ulcer(s)

Enter Code	**Does this resident have one or more unhealed pressure ulcer(s) at Stage 1 or higher?** 0. **No** → Skip to M0900, Healed Pressure Ulcers 1. **Yes** → Continue to M0300, Current Number of Unhealed (non-epithelialized) Pressure Ulcers at Each Stage
☐	

M0300. Current Number of Unhealed (non-epithelialized) Pressure Ulcers at Each Stage

Enter Number	**A. Number of Stage 1 pressure ulcers** **Stage 1:** Intact skin with non-blanchable redness of a localized area usually over a bony prominence. Darkly pigmented skin may not have a visible blanching; in dark skin tones only it may appear with persistent blue or purple hues
☐	

	B. Stage 2: Partial thickness loss of dermis presenting as a shallow open ulcer with a red or pink wound bed, without slough. May also present as an intact or open/ruptured serum-filled blister
Enter Number ☐	**1. Number of Stage 2 pressure ulcers** - If 0 → Skip to M0300C, Stage 3
Enter Number ☐	**2. Number of these Stage 2 pressure ulcers that were present upon admission/reentry** - enter how many were noted at the time of admission
	3. Date of oldest Stage 2 pressure ulcer: ___ - ___ - ___ Month Day Year

	C. Stage 3: Full thickness tissue loss. Subcutaneous fat may be visible but bone, tendon or muscle is not exposed. Slough may be present but does not obscure the depth of tissue loss. May include undermining and tunneling
Enter Number ☐	**1. Number of Stage 3 pressure ulcers** - If 0 → Skip to M0300D, Stage 4
Enter Number ☐	**2. Number of these Stage 3 pressure ulcers that were present upon admission/reentry** - enter how many were noted at the time of admission

	D. Stage 4: Full thickness tissue loss with exposed bone, tendon or muscle. Slough or eschar may be present on some parts of the wound bed. Often includes undermining and tunneling
Enter Number ☐	**1. Number of Stage 4 pressure ulcers** - If 0 → Skip to M0300E, Unstageable: Non-removable dressing
Enter Number ☐	**2. Number of these Stage 4 pressure ulcers that were present upon admission/reentry** - enter how many were noted at the time of admission

M0300 continued on next page

Section M — Skin Conditions

M0300. Current Number of Unhealed (non-epithelialized) Pressure Ulcers at Each Stage - Continued

Enter Number ☐

E. Unstageable - Non-removable dressing: Known but not stageable due to non-removable dressing/device

1. **Number of unstageable pressure ulcers due to non-removable dressing/device** - If 0 → Skip to M0300F, Unstageable: Slough and/or eschar

Enter Number ☐

2. **Number of these unstageable pressure ulcers that were present upon admission/reentry** - enter how many were noted at the time of admission

Enter Number ☐

F. Unstageable - Slough and/or eschar: Known but not stageable due to coverage of wound bed by slough and/or eschar

1. **Number of unstageable pressure ulcers due to coverage of wound bed by slough and/or eschar** - If 0 → Skip to M0300G, Unstageable: Deep tissue

Enter Number ☐

2. **Number of these unstageable pressure ulcers that were present upon admission/reentry** - enter how many were noted at the time of admission

Enter Number ☐

G. Unstageable - Deep tissue: Suspected deep tissue injury in evolution

1. **Number of unstageable pressure ulcers with suspected deep tissue injury in evolution** - If 0 → Skip to M0610, Dimension of Unhealed Stage 3 or 4 Pressure Ulcers or Eschar

Enter Number ☐

2. **Number of these unstageable pressure ulcers that were present upon admission/reentry** - enter how many were noted at the time of admission

M0610. Dimensions of Unhealed Stage 3 or 4 Pressure Ulcers or Eschar
Complete only if M0300C1, M0300D1 or M0300F1 is greater than 0

If the resident has one or more unhealed (non-epithelialized) Stage 3 or 4 pressure ulcers or an unstageable pressure ulcer due to slough or eschar, identify the pressure ulcer with the largest surface area (length x width) and record in centimeters:

☐ . ☐ cm **A. Pressure ulcer length:** Longest length from head to toe

☐ . ☐ cm **B. Pressure ulcer width:** Widest width of the same pressure ulcer, side-to-side perpendicular (90-degree angle) to length

☐ . ☐ cm **C. Pressure ulcer depth:** Depth of the same pressure ulcer from the visible surface to the deepest area (if depth is unknown, enter a dash in each box)

M0700. Most Severe Tissue Type for Any Pressure Ulcer

Enter Code ☐

Select the best description of the most severe type of tissue present in any pressure ulcer bed
1. **Epithelial tissue** - new skin growing in superficial ulcer. It can be light pink and shiny, even in persons with darkly pigmented skin
2. **Granulation tissue** - pink or red tissue with shiny, moist, granular appearance
3. **Slough** - yellow or white tissue that adheres to the ulcer bed in strings or thick clumps, or is mucinous
4. **Necrotic tissue (Eschar)** - black, brown, or tan tissue that adheres firmly to the wound bed or ulcer edges, may be softer or harder than surrounding skin

M0800. Worsening in Pressure Ulcer Status Since Prior Assessment (OBRA, PPS, or Discharge)
Complete only if A0130E = 0

Indicate the number of current pressure ulcers that were **not present or were at a lesser stage** on prior assessment (OBRA, PPS, or Discharge). If no current pressure ulcer at a given stage, enter 0

Enter Number ☐

A. Stage 2

Enter Number ☐

B. Stage 3

Enter Number ☐

C. Stage 4

Section M — Skin Conditions

M0900. Healed Pressure Ulcers
Complete only if A0310E = 0

Enter Code	**A. Were pressure ulcers present on the prior assessment (OBRA, PPS, or Discharge)?**
☐	0. **No** → Skip to M1030, Number of Venous and Arterial Ulcers 1. **Yes** → Continue to M0900B, Stage 2

Indicate the number of pressure ulcers that were noted on the prior assessment (OBRA, PPS, or Discharge) that have completely closed (resurfaced with epithelium). If no healed pressure ulcer at a given stage since the prior assessment (OBRA, PPS, or Discharge), enter 0

Enter Number	
☐	**B. Stage 2**

Enter Number	
☐	**C. Stage 3**

Enter Number	
☐	**D. Stage 4**

M1030. Number of Venous and Arterial Ulcers

Enter Number	
☐	**Enter the total number of venous and arterial ulcers present**

M1040. Other Ulcers, Wounds and Skin Problems

↓ Check all that apply

Foot Problems

☐	**A. Infection of the foot** (e.g., cellulitis, purulent drainage)
☐	**B. Diabetic foot ulcer(s)**
☐	**C. Other open lesion(s) on the foot**

Other Problems

☐	**D. Open lesion(s) other than ulcers, rashes, cuts** (e.g., cancer lesion)
☐	**E. Surgical wound(s)**
☐	**F. Burn(s)** (second or third degree)

None of the Above

☐	**Z. None of the above** were present

M1200. Skin and Ulcer Treatments

↓ Check all that apply

☐	**A. Pressure reducing device for chair**
☐	**B. Pressure reducing device for bed**
☐	**C. Turning/repositioning program**
☐	**D. Nutrition or hydration intervention** to manage skin problems
☐	**E. Ulcer care**
☐	**F. Surgical wound care**
☐	**G. Application of nonsurgical dressings** (with or without topical medications) other than to feet
☐	**H. Applications of ointments/medications** other than to feet
☐	**I. Application of dressings to feet** (with or without topical medications)
☐	**Z. None of the above** were provided

Resident _____ Identifier _____ Date _____

Section N   Medications

N0300. Injections

Enter Days	Record the number of days that injections of any type were received during the last 7 days or since admission/reentry if less than 7 days. If 0 → Skip to N0400, Medications Received

N0350. Insulin

Enter Days	A. Insulin injections - Record the number of days that insulin injections were received during the last 7 days or since admission/reentry if less than 7 days
Enter Days	B. Orders for insulin - Record the number of days the physician (or authorized assistant or practitioner) changed the resident's insulin orders during the last 7 days or since admission/reentry if less than 7 days

N0400. Medications Received

↓ Check all medications the resident received at any time during the last 7 days or since admission/reentry if less than 7 days

☐	A. Antipsychotic
☐	B. Antianxiety
☐	C. Antidepressant
☐	D. Hypnotic
☐	E. Anticoagulant (warfarin, heparin, or low-molecular weight heparin)
☐	F. Antibiotic
☐	G. Diuretic
☐	Z. None of the above were received

Section O — Special Treatments and Procedures

O0100. Special Treatments and Programs

Check all of the following treatments, programs and procedures that were performed during the last **14 days**

	1. While NOT a Resident	2. While a Resident
1. While NOT a Resident Procedure performed *while NOT a resident* of this facility and within the *last 14 days*. Only check column 1 if resident entered (admission or reentry) IN THE LAST 14 DAYS. If resident last entered 14 or more days ago, leave column 1 blank **2. While a Resident** Procedure performed *while a resident* of this facility and within the *last 14 days*	↓ Check all that apply ↓	
Cancer Treatments		
A. Chemotherapy	☐	☐
B. Radiation	☐	☐
Respiratory Treatments		
C. Oxygen therapy	☐	☐
D. Suctioning	☐	☐
E. Tracheostomy care	☐	☐
F. Ventilator or respirator	☐	☐
G. BiPAP/CPAP	☐	☐
Other		
H. IV medications	☐	☐
I. Transfusions	☐	☐
J. Dialysis	☐	☐
K. Hospice care	☐	☐
L. Respite care		☐
M. Isolation or quarantine for active infectious disease (does not include standard body/fluid precautions)	☐	☐
None of the Above		
Z. None of the above	☐	☐

O0250. Influenza Vaccine - Refer to current version of RAI manual for current flu season and reporting period

Enter Code	A. Did the **resident received the Influenza vaccine in this facility** for this year's Influenza season? 0. **No** → Skip to O0250C, If Influenza vaccine not received, state reason 1. **Yes** → Continue to O0250B, Date vaccine received
	B. Date vaccine received → Complete date and skip to O0300A, Is the resident's Pneumococcal vaccination up to date? _____ — _____ — _____ Month Day Year
Enter Code	C. If Influenza vaccine not received, state reason: 1. **Resident not in facility** during this year's flu season 2. **Received outside of this facility** 3. **Not eligible** - medical contraindication 4. **Offered and declined** 5. **Not offered** 6. **Inability to obtain vaccine** due to a declared shortage 9. **None of the above**

O0300. Pneumococcal Vaccine

Enter Code	A. Is the resident's Pneumococcal vaccination up to date? 0. **No** → Continue to O0300B, If Pneumococcal vaccine not received, state reason 1. **Yes** → Skip to O0400, Therapies
Enter Code	B. If Pneumococcal vaccine not received, state reason: 1. **Not eligible** - medical contraindication 2. **Offered and declined** 3. **Not offered**

Section O — Special Treatments and Procedures

O0400. Therapies

A. Speech-Language Pathology and Audiology Services

Enter Number of Minutes

1. **Individual minutes** - record the total number of minutes this therapy was administered to the resident **individually** in the last 7 days

Enter Number of Minutes

2. **Concurrent minutes** - record the total number of minutes this therapy was administered to the resident **concurrently with one other resident** in the last 7 days

Enter Number of Minutes

3. **Group minutes** - record the total number of minutes this therapy was administered to the resident as **part of a group of residents** in the last 7 days

If the sum of individual, concurrent, and group minutes is zero, ➞ skip to O0400B, Occupational Therapy

Enter Number of Days

4. **Days** - record the **number of days** this therapy was administered for **at least 15 minutes** a day in the last 7 days

5. **Therapy start date** - record the date the most recent therapy regimen (since the last assessment) started

6. **Therapy end date** - record the date the most recent therapy regimen (since the last assessment) ended - enter dashes if therapy is ongoing

__ __ - __ __ - ____   __ __ - __ __ - ____
Month   Day   Year   Month   Day   Year

B. Occupational Therapy

Enter Number of Minutes

1. **Individual minutes** - record the total number of minutes this therapy was administered to the resident **individually** in the last 7 days

Enter Number of Minutes

2. **Concurrent minutes** - record the total number of minutes this therapy was administered to the resident **concurrently with one other resident** in the last 7 days

Enter Number of Minutes

3. **Group minutes** - record the total number of minutes this therapy was administered to the resident as **part of a group of residents** in the last 7 days

If the sum of individual, concurrent, and group minutes is zero, ➞ skip to O0400C, Physical Therapy

Enter Number of Days

4. **Days** - record the **number of days** this therapy was administered for **at least 15 minutes** a day in the last 7 days

5. **Therapy start date** - record the date the most recent therapy regimen (since the last assessment) started

6. **Therapy end date** - record the date the most recent therapy regimen (since the last assessment) ended - enter dashes if therapy is ongoing

__ __ - __ __ - ____   __ __ - __ __ - ____
Month   Day   Year   Month   Day   Year

C. Physical Therapy

Enter Number of Minutes

1. **Individual minutes** - record the total number of minutes this therapy was administered to the resident **individually** in the last 7 days

Enter Number of Minutes

2. **Concurrent minutes** - record the total number of minutes this therapy was administered to the resident **concurrently with one other resident** in the last 7 days

Enter Number of Minutes

3. **Group minutes** - record the total number of minutes this therapy was administered to the resident as **part of a group of residents** in the last 7 days

If the sum of individual, concurrent, and group minutes is zero, ➞ skip to O0400D, Respiratory Therapy

Enter Number of Days

4. **Days** - record the **number of days** this therapy was administered for **at least 15 minutes** a day in the last 7 days

5. **Therapy start date** - record the date the most recent therapy regimen (since the last assessment) started

6. **Therapy end date** - record the date the most recent therapy regimen (since the last assessment) ended - enter dashes if therapy is ongoing

__ __ - __ __ - ____   __ __ - __ __ - ____
Month   Day   Year   Month   Day   Year

O0400 continued on next page

Section O   Special Treatments and Procedures

O0400. Therapies - Continued

D. Respiratory Therapy

Enter Number of Minutes

[ ]

1. **Total minutes** - record the total number of minutes this therapy was administered to the resident in the last 7 days

   If zero, → skip to O0400E, Psychological Therapy

Enter Number of Days

[ ]

2. **Days** - record the **number of days** this therapy was administered for **at least 15 minutes** a day in the last 7 days

E. Psychological Therapy (by any licensed mental health professional)

Enter Number of Minutes

[ ]

1. **Total minutes** - record the total number of minutes this therapy was administered to the resident in the last 7 days

   If zero, → skip to O0400F, Recreational Therapy

Enter Number of Days

[ ]

2. **Days** - record the **number of days** this therapy was administered for **at least 15 minutes** a day in the last 7 days

F. Recreational Therapy (includes recreational and music therapy)

Enter Number of Minutes

[ ]

1. **Total minutes** - record the total number of minutes this therapy was administered to the resident in the last 7 days

   If zero, → skip to O0500, Restorative Nursing Programs

Enter Number of Days

[ ]

2. **Days** - record the **number of days** this therapy was administered for **at least 15 minutes** a day in the last 7 days

O0500. Restorative Nursing Programs

Record the **number of days** each of the following restorative programs was performed (for at least 15 minutes a day) in the last 7 calendar days (enter 0 if none or less than 15 minutes daily)

Number of Days	Technique
[ ]	A. Range of motion (passive)
[ ]	B. Range of motion (active)
[ ]	C. Splint or brace assistance

Number of Days	Training and Skill Practice In:
[ ]	D. Bed mobility
[ ]	E. Transfer
[ ]	F. Walking
[ ]	G. Dressing and/or grooming
[ ]	H. Eating and/or swallowing
[ ]	I. Amputation/prostheses care
[ ]	J. Communication

O0600. Physician Examinations

Enter Days

[ ]

Over the last 14 days, **on how many days did the physician (or authorized assistant or practitioner) examine the resident?**

O0700. Physician Orders

Enter Days

[ ]

Over the last 14 days, **on how many days did the physician (or authorized assistant or practitioner) change the resident's orders?**

Section P   Restraints

P0100. Physical Restraints

Physical restraints are any manual method or physical or mechanical device, material or equipment attached or adjacent to the resident's body that the individual cannot remove easily which restricts freedom of movement or normal access to one's body

Coding:
0. **Not used**
1. **Used less than daily**
2. **Used daily**

↓ **Enter Codes in Boxes**

Used in Bed	
☐	A. **Bed rail**
☐	B. **Trunk restraint**
☐	C. **Limb restraint**
☐	D. **Other**
Used in Chair or Out of Bed	
☐	E. **Trunk restraint**
☐	F. **Limb restraint**
☐	G. **Chair prevents rising**
☐	H. **Other**

| **Section Q** | **Participation in Assessment and Goal Setting** |

Q0100. Participation in Assessment

Enter Code	**A. Resident participated in assessment** 0. **No** 1. **Yes**
Enter Code	**B. Family or significant other participated in assessment** 0. **No** 1. **Yes** 9. **No family or significant other**
Enter Code	**C. Guardian or legally authorized representative participated in assessment** 0. **No** 1. **Yes** 9. **No guardian or legally authorized representative**

Q0300. Resident's Overall Expectation

Complete only if A0310E = 1

Enter Code	**A. Resident's overall goal established during assessment process** 1. Expects to be **discharged to the community** 2. Expects to **remain in this facility** 3. Expects to be **discharged to another facility/institution** 9. **Unknown or uncertain**
Enter Code	**B. Indicate information source for Q0300A** 1. **Resident** 2. If not resident, then **family or significant other** 3. If not resident, family, or significant other, then **guardian or legally authorized representative** 9. **None of the above**

Q0400. Discharge Plan

Enter Code	**A. Is there an active discharge plan in place for the resident to return to the community?** 0. **No** 1. **Yes** → Skip to Q0600, Referral
Enter Code	**B. What determination was made by the resident and the care planning team regarding discharge to the community?** 0. **Determination not made** 1. **Discharge to community determined to be feasible** → Skip to Q0600, Referral 2. **Discharge to community determined to be not feasible** → Skip to next active section (V or X)

Q0500. Return to Community

Enter Code	**A. Has the resident been asked about returning to the community?** 0. **No** 1. **Yes** - previous response was **"no"** 2. **Yes** - previous response was **"yes"** → Skip to Q0600, Referral 3. **Yes** - previous response was **"unknown"**
Enter Code	**B. Ask the resident** (or family or significant other if resident is unable to respond): **"Do you want to talk to someone about the possibility of returning to the community?"** 0. **No** 1. **Yes** 9. **Unknown or uncertain**

Q0600. Referral

Enter Code	**Has a referral been made to the local contact agency?** 0. **No** - determination has been made by the resident and the care planning team that contact is not required 1. **No** - referral not made 2. **Yes**

Section V	**Care Area Assessment (CAA) Summary**

V0100. Items From the Most Recent Prior OBRA or Scheduled PPS Assessment

Complete only if A0310E = 0 and if the following is true for the **prior assessment**: A0310A = 01- 06 or A0310B = 01- 06

Enter Code	**A.** **Prior Assessment Federal OBRA Reason for Assessment** (A0310A value from prior assessment)
	01. **Admission** assessment (required by day 14)
	02. **Quarterly** review assessment
	03. **Annual** assessment
	04. **Significant change in status** assessment
	05. **Significant correction** to **prior comprehensive** assessment
	06. **Significant correction** to **prior quarterly** assessment
	99. **Not OBRA required** assessment

Enter Code	**B.** **Prior Assessment PPS Reason for Assessment** (A0310B value from prior assessment)
	01. **5-day** scheduled assessment
	02. **14-day** scheduled assessment
	03. **30-day** scheduled assessment
	04. **60-day** scheduled assessment
	05. **90-day** scheduled assessment
	06. **Readmission/return** assessment
	07. **Unscheduled assessment used for PPS** (OMRA, significant or clinical change, or significant correction assessment)
	99. **Not PPS** assessment

	C. **Prior Assessment Reference Date** (A2300 value from prior assessment)
	___ ___ – ___ ___ – ___ ___ ___ ___
	Month Day Year

Enter Score	**D.** **Prior Assessment Brief Interview for Mental Status (BIMS) Summary Score** (C0500 value from prior assessment)

Enter Score	**E.** **Prior Assessment Resident Mood Interview (PHQ-9©) Total Severity Score** (D0300 value from prior assessment)

Enter Score	**F.** **Prior Assessment Staff Assessment of Resident Mood (PHQ-9-OV) Total Severity Score** (D0600 value from prior assessment)

Section V — Care Area Assessment (CAA) Summary

V0200. CAAs and Care Planning

1. Check column A if Care Area is triggered.
2. For each triggered Care Area, indicate whether a new care plan, care plan revision, or continuation of current care plan is necessary to address the problem(s) identified in your assessment of the care area. The Addressed in Care Plan column must be completed within 7 days of completing the RAI (MDS and CAA(s)). Check column B if the triggered care area is addressed in the care plan.
3. Indicate in the Location and Date of CAA Information column where information related to the CAA can be found. CAA documentation should include information on the complicating factors, risks, and any referrals for this resident for this care area.

A. CAA Results

Care Area	A. Care Area Triggered	B. Addressed in Care Plan	Location and Date of CAA Information
	↓ Check all that apply ↓		
01. Delirium	☐	☐	
02. Cognitive Loss/Dementia	☐	☐	
03. Visual Function	☐	☐	
04. Communication	☐	☐	
05. ADL Functional/Rehabilitation Potential	☐	☐	
06. Urinary Incontinence and Indwelling Catheter	☐	☐	
07. Psychosocial Well-Being	☐	☐	
08. Mood State	☐	☐	
09. Behavioral Symptoms	☐	☐	
10. Activities	☐	☐	
11. Falls	☐	☐	
12. Nutritional Status	☐	☐	
13. Feeding Tube	☐	☐	
14. Dehydration/Fluid Maintenance	☐	☐	
15. Dental Care	☐	☐	
16. Pressure Ulcer	☐	☐	
17. Psychotropic Drug Use	☐	☐	
18. Physical Restraints	☐	☐	
19. Pain	☐	☐	
20. Return to Community Referral	☐	☐	

B. Signature of RN Coordinator for CAA Process and Date Signed

1. Signature

2. Date ___ — ___ — ___
   Month   Day   Year

C. Signature of Person Completing Care Plan and Date Signed

1. Signature

2. Date ___ — ___ — ___
   Month   Day   Year

Section X	Correction Request

X0100. Type of Record

Enter Code	1. **Add new record** → Skip to Z0100, Medicare Part A Billing
	2. **Modify existing record** → Continue to X0150, Type of Provider
	3. **Inactivate existing record** → Continue to X0150, Type of Provider

Identification of Record to be Modified/Inactivated - The following items identify the existing assessment record that is in error. In this section, reproduce the information EXACTLY as it appeared on the existing erroneous record, even if the information is incorrect. This information is necessary to locate the existing record in the National MDS Database.

X0150. Type of Provider

Enter Code	**Type of provider**
	1. **Nursing home (SNF/NF)**
	2. **Swing Bed**

X0200. Name of Resident on existing record to be modified/inactivated

A. First name:

C. Last name:

X0300. Gender on existing record to be modified/inactivated

Enter Code	1. **Male**
	2. **Female**

X0400. Birth Date on existing record to be modified/inactivated

— —		— —
Month	Day	Year

X0500. Social Security Number on existing record to be modified/inactivated

— —	— —	

X0600. Type of Assessment on existing record to be modified/inactivated

Enter Code	A. **Federal OBRA Reason for Assessment**
	01. **Admission** assessment (required by day 14)
	02. **Quarterly** review assessment
	03. **Annual** assessment
	04. **Significant change in status** assessment
	05. **Significant correction** to **prior comprehensive** assessment
	06. **Significant correction** to **prior quarterly** assessment
	99. **Not OBRA required** assessment
Enter Code	B. **PPS Assessment**
	PPS Scheduled Assessments for a Medicare Part A Stay
	01. **5-day** scheduled assessment
	02. **14-day** scheduled assessment
	03. **30-day** scheduled assessment
	04. **60-day** scheduled assessment
	05. **90-day** scheduled assessment
	06. **Readmission/return** assessment
	PPS Unscheduled Assessments for a Medicare Part A Stay
	07. **Unscheduled assessment used for PPS** (OMRA, significant or clinical change, or significant correction assessment)
	Not PPS Assessment
	99. **Not PPS** assessment
Enter Code	C. **PPS Other Medicare Required Assessment - OMRA**
	0. **No**
	1. **Start of therapy** assessment
	2. **End of therapy** assessment
	3. **Both Start and End of therapy** assessment

X0600 continued on next page

Section X	Correction Request

X0600. Type of Assessment - Continued

Enter Code	**D. Is this a Swing Bed clinical change assessment?** Complete only if X0150 = 2 0. **No** 1. **Yes**
Enter Code	**F. Entry/discharge reporting** 01. **Entry** record 10. **Discharge** assessment-**return not anticipated** 11. **Discharge** assessment-**return anticipated** 12. **Death in facility** record 99. **Not entry/discharge** record

X0700. Date on existing record to be modified/inactivated - **Complete one only**

A. Assessment Reference Date - Complete only if X0600F = 99

__ __ — __ __ — __ __ __ __
Month   Day   Year

B. Discharge Date - Complete only if X0600F = 10, 11, or 12

__ __ — __ __ — __ __ __ __
Month   Day   Year

C. Entry Date - Complete only if X0600F = 01

__ __ — __ __ — __ __ __ __
Month   Day   Year

Correction Attestation Section - Complete this section to explain and attest to the modification/inactivation request

X0800. Correction Number

Enter Number	**Enter the number of correction requests to modify/inactivate the existing record, including the present one**

X0900. Reasons for Modification - Complete only if Type of Record is to modify a record in error (X0100 = 2)

↓ **Check all that apply**

☐	**A. Transcription error**
☐	**B. Data entry error**
☐	**C. Software product error**
☐	**D. Item coding error**
☐	**Z. Other error requiring modification** If "Other" checked, please specify: _____

X1050. Reasons for Inactivation - Complete only if Type of Record is to inactivate a record in error (X0100 = 3)

↓ **Check all that apply**

☐	**A. Event did not occur**
☐	**Z. Other error requiring inactivation** If "Other" checked, please specify: _____

Section X Correction Request

X1100. RN Assessment Coordinator Attestation of Completion

A. Attesting individual's first name:

B. Attesting individual's last name:

C. Attesting individual's title:

D. Signature

E. Attestation date

        —   —

    Month   Day   Year

Section Z   Assessment Administration

Z0100. Medicare Part A Billing

	A. **Medicare Part A HIPPS code** (RUG group followed by assessment type indicator):
	B. **RUG version code:**
Enter Code	C. **Is this a Medicare Short Stay assessment?** 0. **No** 1. **Yes**

Z0150. Medicare Non-Therapy Part A Billing

	A. **Medicare non-therapy Part A HIPPS code** (RUG group followed by assessment type indicator):
	B. **RUG version code:**

Z0200. State Medicaid Billing (if required by the state)

	A. **RUG Case Mix group:**
	B. **RUG version code:**

Z0250. Alternate State Medicaid Billing (if required by the state)

	A. **RUG Case Mix group:**
	B. **RUG version code:**

Z0300. Insurance Billing

	A. **RUG Case Mix group:**
	B. **RUG version code:**

Section Z — Assessment Administration

Z0400. Signature of Persons Completing the Assessment or Entry/Death Reporting

I certify that the accompanying information accurately reflects resident assessment information for this resident and that I collected or coordinated collection of this information on the dates specified. To the best of my knowledge, this information was collected in accordance with applicable Medicare and Medicaid requirements. I understand that this information is used as a basis for ensuring that residents receive appropriate and quality care, and as a basis for payment from federal funds. I further understand that payment of such federal funds and continued participation in the government-funded health care programs is conditioned on the accuracy and truthfulness of this information, and that I may be personally subject to or may subject my organization to substantial criminal, civil, and/or administrative penalties for submitting false information. I also certify that I am authorized to submit this information by this facility on its behalf.

Signature	Title	Sections	Date Section Completed
A.			
B.			
C.			
D.			
E.			
F.			
G.			
H.			
I.			
J.			
K.			
L.			

Z0500. Signature of RN Assessment Coordinator Verifying Assessment Completion

A. Signature:

B. Date RN Assessment Coordinator signed assessment as complete:

_____ — _____ — _____
Month   Day   Year

3252674R00230

Made in the USA
San Bernardino, CA
19 July 2013